Handbook of Local Anesthetics

Handbook of Local Anesthetics

Editor: Chris Headley

AMERICAN
MEDICAL PUBLISHERS
www.americanmedicalpublishers.com

AMERICAN
MEDICAL PUBLISHERS
www.americanmedicalpublishers.com

Cataloging-in-publication Data

Handbook of local anesthetics / edited by Chris Headley.
p. cm.
Includes bibliographical references and index.
ISBN 979-8-88740-149-2
1. Local anesthesia. 2. Anesthesia. 3. Local anesthetics--Guidebooks. 2. Anesthetics--Guidebooks.
I. Headley, Chris.
RD84 .H36 2023
617.964--dc23

American Medical Publishers,
41 Flatbush Avenue,
1st Floor, New York,
NY 11217, USA

ISBN 979-8-88740-149-2 (Hardback)

Contents

Preface

A local anaesthetic (LA) is a drug that prevents the body from feeling any sensation of pain. In contrast to a general anaesthetic, a local anaesthetic causes pain to disappear in a specific body area without causing loss of consciousness. Almost every nerve between the peripheral nerve terminals and the central nervous system can be blocked with local anaesthetics. Paralysis (loss of muscle power) can be induced if LA is applied to specific nerve pathways, a phenomenon known as local anaesthetic nerve block. LA are used in acute pain, chronic pain and surgery. As a result of the local anaesthetic, edema of the tongue, throat and larynx might occur. During the administration of LA injection, there is a risk of accidental injury to local blood vessels. Also, there are chances of excitatory or depressant effects on the central nervous system, along with cardiac toxicity and allergy. This book presents various works that consist of contributions made by international experts. Its objective is to present upcoming studies on local anaesthetics. The book is appropriate for students seeking detailed information in this area of study as well as for experts.

After months of intensive research and writing, this book is the end result of all who devoted their time and efforts in the initiation and progress of this book. It will surely be a source of reference in enhancing the required knowledge of the new developments in the area. During the course of developing this book, certain measures such as accuracy, authenticity and research focused analytical studies were given preference in order to produce a comprehensive book in the area of study.

This book would not have been possible without the efforts of the authors and the publisher. I extend my sincere thanks to them. Secondly, I express my gratitude to my family and well-wishers. And most importantly, I thank my students for constantly expressing their willingness and curiosity in enhancing their knowledge in the field, which encourages me to take up further research projects for the advancement of the area.

Editor

1

Current Local Anesthetic Applications in Regional Anesthesia

Jeffrey M. Carness and Mark J. Lenart

Abstract

Complete anesthesia is often described using terminology that pertains to the pharmacodynamic effects of the medications administered. This vocabulary often includes akinesia, analgesia, amnesia and hypnosis. Local anesthesia is more specific and represents the administration of an amide or ester local anesthetic, to affect analgesia, at or around the site of administra-tion. Anesthesiologists employ a breadth of different clinical techniques that utilize local anesthetic medications. These techniques include topical, mucosal, endotracheal, intravenous, peripheral nerve block, epidural, and intrathecal (spinal) administration. Unique to the fields of anesthesiology and pain medicine, however, is the administration of epidural and intrathecal local anesthetic. Together, these routes are jointly referred to as neuraxial anesthesia and are often utilized to facilitate surgical intervention, labor analgesia, or pain therapy. The history of neuraxial local anesthetic administration is rich and intriguing. The anatomy of the spinal cord and surrounding structures is complex and pertinent to the pharmacologic discussion of neuraxial local anesthetic administration. The pharmacodynamic and pharmacokinetic interactions of local anesthetics, when administered via the neuraxial route, are unique and worthy of continued investigation. Much has been studied, but there is still more to be discovered. These topics will be the focus of our discussion.

Keywords: anesthetics, local, anesthesia, conduction, pharmacology, administration and dosage pharmacokinetics, drug-related side effects and adverse reactions, injections, spinal, injections, epidural, epidural space, analgesia, epidural, anesthesia, epidural, ropivacaine, bupivacaine, lidocaine, chloroprocaine

1. Introduction

Anesthesia is often described using terminology that references the pharmacodynamic effects of a medication. This terminology often includes akinesia (loss or impairment of voluntary movement), analgesia (insensibility to pain), amnesia (loss of memory) and hypnosis (any of various conditions that resemble sleep). Local anesthesia is more specific and represents the administration of a medication, typically an amide or ester local anesthetic, to affect analgesia, and possibly akinesia, at or around the site of administration. Anesthesiologists employ a breadth of different clinical techniques that utilize local anesthetic medications. These techniques include topical, mucosal, endotracheal, intravenous, peripheral nerve block, epidural, and intrathecal (spinal) administration. Unique to the fields of anesthesiology and pain medicine, however, is the administration of local anesthetics via the epidural and intrathecal routes. Together, these routes are jointly referred to as neuraxial anesthesia and are often utilized to facilitate surgical intervention, labor analgesia, or pain therapy. Much has been studied, but there is still more to be discovered. These topics will be the focus of our discussion.

2. Neuraxial anesthesia

2.1 Basic anatomy

To understand the pharmacokinetic, pharmacodynamic, and pharmacotherapeutic activity of local anesthetics in this region, one needs a thorough understanding of neuraxial anatomy. The term neuraxis refers to the axial unpaired portion of the central nervous system. Of great importance to the discussion of neuraxial anesthesia is the spinal cord, nerve roots, and the meninges and vertebral bodies that house and protect them.

2.1.1 Membranes

The spinal cord is surrounded by three protective membranes which delineate potential and actual neuraxial spaces. Listed from outermost to innermost, these membranes are termed meninges and refer to the dura mater, the arachnoid mater and the pia mater. The pia mater directly envelops the spinal cord (**Figure 1**). Epidural refers to the potential space between the ligamentum flavum and the outer surface of the dura mater. Subdural refers to a potential space between the dura mater and the arachnoid mater. The term intrathecal refers to the thecal sac or the dura mater enclosure of the cerebrospinal fluid-filled sub-arachnoid (i.e., sub-arachnoid mater) space. This space remains outside of the pia mater. These spaces are surrounded by the bony architecture created by the vertebrae.

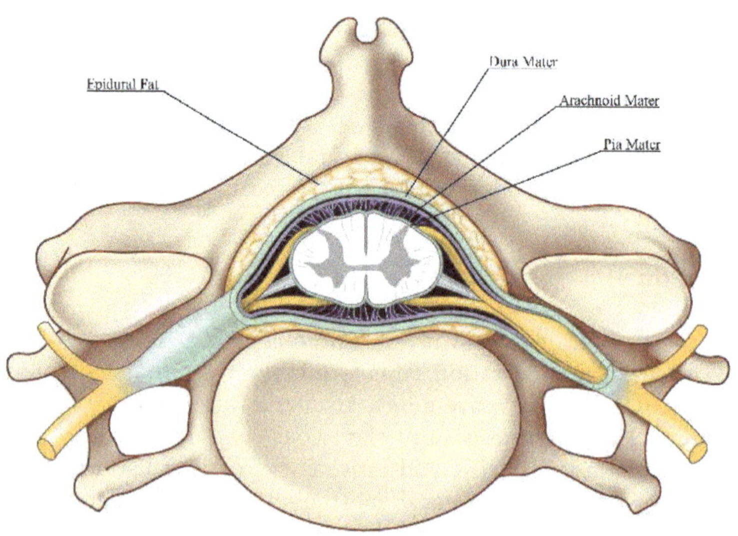

Figure 1.
Meninges—protective membranes of the spinal cord.

2.1.2 Bones and ligaments

The vertebral column protects the spinal cord and provides support for standing and walking. The vertebral column is easily recognized by its three curvatures (cervical lordosis, thoracic kyphosis, and lumbar lordosis) and five sections, to include the cervical, thoracic, lumbar, sacral and coccygeal regions. Each region consists of seven, twelve, five, five, and four vertebrae respectively for a total of 33. Each vertebra consists of two components: a vertebral body and the remaining vertebral arch. The vertebral arch is composed of several components to include laminae, pedicles, spinous, and transverse processes (**Figure 2**). Access to the epidural and intrathecal space for neuraxial local anesthetic administration is obtained via the spaces between each vertebra. Variation in bony structure between lumbar, thoracic, and cervical vertebrae will dictate the approach to these specific regions (e.g., the greater downward angle of the thoracic spinous processes necessitates a steeper midline approach). Between each of the vertebra are several ligaments that are also typically traversed when administering neuraxial local anesthetics. From superficial to deep are the supraspinous ligament, interspinous ligament, and the ligamentum flavum (named for its yellow pigmentation). The interspinous ligament is affixed to the inferior and superior aspect of the spinous processes. The supraspinous ligament attaches to the tips of the vertebral spinous processes (**Figure 3**) and runs from the level of C7 to the sacrum.

2.1.3 Vasculature/adipose tissue

The epidural space contains several anatomic structures and tissues to include vasculature, nerve roots, and adipose tissue. The internal vertebral venous plexus, also known as the epidural venous plexus, assists with vertebral venous drainage and serves as an alternate conduit for venous return in the setting of compro-mised caval blood flow. The plexus consists of two larger anterior longitudinal veins, located in the anterior aspect of the spinal canal, and two smaller posterior longitudinal veins. These veins are connected by transverse veins, completing the plexus. The longitudinal veins are located more posteriorly at the level of the cervical and lumbar vertebrae, and more posterolaterally at the level of the thorax [1]. The plexus is surrounded by epidural adipose tissue. Combined with reported

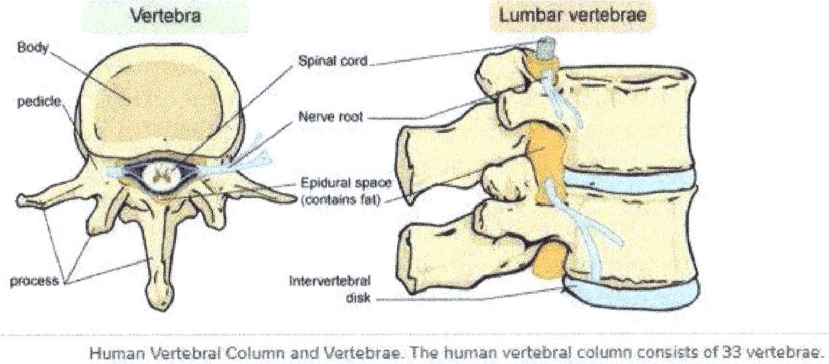

Human Vertebral Column and Vertebrae. The human vertebral column consists of 33 vertebrae.

Figure 2.
Human vertebral column and vertebrae. The human vertebral column consists of 33 vertebrae.

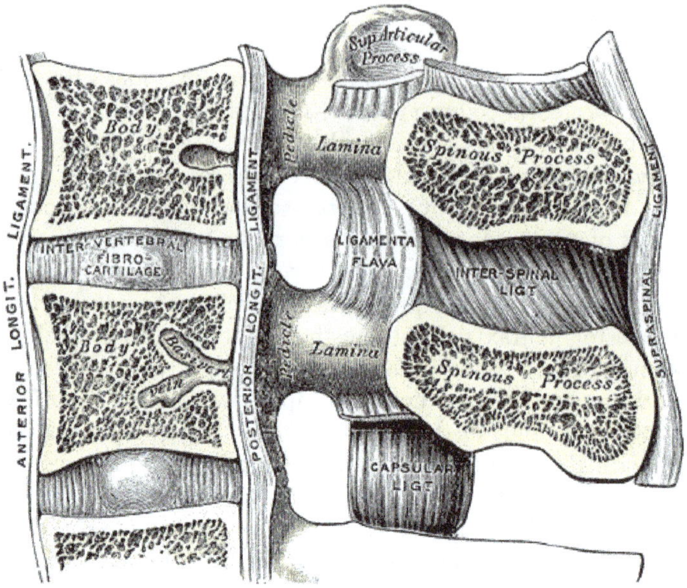

Figure 3.
Spinal ligaments—this file is licensed under the Creative Commons Public Domain Mark 1.0—https://commons.wikimedia.org/wiki/File:Gray301.png.

disruptions in the posterior fusions of the left and right ligamentum flavum, the adipose tissue and vasculature serve to provide variation in the construct of this potential space when expanded by local anesthetic.

2.2 Intrathecal administration

2.2.1 History of spinal anesthesia

Various local anesthetics have been investigated for surgical anesthesia (**Table 1**). These are divided into two primary categories of local anesthetics (i.e., esters and amides). Initial studies began with the investigation of the spinal effects of esters such as cocaine. This was followed by investigation of amylocaine (no longer utilized in clinical practice), procaine (also known as Novocain), dibucaine and tetracaine. Of note, amylocaine was first synthesized circa 1903 and is referenced as the first synthetic local anesthetic to be utilized in spinal anesthesia [2]. This was followed by the synthesis of procaine (circa 1904) with subsequent early twentieth-century investigation into its intrathecal administration. Procaine likely found greater clinical application as a result of the presumed systemic effects (to include physical dependence) and presumed neurotoxic effects of spinal cocaine administration [3]. Of note, however, is the side effect profile of procaine, which commonly includes nausea, vasomotor paralysis, and a greater risk for anaphylaxis associated with its metabolite para-aminobenzoic acid (PABA) [3, 4]. The period of 1930 through the early 1940s saw the discovery and intrathecal employment of longer acting local anesthetics (i.e., dibucaine and tetracaine). In 1930, Jones described his experiences with the administration of dibucaine (also known as cinchocaine or nupercaine) [5, 6]. With a shorter duration of action compared to dibucaine, a more favorable ratio of sensory to motor fiber blockade, less sympathetic blockade than procaine, and less perceived toxicity, initial studies into the administration of tetracaine showed significant promise [7, 8]. In 1945, lidocaine (originally called Xylocaine as it is a xylidine derivative) was initially administered as a spinal anesthetic. As a

Esters	
	Cocaine
	Amylocaine
	Procaine
	Tetracaine
	Chloroprocaine
Amides	
	Dibucaine
	Lidocaine
	Mepivacaine
	Prilocaine
	Bupivacaine
	Articaine
	Ropivacaine
	Levobupivacaine

Table 1.
Local anesthetics for spinal anesthesia.

short-acting amide local anesthetic, its pharmacologic profile was deemed ideal for short to moderate duration operative procedures [9]. Subsequently, in 1946, procaine was used to synthesize chloroprocaine. Initial reports for the use of chloroprocaine for spinal anesthesia were positive [10], and chloroprocaine was approved for spinal anesthesia by the United States Food and Drug Administration in 1955. With rapid ester hydrolysis neutralizing the effects of chloroprocaine, it became the local anesthetic of choice for the fastest onset and fastest resolution of spinal blockade. The rapid ester hydrolysis also created an environment in which almost twice the amount of chloroprocaine could be administered, compared to procaine, without toxicity. The improved safety profile also likely contributed to the popularity of this medication [10]. Despite investigations into other spinally administered local anesthetics, these three local anesthetics (i.e., chloroprocaine, lidocaine, and tetracaine) would find widespread use for short duration, moderate duration, and long duration operative procedures for the next half of a century. Shortly after the approval of chloroprocaine, mepivacaine (1956) [11] and prilocaine (1965) [12] would see their first usage in spinal anesthesia. These two medications, both xylidine derivatives as well, demonstrate similar potency when compared to lidocaine [9]. With subsequent studies demonstrating a risk for the development of transient neurologic symptoms associated with intrathecal lidocaine administration, it would seem that mepivacaine and prilocaine are currently undergoing further investigation and may serve as alternatives to lidocaine for ambulatory or surgical procedures of short to moderate duration [13–15]. The mid-1960s discovery, synthesis, and spinal administration of bupivacaine, an intermediate to long-acting amide local anesthetic, resulted in widespread popular clinical application [16, 17]. When evidence surfaced regarding the potential for racemic bupivacaine toxicity, two (S)-enantiomers of bupivacaine were researched and scrutinized for spinal anesthesia administration. Initial studies utilizing spinal ropivacaine (S-enantiomer of bupivacaine) were conducted in the early 1990s [18–20]. Additional studies regarding the other pure (S)-enantiomer of bupivacaine, levobupivacaine, were initiated in 1999 [21–23]. Intrathecal administration of both levobupivacaine and ropivacaine continue.

2.2.2 Pharmacokinetics of intrathecal local anesthetic administration

The exact mechanism and site of action of local anesthetics in the intrathecal space are not clear. Some evidence suggest that local anesthetics work to directly inhibit Na $^+$ and K^+ ion channel conduction at the peripheral dorsal nerve root and the spinal cord within the thecal sac [9, 24]. For this to occur, the local anesthetic must be absorbed by the neuron and bind to an intracellular site on the Na^+/K^+ ion channels. This may only occur when the channels are seen in a conformation associated with depolarization. Thus, the activity of local anesthetics is referred to as "use-dependent" activity [25, 26]. Understandably, there are a minimum number of axonal Na^+/K^+ channels which must depolarize to continue the propagation of the neuronal impulse. The term "conduction safety" has been utilized to refer to the overabundance of sum-mation action potential necessary at the axonal regional level to facilitate continued propagation of this impulse. Due to the decreased conduction safety at the telodendron of the axon, as compared to the trunk, it is believed that the local anesthetic blockade has a greater effect in this region [27]. Recognizing the complexity of the neuro-physiology of pain, this view of an isolated Na^+/K^+ channel mechanism may be too simplistic [24]. Primary, secondary, and tertiary synaptic activity occurs as sensory input is transmitted from the peripheral nervous system to the central nervous system and ultimately to the primary sensory cortex of the brain. It is widely recognized that neuronal transmission relies on both excitatory and inhibitory post-synaptic potentials for inter-neuronal transmission. Liu et al. summarized the current understanding of the research, which considers a multitude of potential sites for the activity of spinally administered local anesthetics, to include neuronal transmission at the level of the dorsal and anterior horn of the spinal cord [9]. It has been postulated that there may be a role for calcium ion channel manipulation (low voltage and high voltage L-type calcium channels) in this region [28]. Furthermore, it has been proposed that local anesthetics administered in the intrathecal space may contribute to the inhibition of substance P activity at the level of the dorsal root ganglion and the dorsal horn of the spinal cord [29]. Local anesthetics may also contribute to γ-aminobutyric acid inhibi-tory potentiation resulting in the inhibition of sensory transmission [30].

Even more fascinating is the discussion and research regarding alteration in electrical "coding" by disruption or alteration in "after-potentials" or "after-oscillations." This begins with interruption in neuronal transmission by an incomplete local anesthetic neuronal blockade due to sub-blocking concentrations of local anesthetic. Inhibition of sequential firing, or the depolarization of specific neurons, or disruption of weighted telodendron discharge patterns on a single neuron may contribute to changes in temporal excitability patterns sufficient to disrupt sensory input [27].

The extent of clinical activity depends upon several pharmacokinetic factors which can modify the overall visible clinical effects of the local anesthetic. By report, there are over 25 different factors, some theoretical, which can affect the spread and distribution of local anesthetics within the neuraxis [31]. Patient characteristics include age, height, intra-abdominal pressure, patient position, CSF currents, and CSF volume. Local anesthetic characteristics include potency, dosage, baricity, lipid solubility, degree of protein binding, and the log of the acid dissociation constant (i.e., the pK_a). These local anesthetic characteristics further determine the amount of local anesthetic absorption (neuronal, myelin, adipose, or vasculature) and will ultimately contribute to the observed clinical effect.

2.2.2.1 Cerebrospinal fluid

The intrathecal route of local anesthetic administration is unique in that it bypasses first pass metabolism by the liver and mechanically penetrates the blood-brain barrier. This deposition into the cerebrospinal fluid generates unique pharmacokinetic considerations. As Greene et al. states, "Uptake of local anesthetic injected into the CSF determines which neuronal functions are affected, elimination from the CSF determines the duration, and distribution within the CSF determines the extent of altered neuronal function" [31]. A discussion of CSF is therefore critical.

Cerebrospinal fluid is maintained within the ventricular system of the brain, to include the cisterns and the intracranial subarachnoid space, as well as the spinal subarachnoid space (i.e., the thecal sac). There is approximately 150 ml of cerebrospinal fluid in the healthy, adult patient. CSF is continuously produced by the choroid plexus, and absorbed via arachnoid villi, at a rate of ~20 ml/h with 400–600 ml of CSF generated daily [32]. Decreased CSF volume at the time of injection increases the concentration of local anesthetic in the administered region and influences the clinical effect. Conditions which increase intra-abdominal pressure, and redistribute CSF, will mimic CSF volume depletion (i.e., obesity, pregnancy, etc.), amplify CSF oscillation, and potentially modify the effects of the local anesthetic as well [33].

2.2.2.2 Absorption, mechanism, onset and duration of action of spinal local anesthetics

The uptake or absorption of local anesthetic into the vasculature also limits the distribution and clinical effects of spinal anesthesia. As vascular absorption is greatest in the epidural space, and the meninges are permeable to local anesthetic, a concentration gradient is established between the spinal cord, intrathecal space, and the epidural space [34]. While there is little intrathecal vascular absorption, some local anesthetic may penetrate the pia mater and be absorbed by vasculature in the spinal cord directly. It is also believed that a more efficient mechanism is vascular absorption via the increased surface area in the perivascular space (where blood vessels perforate the pia mater) [24, 34]. Of additional interest is consideration of the effects that local anesthetics have on spinal vasculature. Bupivacaine and ropivacaine have been shown to decrease spinal blood flow, whereas tetracaine and lidocaine have been shown to increase spinal blood flow [35, 36].

With regard to absorption, local anesthetic must be in an electrically neutral configuration (i.e., as an uncharged hydrophobic form of the medication) to penetrate neuronal tissue. This concept necessitates further discussion of acid dissociation. Becker and Reed provide a summary for reference [37]. In order to maintain stability in solution, local anesthetics are formulated as a hydrochloride salt creating a quaternary amine formulation that is electrically charged to enable water solubility (hydrophilic). The local anesthetic must, therefore, revert to the uncharged lipophilic (hydrophobic) tertiary amine form for neuronal penetration (i.e., the electrically neutral form). The more a local anesthetic dissociates and releases hydrogen ions at the body's physiologically neutral pH of 7.4, the more local anesthetic will remain in the tertiary form and the greater the neuronal absorption (**Figure 4**). Understanding the resting pH of the medication is useful, as is under-standing hydrogen ion dissociation. The dissociation equilibrium between hydrogen ions and the deprotonated local anesthetic constitutes the equilibrium that deter-mines the K_a (acid dissociation constant) of the drug. It is expressed as a ratio of hydrogen ion dissociation at equilibrium by the following equation:

$$K_a = \frac{[B][H+]}{BH+} \tag{1}$$

K_a values are typically very small (i.e., 1×10^{-3}), making comparison and manipulation more challenging. However, the inverse logarithmic value of the K_a can be utilized to express pK_a. These pK_a values represent the log of the K_a

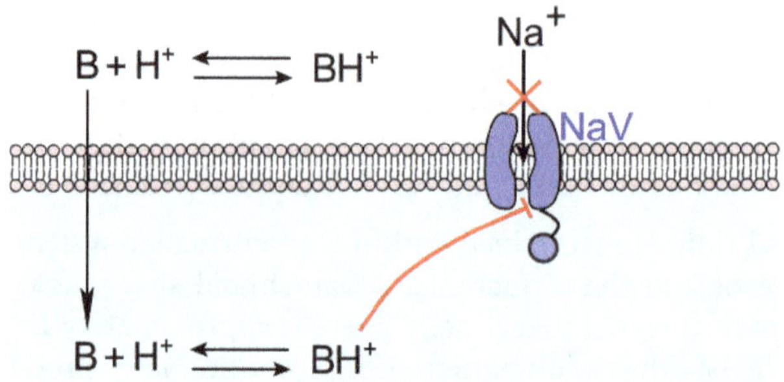

Figure 4.
Mechanism of action of local anesthetics—this file is licensed under the Creative Commons Attribution-Share Alike 3.0 Unported license. https://commons.wikimedia.org/wiki/File:LA_andNaV.svg.

(acid dissociation constant), or the pH at which 50% of the drug is in the protonated electrically charged hydrophilic quaternary amine form, and 50% is in the uncharged, lipophilic tertiary amine form. Values range from 7.6 → ~9.0, meaning that no local anesthetics reach complete equilibrium within the body's normal pH range of 7.35–7.45. The pK_a values for mepivacaine (~7.6), prilocaine (~7.9) and lidocaine (~7.9) most closely approximate physiologic pH, suggesting that their neuronal absorption occurs more quickly, leading to faster onset of clinical symp-toms. The pK_a values of bupivacaine (~8.1) and ropivacaine (~8.1) have a somewhat slower onset of clinical effect [37].

In addition to neuronal and vascular absorption, the lipid absorption of a local anesthetic also plays a role in the time of onset—the greater the lipid solubility, the faster the myelin/neuronal penetration. As reported by Becker and Reed, however, this appears only to be true in vitro. They hypothesize that the higher lipid solubility "may impede dispersion throughout tissue fluids." When applied in vivo, the lipid solubility appears to promote adipose tissue absorption over neuronal absorption leading to a delayed onset of clinical effect [37]. This helps to explain the clinically observed pharmacologic effects of long-acting local anesthetics (i.e., bupivacaine/ropivacaine/tetracaine) versus shorter-acting local anesthetics such as lidocaine and mepivacaine. Lidocaine and mepivacaine have a much faster onset of action compared to bupivacaine and ropivacaine when administered intrathecally (despite the increased lipid solubility of bupivacaine/ropivacaine).

The pharmacokinetic variable that appears to have the greatest influence on the duration of action is the degree of intrathecal protein binding. Clement et al. demonstrated that the non-protein bound or unbound fraction of intrathecal bupivacaine is lower than lidocaine. Because bupivacaine has a higher degree of protein binding, it has a longer observed clinical effect [38].

2.2.3 Pharmacodynamics of intrathecal local anesthetic administration

The nature of the surgical procedure, or site of pain origination, will dictate pursuit of a specific distribution of anesthesia. The distributed effect of intrathe-cal local anesthetic administration is often measured via perceived differences in sensation of temperature or sharp tactile stimulation. Each spinal nerve provides a specific anatomic distribution of sensation, or dermatome, which may be measured. In addition to the desired clinical sensory blockade, pharmacodynamic effects may be seen throughout several organ systems to include the cardiovascular, respiratory, gastrointestinal, renal, and immune systems.

2.2.3.1 Cardiovascular

Undoubtedly, the spinal administration of local anesthesia can result in hypotension. This is largely believed to be secondary to a sympathetic nervous system blockade in the region of the pre-ganglionic neuron prior to its synapse on the sympathetic chain ganglion. This blockade results in vascular dilation, which produces a decrease in systemic vascular resistance (SVR) (venous > arterial). This decrease in SVR, and the associated decrease in preload, may stimulate a reflexive baroreceptor response increasing the heart rate to maintain cardiac output. However, it has been well reported that patients may also experience a different type of cardiac reflex known as the Reverse Bainbridge (atrial), or Bezold-Jarisch reflex (ventricular). These reflexes stem from the recognition of a decreased preload to either the atria or ventricle, which results in reflexive bradycardia to slow the heart and allow for increased filling time. This ultimately results in a lower cardiac output.

Additionally, the distribution of local anesthetic can block cardiac accelerator fibers which stem from thoracic sympathetic ganglia T1-T4, further preventing the reflexive cardiac baroreceptor response. Due to the complexity of these interacting variables, changes to cardiac output with spinal anesthesia are also variable. Ultimately, spinal anesthesia often results in a decrease in mean arterial pressure (MAP), though this is not necessarily true for pre-eclamptic patients with non-sympathetically mediated elevations in blood pressure. When untreated, depressed cardiovascular effects may result in decreased cerebral perfusion, nausea/vomiting, and cardiovascular collapse.

2.2.3.2 Respiratory

In 1991, Steinbrook et al. investigated the effects of spinal lidocaine and bupivacaine on resting pulmonary function in eleven volunteers. They identified a slight decrease in end-tidal CO_2 (34 mmHg → 31 mmHg) with an inverse age correlation (i.e., younger patients had a greater drop in end-tidal CO_2). They reported the absence of significant change in tidal volume, respiratory rate, and minute ventilation, hypothesizing instead an increase in dead space ventilation associated with spinal administration. They further comment on the paralysis of abdominal musculature leading to an increase in chest wall compliance and a decrease in mechanical work of breathing. It is interesting to note their comments regarding increased chest wall compliance and increased respiratory frequency variation [39]. Of note, they also allude to spinal level deafferentation of the chest wall receptors, but make no specific reference to intercostal involvement.

2.2.3.3 Renal

It is well recognized that the kidney receives direct sympathetic innervation from renal sympathetic nerve fibers derived from the sympathetic chain ganglia. In addition, the kidney auto-regulates its blood flow utilizing humoral/endocrine factors released as a result of changes sensed in the macula densa. It is believed that this mechanism functions both interdependently and independently from sympathetic function, enabling the preservation of renal blood flow in the absence of sympathetic directive. As described by Smith et al. [40], "It is possible to assume that the renal vascular bed acquires autonomy de novo only as a consequence of denervation, but in view of the rapidity and smoothness of anesthetic denervation any such assumption seems quite superfluous." It is now understood that there is little effect on overall renal function as a result of spinal or epidural sympathetic blockade from local anesthetic administration. Glomerular filtration and renal blood flow are recognized to only decrease slightly in direct relation to decreases in mean arterial pressure associated with the sympathetic blockade [40–42].

2.2.3.4 Digestive

Sympathetic nervous system blockade as a consequence of spinal local anesthetic administration leads to unimpeded parasympathetic nervous system activity and gastrointestinal hyperactivity. Hypotension encountered as a result of spinal local anesthesia may lead to gastrointestinal ischemia and the release of emetogenic substances such as serotonin. Furthermore, hypotension may lead to hypoperfusion of the area postrema of the medulla (brain stem—known chemoreceptor trigger zone for vomiting) resulting in increased serotonin release. The combination of these factors may contribute to intraoperative/postoperative nausea and vomiting. It is also important to recognize that hypotension associated with spinal local anesthetic administration may result in hypoperfusion of the liver. Because hepatic blood flow is not auto-regulated, this low perfusion pressure may result in impairment of metabolic functions to include subsequent drug metabolism [43].

2.2.3.5 Immune

Regarding the anti-inflammatory and immunomodulatory effects of local anesthetics, Cassuto et al. wrote that it is well recognized that the innate and adaptive immune systems contribute to the destruction of foreign substances and tissue repair following injury. The immune cells involved in these processes include neutrophils, macrophages, monocytes, mast cells, T-cells, and B-cells. These cells must undergo chemotactic targeting to the area of injury, adhere to blood vessel walls, traverse the blood vessel wall into the tissue, engulf the offending agent, and destroy it. Local anesthetics have been thought to interfere with every step of this process. They inhibit leukocyte adherence to the vascular endothelium by possibly interrupting interactions between leukocyte cell membrane integrins and their receptors (cellular adhesion molecules—CAMs) expressed on the vascular endothelium. Similarly, they inhibit the trans-endothelial migration and motility of leukocytes and may interfere with the "priming" of leukocytes, preventing their full pathogen-destroying capability by decreasing their free radical production. It has been suggested that local anesthetics further interrupt the normal cellular actomyosin filament activity resulting in disruption of the ability of the leukocyte to modulate the cell membrane to engulf the offending agent for lysosomal destruction. Furthermore, local anesthetics are responsible for a dose-dependent decrease in the release of lysosomal enzymes [44, 45].

Of additional interest are the anti-inflammatory properties of local anesthetics that are believed to stem from their inhibition of arachidonic acid derivative synthesis, their release of histamine, and their attenuation of cytokine release (i.e., IL-1, IL-6, IL-8, TNF-alpha, etc.). Inhibition of phospholipase A2 synthesis prevents arachidonic acid cleavage; inhibition of prostaglandin E1/E2 synthesis has been attributed to a potential reduction in inflammatory pain; inhibition of thromboxane A2 synthesis results in decreased platelet aggregation; and inhibition of leukotriene B4 synthesis has been implicated in the reduction of capillary hyper-permeability, resulting in decreased edema formation due to inflammatory plasma extravasation. Based on this aggregate model of cell membrane interference (i.e., ion channel inhibition, cell membrane protein cleavage, cell membrane receptor binding and inhibition, cell membrane actomyosin function disruption, etc.) researchers have targeted investiga-tion of specific local anesthetics for their antibacterial and antiviral effects [44, 46].

2.2.3.6 Factors which effect intrathecal spread

Several factors are considered relevant to the intrathecal spread of local anesthetic. These factors may be divided into three categories: factors specific to the local anesthetic solution, factors specific to the patient, and factors specific to the procedure itself. All of these have been described in an article by Hocking and Wildsmith which may be referenced for additional information [47].

With regard to the local anesthetic solution, the degree of intrathecal spread is related to the baricity, temperature, viscosity, and dosage of local anesthetic administered. Baricity is the ratio of substance density to CSF density. As such, there are hyperbaric, hypobaric or isobaric (i.e., denser than cerebrospinal fluid, less dense than cerebrospinal fluid, or similar density to cerebrospinal fluid) formulations of local anesthetic solution. Upon injection, baricity affects the caudal versus cephalad spread of solution within the CSF. Baricity, in combination with patient position-ing, will ultimately determine the spread and distribution of local anesthetic within the thecal sac. Temperature also affects the density of a local anesthetic solution such that a refrigerated or warmed solution may possess a baricity different from its manufactured specification. Investigations evaluating the additional effect of local anesthetic solution viscosity on intrathecal spread suggest that increased viscosity is associated with increased local anesthetic distribution within the intrathecal space [48]. Finally, there is a relationship between dosage, volume, and concentration. Recognizably, changes in any of these variables influence the others as they pertain to the specific mixture of a local anesthetic solution prepared for administration. Though several studies have been performed to evaluate these factors, dosage seems to have the most significant impact on the intrathecal spread of local anesthetic.

In discussing patient factors, patient height, position, and age all contribute to the spread of intrathecal local anesthetic. Though it may affect spread, gross height is not a reliable characteristic for determination of local anesthetic dosing. Hartwell et al. demonstrated a correlation between vertebral column length and the level of local anesthetic sensory blockade. As a surrogate for height, the authors suggest the use of vertebral column length instead. This recommendation is based on the recognition that there may be patient height differences attributed to differ-ences in extremity length, which have no reference value with regard to thecal sac dimensions or cerebrospinal fluid volume. Regarding thecal sac characteristics, it is recognized that the vertebral column curvatures (and thus variations in thecal sac positioning) influence the intrathecal spread of local anesthetic. The interplay between lumbar lordosis, thoracic kyphosis, and baricity helps to explain the largely "dependent" thoracic distribution of hyperbaric local anesthetic solutions after intrathecal injection and positioning of a patient in the supine position. With regard to baricity, it was demonstrated that the density of CSF varies between patients. CSF in women is less dense than in men. It is less dense in pregnant women than in non-pregnant women and is less dense in pre-menopausal women than in post-menopausal women. This fact has unique importance in that a significant portion of surgeries performed under spinal anesthesia are cesarean sections in pre-menopausal, pregnant women who can be expected to have decreased CSF density. It has been further demonstrated that extremes of age can impact the spread of intrathecal local anesthetic. Veering et al. reported on the increasing length of time required for the maximum upper level of analgesia to be seen with advancing age. This was associated with an inverse onset of motor blockade relationship such that a faster onset of motor blockade was seen with advancing age. Furthermore, the time to peak plasma concentration of local anesthetic was increased, and the total plasma clearance decreased with advancing age [49–52].

Finally, procedural components may have an impact on the distribution of local anesthetic. It is known that the initial pressure generated by the injection of local anesthetic creates waves within the CSF. It was previously believed that generation of additional fluid waves, via a technique known as barbotage, would facilitate greater spread. Several investigations have demonstrated that barbotage does not affect the ultimate height of the sensory blockade. It may, however, slightly decrease the time to achieve maximum sensory and motor blockade, though this may be of limited clinical value [53–55]. Regarding injection speed and pressure itself, studies have been mixed. It would seem that utilizing increasing speed, and pressure of injection potentially facilitates a greater spread of isobaric local anesthetic with diminishing effects seen with hyperbaric local anesthetic [47, 56]. Lastly, the needle orientation and approach (midline versus paramedian) to the neuraxis may alter local anesthetic distribution. James et al. demonstrated a faster onset of T4 block when the Sprotte needle was inserted with the side eye facing cephalad [57]. Urmey et al., similar to Neigh et al., also reported a higher dermatomal distribution when the side aperture of the needle was oriented in a cephalad manner [58, 59]. To the contrary, Masse et al. reported that the orientation of the aperture of the Whitacre needle did not influence the cephalad spread of hyperbaric bupivacaine in parturients [60]. Stienstra et al. demonstrated that a paramedian approach with steep angle (70–100 degrees from level) was also associated with a greater cephalad sensory blockade [61].

2.2.4 Adverse effects

2.2.4.1 Local anesthetic systemic toxicity

Each local anesthetic has a unique pharmacokinetic profile. This profile dictates the potential for adverse events that may be seen with local anesthetic administration. One of the most concerning adverse effects is local anesthetic systemic toxicity (LAST). Inadvertent vascular administration or changes in vascular absorption may result in a constellation of symptoms, dependent upon the rate of increase in serum concentration and the injection location. Symptoms are typically classified into two groups: central nervous system or cardiovascular. Central nervous system (CNS) symptoms may include dizziness, perioral numbness, tinnitus, metallic taste, agitation, seizures, and coma. Cardiovascular (CV) symptoms, usually seen with increasing serum concentrations, may include dysrhythmias (i.e., tachycardia, bradycardia, and ventricular ectopy), myocardial depression, hypotension, and asystole. It is important to note, however, that CNS symptoms may not be noted prior to the onset of cardiovascular collapse. The potential for local anesthetic toxicity may be conceptualized using a metric estimation of the ratio of CV toxic dose: CNS toxic dose. This ratio is lower (i.e., more potential for cardiac toxicity) for amide anesthetics such as ropivacaine and bupivacaine (with bupivacaine having the lowest ratio and greatest potential for toxicity). This is due in part to its lipid solubility, greater protein binding, and hepatic metabolism [62, 63]. An exact mechanism for LAST has yet to be fully elucidated, but it has been suggested that the ultimate cause is likely a combination of $Na^+/K^+/Ca^{2+}$ ion channel blockade (resulting in myocardial depression) in conjunction with metabotropic intracellular effects. These intracellular effects include a potential mitochondrial translocase inhibition, which may prevent the movement of the acyl portion of fats and ketones into the inner mitochondria for energy processing. This substrate reduction may create a synergistic depression of cardiac function as a consequence of the myocar-dial reliance on mitochondrial oxidation of fatty acids and ketones for energy [63].

It is important to recognize that certain pathophysiologic states will also affect the toxicity of local anesthetics. These include renal dysfunction, cardiac dysfunction, and hepatic dysfunction. In patients with renal dysfunction, a greater volume of distribution and greater alpha-1 glycoprotein binding would portend a lower free fraction serum concentration. However, there is often a hyperdynamic circulation associated with diminished elimination of the agent leading to a variable serum concentration and recommendations for reduced dosages [63]. Patients with severe heart failure experience a decreased intravascular uptake portending a lower serum concentration. However, they often experience diminished renal and hepatic perfusion leading to a decreased rate of metabolism and elimination necessitating recommendations for reduced dosages as well. Finally, severe hepatic disease, with its associated decreased hepatic metabolism, necessitates decreased local anesthetic administration to offset the delayed metabolism and elimination of the local anesthetic from the body [63].

Regardless of the manifestation, the key to successful treatment is early consideration of the diagnosis. The development and widespread distribution of lipid emulsion has improved the survival of such cases via a mechanism that includes a combination of reduced tissue binding and improved energetic-metabolic effects. Since the first report of a patient saved by lipid rescue in 2006 [64] case reports and clinical experience have continued to add to the body of evidence suggesting its efficacy.

2.2.4.2 Neurotoxicity

Initial concerns regarding the administration of lidocaine for spinal anesthesia surfaced in the early 1990s. At that time, microcatheters were being employed for the continuous intrathecal administration of lidocaine. A case report in 1991 brought to light the potential for cauda equina syndrome associated with intrathecal lidocaine administration. This was believed to be a result of pooling of high concentration (5%) lidocaine inside the caudal dural sac [65]. Ongoing surveillance and reporting, however, indicated a continuum of symptoms. This was described at the time as Transient Radicular Irritation (TRI) associated with intrathecal bolus lidocaine administration for spinal anesthesia. These symptoms were later reclassified and have come to be better known as Transient Neurologic Symptoms (i.e., the occurrence of sensory radicular neuropathic pain in the absence of motor dysfunction that resolves within 72 h) [66]. Additional studies were performed to evaluate for contributing causes to include concentration, baricity, dosage, and adjuncts (i.e., epinephrine, dextrose, etc.). Furthermore, the occurrence of TNS with alternative local anesthetics, such as bupivacaine, mepivacaine, etc., have been investigated as well.

2.2.4.2.1 Reported incidence of neurotoxicity

According to data presented by Brull et al., the incidence of radiculopathy or neuropathy following contemporary spinal local anesthetic administration is believed to occur in 3.78 out of 10,000 spinal esthetics. They further report that the risk of cauda equina syndrome with spinal anesthesia is less frequent, occurring in ~0.11/10,000, and the risk of permanent neurologic injury is reportedly exceedingly rare [67].

2.2.4.2.2 Neurotoxicity mechanism

The exact mechanism for the occurrence of neurologic injury or production of transient neurologic symptoms is unknown. Recognizably, each local anesthetic has a different pharmacodynamic profile resulting in greater frequency (i.e., lidocaine) versus lesser frequency (i.e., bupivacaine) of neurologic symptoms believed to be secondary to neuronal insult. There has been a suggestion that neurologic symptoms following spinal local anesthetic administration may stem from the local vasoconstrictive properties of the local anesthetic [68]. It is understood that different local anesthetics have different vasoconstrictive effects and that these effects are also dose-dependent. High concentrations of local anesthetic result in vasodila-tion, whereas low concentrations have a more vasoconstrictive effect [68]. This vasoconstrictive effect at low dose may result in neuronal ischemia. Certainly, there is always the potential for mechanical trauma from the needle or intrafascicular injection with increased intrafascicular administration pressures leading to neuronal ischemia and injury [65]. This, however, is rare. There is research that suggests the effects of local anesthetics are the result of their impact on intracellular metabolism, such as on the mitogen-activated protein kinase (MAPK) and caspase pathways. It is interesting to note the activation of different MAPK pathways with specific local anesthetics (i.e., tetracaine activates the c-Jun N-terminal kinase pathway versus lidocaine activation of the p38 MAPK pathway) [69]. Furthermore, use of lipoxygenase inhibitors seems to diminish the degree of neuronal apoptosis in response to lidocaine administration suggesting a potential role for inflammatory mediators in the generation of neurotoxicity [69]. Kan et al. further investigated an inflammatory component by demonstrating the ability to regulate levels of caspase-9 and matrix-metalloprotease-3 expression via preemptive incubation with subsequent inflammatory signaling pathway modification. This resulted in decreased apoptosis in response to in vitro neuronal lidocaine administration [70].

2.2.4.3 *Other adverse effects*

2.2.4.3.1 *Hypotension*

Hypotension after spinal local anesthetic administration is a well-known direct effect of sympathetic nervous system blockade with venous pooling of blood in the lower extremities. Defining hypotension is as challenging as determining treatment since the literature utilizes different definitions (i.e. <100 mmHg, <90 mmHg, <80% of baseline, etc.) [71]. Numerous studies have evaluated different methodologies for treating this hypotension. Definition and treatment are beyond the scope of this chapter.

2.2.4.3.2 *Infectious complications*

Historically, and anecdotally, spinal local anesthetic administration has a low reported incidence of infectious complications, and include, but are not limited to paraspinal abscesses, spinal/epidural abscesses, meningitis, arachnoiditis, and systemic inflammation with sepsis. In reviewing the literature for infectious complications, a very low correlating incidence was discovered. Moore and Bridenbaugh, after reviewing 52,112 spinal anesthetics, reported the occurrence of three central nervous system infections (i.e., 0.06 cases per 1000) [72]. In a more recent review, Horlocker et al. reported on the occurrence of two infectious complications out of 4767 consecutive spinal anesthetics which were reviewed (i.e., 0.4 cases per 1000). One case was a disc abscess and the other a paraspinal abscess. Both patients remained neurologically intact after appropriate treatment. Infections associated with spinal local anesthetic injection are infrequent and, as discussed previously, may be due in part to the concentration-dependent antibacterial effects of local anesthetic administration [73].

2.2.4.3.3 *Vertebral canal hematoma*

The etiology of vertebral canal hematoma after neuraxial local anesthetic administration appears multifactorial with patient-related (i.e., demographics, comorbidities, etc.), medication-related and procedural contributions [74]. Historical demographic data portrays a potential predisposition based upon age and gender [75]. The retrospectively reported incidence of vertebral canal hematoma varies widely and ranges from 1:3600 (seen in patients receiving a spinal local anesthetic for total knee arthroplasty), to 1:200,000 (as seen in obstetric patients receiving an epidural local anesthetic for labor analgesia) [74, 76, 77]. The report on the Third National Audit Project of the Royal College of Anesthetists further suggests a prospective incidence of 8 vertebral canal hematomas in 707,425 (~ 1:88,000). Interestingly, 46% of these neuraxial blocks were spinals, and there were zero vertebral canal hematomas associated with spinal instrumentation. Recognizably, this complication portends a notably poor prognosis associated with persistent neurologic deficit [78].

2.2.4.3.4 Thermoregulatory disruption

Administration of spinal anesthesia is associated with a disruption in thermoregulation. The threshold for vasoconstriction and shivering in response to hypothermia becomes dysregulated. According to Kurz et al., the threshold for triggering a thermoregulatory response to hypothermia is decreased by ~0.5°C. Temperature is lost more quickly during the initial 30 min after spinal anesthesia (as a result of core-to-peripheral redistribution of heat) when compared to epidural local anesthetic administration. This is believed to be secondary to a lesser degree of autonomic thermal dysregulation in the lower extremities with epidural local anesthesia administration (i.e., failure to obtain a complete blockade with epidural versus spinal local anesthesia administration). This clinical effect garners greater importance when considering the detrimental effects of hypothermia (i.e., wound infection, coagulopathy, delayed arousal from anesthesia, etc.). Though beyond the scope of this chapter, yet still of clinical importance, is the potential additive effect of intrathecal opioid administration on the disruptive thermoregulatory effect of spinal local anesthetic administration [79–81].

2.2.4.3.5 Post-dural puncture headache

The term post-dural puncture headache often refers to a clinical constellation of symptoms seen after penetration of the dura mater. Symptoms include the presence of a transient, self-limited, positional, frontal-occipital headache tradi-tionally believed to occur within 72 h of dural penetration. In addition, patients may complain of nausea (+/− vomiting), dizziness, tinnitus, neck stiffness, or photophobia. Studies indicate a significant association with specific types of needles used for spinal local anesthetic administration. Smaller gauge, pencil point needles (i.e., spinal needles) are less often associated with post-dural puncture headaches, as compared to larger gauge cutting needles (i.e., epidural needles). For this reason, post-dural puncture headache is less often associated with spinal local anesthetic administration, as compared to inadvertent puncture with epidural catheter placement. Historically, treatments focused on bed rest, hydration, caffeine, and analgesics to include acetaminophen and NSAIDs. These conservative treatments are not currently supported by evidence of efficacy. The sterile epidural injection of blood (i.e., an epidural blood patch), is recognized as traditional therapy and is effective in providing adequate pain relief in ~65–70% of patients. Optimally, in light of the challenges with treating post-dural puncture headaches, it is best to avoid inadvertent dural puncture. If inadvertent dural puncture occurs, techniques to minimize the likelihood of post-dural puncture headache should be considered [82].

2.2.4.3.6 Hearing loss

Hearing loss after neuraxial local anesthetic administration deserves special consideration. Some providers remain unaware of the potential for this type of transient, self-limited low-frequency sensorineural hearing loss. This type of hearing loss may be as prevalent as 10–50% of all spinal local anesthetic administra-tions (with such variable reported prevalence due to the limited degree of patient/clinician awareness). Interestingly, it seems the same risk factors for a post-dural puncture headache apply in the setting of post-spinal local anesthesia hearing loss. According to Sprung et al., the subarachnoid space is contiguous with a small canal in the ear (i.e., the cochlear aqueduct) that transmits cerebrospinal fluid pressure to the inner ear. Sound waves are theorized to be transmitted through the fluid in the middle ear onto the basilar membrane. Changes in transmitted pressure to the middle ear are hypothesized to distort the interpretation of these sound waves through the basilar membrane. Decreases in cerebrospinal fluid pressure, as transmitted through the cochlear canal and into the fluid of the inner ear, is believed to be the mechanism by which patients suffer a loss of low-frequency sensorineural hearing after spinal anesthesia administration [83].

2.3 Epidural administration

2.3.1 Contents and structure of the epidural space

Transitioning to a discussion of epidural local anesthetic administration generates an opportunity for a brief discussion of the epidural anatomy to supplement the anatomy discussed at the beginning of the chapter.

2.3.1.1 Definition/surrounding bony construct

The epidural space is widest posteriorly in the midline and averages about 5 mm between the ligamentum flavum and the dura in the lumbar region. The boundaries of the epidural space are:

Above: the foramen magnum where the periosteal and spinal layers of the dura fuse

Below: the sacrococcygeal membrane

Anteriorly: the posterior longitudinal ligament covering the posterior aspect of the vertebral bodies and the intervertebral discs

Posteriorly: the anterior surfaces of the vertebral lamina and the ligamentum flavum

Laterally: the pedicles of the vertebrae and the intervertebral foramina [1, 84]

Interestingly, spinal nerve root cuffs are identified along the lateral aspect of the epidural space. These have previously been defined as "prolongations of the dura and arachnoid lamina" and are believed to enclose spinal nerve roots within this space. Previously referred to as "dural cuffs," it is now believed that the cuffs include not only the dura mater but the arachnoid mater as well, thus making this previous term inaccurate [85]. This construct may influence the spread of local anesthetic when administered via the epidural route.

2.3.1.2 Adipose tissue

The contents of the spinal canal are cushioned in a packing of fat, through which injected solutions track while spreading to target receptors. This adipose tissue is richly vascularized [86, 87] yet lies mostly unattached in the spinal canal. In the region of nerve roots, collagen concentration increases and coalesces with the fat in the intervertebral foramina. Adipose tissue "competes" for its share of the drug, along with nervous tissue and vasculature, and is an important pharmacologic space and repository. Medications with high lipid solubility and/or lipoprotein binding tend to enter and remain in this tissue, depending on local blood flow, and can impact drug behavior in the epidural space profoundly. This competition with extraneural tissue then generates, when compared to spinal doses, a higher epidural medication dosage requirement [88].

2.3.1.3 Vasculature

Spinal arteries, epidural veins, and lymphatics are all co-inhabitors of this space. Spinal arteries derive from the vertebral, ascending cervical, deep cervical, intercostal, lumbar, and iliolumbar arteries. They lie chiefly in the lateral epidural space. Epidural veins arise from the internal vertebral venous plexus and drain both the spinal cord and the spinal canal. Lying mainly anterolaterally, they pass through the intervertebral foramina on their journey toward the vertebral, posterior intercostal, lumbar and lateral sacral veins. It is through this network that increased pressures (intra-abdominal and intrathoracic) are transmitted to the epidural space [84]. The lack of valves in this system results in the distention of these vessels and a consequent reduction in epidural space volume. The lymphatic network is located anteriorly to the intervertebral foramen and aid in the cleansing of the subarach-noid space, draining to the regional lymph nodes.

2.3.1.4 Rivulets

The interrelationship between the factors that influence epidural blockade and the clinical effect is surprisingly complex. Epidural analgesia is not a simple matter of spinal root or ganglion blockade, but rather is the end state of action at various sites after passage through multiple sites. Unique to epidural local anesthetic administra-tion is the concept of rivulets. Hogan reported the spread of injected ink as "rivulets" through numerous small channels rather than as a unified advancing front [89]. Injection results in circumferential spread anteriorly and posteriorly around the thecal sac. Laterally, epidural solution extrudes beyond the intervertebral foramen following a parallel path along the paraspinous musculature fascial plane [89]. Hogan et al. also noted that the lateral spread of epidural solution sporadically encompassed the more proximal dorsal nerve root prior to the dorsal root ganglion in the "axilla" of the nerve root. This non-uniform distribution of solution, within the epidural space, may then correlate with clinical data suggesting that slow, not fast, injection rates (0.3–0.75 ml/s) result in the most effective spread of analgesia [89]. Undoubtedly, this variation in epidural space content combined with varying spread contributes to the somewhat unpredictable clinical effects seen with epidural local anesthetic administration.

2.3.2 Pharmacokinetics of epidural local anesthetic administration

2.3.2.1 Factors which affect epidural spread

As mentioned above, and contrary to the effects of intrathecal local anesthetic, the complex nature of epidural analgesia is suggested by the lack of relevance of physical factors affecting anatomical spread when compared to the clinically present segmental analgesia.

2.3.2.2 Absorption, potency, duration, onset

Local anesthetics stabilize excitable cell membranes and block sodium and potassium flux through the axonal membrane ion pores. The anesthetic profile and clinical characteristics of a local anesthetic depends on its lipid solubility, protein binding, and dissociation constant (pK_a). Lipid solubility is generally agreed to be the primary determinant of intrinsic anesthetic potency. Protein binding is the characteristic associated with duration of action of the agent since those that attach to protein components of nerve membranes are less likely to diffuse from the site of action to enter the systemic circulation. The pK_a of a compound, as discussed earlier in detail and defined as the pH at which there is equilibrium between the ionized and unionized states of the molecule, impacts the rate of onset of clinical effect. This value is important for effective anesthesia because the uncharged form of the molecule is essential for epineural diffusion across lipid nerve sheaths and cell membranes. Conversely, only the charged form can dissociate in water and diffuse through cellular fluid and intracellular metabolism [90, 91].

2.3.2.3 Metabolism

The metabolic mechanism of local anesthetics depends on their chemical classification. Amide-type local anesthetics, including ropivacaine, are primarily metabolized by the hepatic esterase activity seen in the P450 system in the liver [92, 93]. Ester-type local anesthetics (procaine, benzocaine, tetracaine) are predomi-nantly hydrolyzed by plasma pseudocholinesterase.

2.3.3 Pharmacodynamics of epidural local anesthetic administration

2.3.3.1 Measuring effects

A discussion of clinical effect should include a comment on the differential blockade. Independent of differences in nerve fiber size and resistance to blockade, local anesthetics have varied differential blockade characteristics. Even within a single agent, the differential blockade can vary. As an example, bupivacaine, one of the best agents at producing effective analgesia while sparing motor loss, loses its motor-sparing characteristics as the bupivacaine concentration is increased from 0.5 to 0.75%.

The mode of action of epidural analgesia is far from clear. Proposed sites of action have included: (1) mixed spinal nerves in the paravertebral space, (2) dorsal root ganglia, (3) spinal roots, and (4) the periphery of the spinal cord. Regardless, blockade of a nerve fiber varies based on the duration of exposure, the exposed length of the axon, the type and site of the axon, and the concentration of local anesthetic at the axonal membrane.

Tachyphylaxis describes the condition of acute tolerance to local anesthetic drugs, though its mechanism is not well understood. The relationship between the change of response and interval between injections is complicated. However, it is likely the interval between the disappearance of analgesia and the subsequently repeated injection of local anesthetic is primary. When it occurs, decreasing analgesic effectiveness is noted, including a decrease in the number of dermatomes blocked as well as a decrease in motor block, showing that all measurable components of anesthesia are affected. Simply, with repeated doses, fewer segments are anesthetized, the duration of action is decreased, and both motor and sensory blockade are less intense [94].

The response to epidural blockade includes both autonomic blockade as a result of sympathetic interruption and somatic pain blockade (similar to intrathecal injection of local anesthetic, but with a greater duration of time to achieve clinical effect). The sympathetic blockade has consequent effects on vascular beds, cardiac functioning, and other visceral structures as discussed previously. Somatic pain blockade provides for the potential of anatomic functional restoration secondary to pain responses. Both results can occur as a consequence of epidural blockade and may be utilized in the operating room, in the labor suite or the pain clinic.

3. Conclusions

In conclusion, the administration of local anesthetic via the intrathecal or epidural route possesses unique pharmacokinetic and pharmacodynamic properties. These properties are influenced by the complex anatomy of bones, ligaments, membranes, vasculature, and adipose tissue. Understandably, the mechanism of action of local anesthetics is complex with primary Na^+ and K^+ ion channel activity. Additional involvement of Ca^{2+} ion channels, γ-aminobutyric acid, and substance P have been proposed.

Pharmacokinetic variables affecting the clinical picture associated with local anesthetic administration include the protein binding, lipid solubility, and pK_a. Spinal local anesthetic pharmacodynamic effects are variable and influenced by factors that are unique to the local anesthetic solution, factors that are unique to the patient, and factors that are associated with the method of local anesthetic administra-tion. Epidural pharmacodynamic effects are characterized by a lack of relevance of physical factors affecting anatomical spread when compared to the clinically present segmental analgesia. Both spinal and epidural local anesthetic administration are associated with clinical effects that involve the cardiovascular, pulmonary, digestive, renal, and immune systems to varying degrees of significance. Local anesthetic toxic-ity affects the nervous system and cardiovascular system to varying degrees based on the properties of the individual local anesthetic (i.e., lipid solubility, CV: CNS toxicity ratio, etc.) and the toxic dosage administered. Regardless of the manifestations of toxicity, the key to successful treatment is early consideration of the diagnosis. The development and widespread distribution of lipid emulsion has improved survival and should be considered in all cases where local anesthetic toxicity is a concern.

Conflict of interest

The views expressed in the manuscript are those of the authors and do not reflect the official policy or position of the Department of the Navy, Department of Defense, or the U.S. Government.

We are military service members. This work was prepared as part of our official duties. Title 17 U.S.C. 105 provides that "Copyright protection under this title is not available for any work of the United States Government." Title 17 U.S.C. 101 defines a United States Government work as a work prepared by a military service member as part of that person's official duties.

The authors have no conflict of interest or financial disclosure to report.

Author details

Jeffrey M. Carness[1*] and Mark J. Lenart[2]

1 United States Naval Hospital, Bremerton, Washington, USA

2 Naval Medical Center, Portsmouth, Virginia, USA

*Address all correspondence to: jeffrey.m.carness.mil@mail.mil

References

[1] Richardson J, Groen GJ. Applied epidural anatomy. Continuing Education in Anaesthesia Critical Care & Pain. 2005;**5**(3):98-100

[2] Barker AE. A report on clinical experiences with spinal analgesia in 100 cases, and some reflections on the procedure. British Medical Journal. 1907;**1**(2412):665-674

[3] Axelrod EH, Alexander GD, Brown M, Schork MA. Procaine spinal anesthesia: A pilot study of the incidence of transient neurologic symptoms. Journal of Clinical Anesthesia. 1998;**10**(5):404-409

[4] Johnson S. Cocaine to procaine: An unexpected history of local anaesthesia. Biomedical Journal of Scientific & Technical Research. 2018;**7**(2):1-4. DOI: 10.26717/BJSTR.2018.07.001467

[5] Jones WH. Percaine: A new regional and spinal analgesic, with special reference to high thoracic nerve root block and a new technique. Proceedings of the Royal Society of Medicine. 1930;**23**(7):919-928

[6] No authors listed. Dibucaine, cinchocaine, or nupercaine? CIBA's Trademarked long-acting amide local anesthetic. Anesthesiology. 2018;**128**(4):753. DOI:10.1097/ALN.0000000000002165

[7] Lund PC, Rumball AC. Hypobaric pontocaine spinal anaesthesia; 1,640 consecutive cases. Anesthesiology. 1947;**8**(2):181-199

[8] Garth WL. Subarachnoid block with crystalline pontocaine. Anesthesiology. 1941;**2**(2):205-206

[9] Liu SS, McDonald SB. Current issues in spinal anesthesia. Anesthesiology. 2001;**94**(5):888-906

[10] Foldes FF, McNall PG. 2-Chloroprocaine: A new local anesthetic agent. Anesthesiology. 1952;**13**(3):287-296

[11] Dhuner KG, Egner B, Ekenstam BA, Oljelund O, Ulfendahl LR. Trials with carbocaine; a new local anaesthetic drug. British Journal of Anaesthesia. 1956;**28**(11):503-506

[12] Crankshaw TP. Citanest(prilocaine) in spinal analgesia. Acta Anaesthesiologica Scandinavica. Supplementum. 1965;**16**:287-290

[13] Liguori GA, Zayas VM, Chisholm MF. Transient neurologic symptoms after spinal anesthesia with mepivacaine and lidocaine. Anesthesiology. 1998; **88**(3):619-623

[14] Hampl KF, Heinzmann-Wiedmer S, Luginbuehl I, Harms C, Seeberger M, Schneider MC, et al. Transient neurologic symptoms after spinal anesthesia: A lower incidence with prilocaine and bupivacaine than with lidocaine. Anesthesiology. 1998;**88**(3):629-633

[15] Manassero A, Fanelli A. Prilocaine hydrochloride 2% hyperbaric solution for intrathecal injection: A clinical review. Local and Regional Anesthesia. 2017;**10**:15-24. DOI: 10.2147/LRA.S112756

[16] Ekblom L, Widman B. LAC-43 and tetracaine in spinal anaesthesia. A controlled clinical study. Acta Anaesthesiologica Scandinavica. Supplementum. 1966;**23**:419-425

[17] Lund PC, Cwik JC, Vallesteros F. Bupivacaine—A new long-acting local anesthetic agent. A preliminary clinical and laboratory report. Anesthesia and Analgesia. 1970;**49**(1):103-114

[18] van Kleef JW, Veering BT, Burm AG. Spinal anesthesia with ropivacaine: A double-blind study on the efficacy and safety of 0.5% and 0.75% solutions in patients undergoing minor lower limb surgery. Anesthesia and Analgesia. 1994;**78**(6):1125-1130

[19] Wahedi W, Nolte H, Klein P. Ropivacaine for spinal anesthesia. A dose-finding study. Der Anaesthesist. 1996;**45**(8):737-744. DOI: 10.1097/00000542-199801000-00025

[20] Gautier PE, De Kock M, Van Steenberge A, Poth N, Lahaye-Goffart B, Fanard L, et al. Intrathecal ropivacaine for ambulatory surgery. Anesthesiology. 1999; **91**(5):1239-1245. DOI: 10.1097/00000542-199911000-00013

[21] Burlacu CL, Buggy DJ. Update on local anesthetics: Focus on levobupivacaine. Therapeutics and Clinical Risk Management. 2008;**4**(2):381-392. DOI: 10.2147/tcrm. s1433

[22] Alley EA, Kopacz DJ, McDonald SB, Liu SS. Hyperbaric spinal levobupivacaine: A comparison to racemic bupivacaine in volunteers. Anesthesia and Analgesia. 2002;**94**(1):188-193

[23] Glaser C, Marhofer P, Zimpfer G, Heinz MT, Sitzwohl C, Kapral S, et al. Levobupivacaine versus racemic bupivacaine for spinal anesthesia. Anesthesia and Analgesia. 2002;**94**(1):194-198

[24] Olschewski A, Hempelmann G, Vogel W, Safronov BV. Blockade of Na+ and K+ currents by local anesthetics in the dorsal horn neurons of the spinal cord. Anesthesiology. 1998;**88**(1):172-179. DOI: 10.1097/00000542-199801000-00025

[25] Lirk P, Picardi S, Hollmann MW. Local anaesthetics: 10 essentials. European Journal of Anaesthesiology. 2014;**31**(11):575-585. DOI: 10.1097/EJA.0000000000000137

[26] Swadlow HA, Kocsis JD, Waxman SG. Modulation of impulse conduction along the axonal tree. Annual Review of Biophysics and Bioengineering. 1980; **9**:143-179

[27] Raymond SA. Subblocking concentrations of local anesthetics: Effects on impulse generation and conduction in single myelinated sciatic nerve axons in frog. Anesthesia and Analgesia. 1992;**75**(6):906-921. DOI: 10.1213/00000539-199212000-00008

[28] Sugiyama K, Muteki T. Local anesthetics depress the calcium current of rat sensory neurons in culture. Anesthesiology. 1994;**80**(6):1369-1378. DOI: 10.1097/00000542-199406000-00025

[29] Li YM, Wingrove DE, Too HP, Marnerakis M, Stimson ER, Strichartz GR, et al. Local anesthetics inhibit substance P binding and evoked increases in intracellular Ca2+. Anesthesiology. 1995;**82**(1): 166-173. DOI: 10.1097/00000542- 199501000-00021

[30] Nordmark J, Rydqvist B. Local anaesthetics potentiate GABA-mediated Cl- currents by inhibiting GABA uptake. Neuroreport. 1997;**8**(2):465-468

[31] Greene NM. Distribution of local anesthetic solutions within the subarachnoid space. Anesthesia and Analgesia. 1985;**64**(7):715-730

[32] Sakka L, Coll G, Chazal J. Anatomy and physiology of cerebrospinal fluid. European Annals of Otorhinolaryngology, Head and Neck Diseases. 2011;**128**(6):309-316. DOI: 10.1016/j.anorl.2011.03.002

[33] Higuchi H, Hirata J, Adachi Y, Kazama T. Influence of lumbosacral

cerebrospinal fluid density, velocity, and volume on extent and duration of plain bupivacaine spinal anesthesia. Anesthesiology. 2004;**100**(1):106-114. DOI: 10.1097/00000542-200401000-00019

[34] Greene NM. Uptake and elimination of local anesthetics during spinal anesthesia. Anesthesia and Analgesia. 1983;**62**(11):1013-1024

[35] Kozody R, Swartz J, Palahniuk RJ, Biehl DR, Wade JG. Spinal cord blood flow following sub-arachnoid lidocaine. Canadian Anaesthetists' Society Journal. 1985;**32**(5):472-478

[36] Kristensen JD, Karlsten R, Gordh T. Spinal cord blood flow after intrathecal injection of ropivacaine and bupivacaine with or without epinephrine in rats. Acta Anaesthesiologica Scandinavica. 1998;**42**(6):685-690

[37] Becker DE, Reed KL. Essentials of local anesthetic pharmacology. Anesthesia Progress. 2006l;**53**(3): 98-108. DOI: 10.2344/0003- 3006(2006)53[98:EOLAP]2.0.CO;2

[38] Clement R, Malinovsky JM, Le Corre P, Dollo G, Chevanne F, Le Verge R. Cerebrospinal fluid bioavailability and pharmacokinetics of bupivacaine and lidocaine after intrathecal and epidural administrations in rabbits using microdialysis. The Journal of Pharmacology and Experimental Therapeutics. 1999;**289**(2):1015-1021

[39] Steinbrook RA, Concepcion M. Respiratory effects of spinal anesthesia: Resting ventilation and single-breath CO_2 response. Anesthesia and Analgesia. 1991;**72**(2):182-186

[40] Smith HW, Rovenstine EA, Goldring W, Chasis H, Ranges HA. The effects of spinal anesthesia on the circulation in normal, unoperated man with reference to the autonomy of the arterioles, and especially those of the renal circulation. The Journal of Clinical Investigation. 1939;**18**(3):319-341

[41] Mercatello A. Changes in renal function induced by anesthesia. Annales Françaises d'Anesthèsie et de Rèanimation. 1990;**9**(6):507-524

[42] Suleiman MY, Passannante AN, Onder RL, Greene-Helms WF, Perretta SG. Alteration of renal blood flow during epidural anesthesia in normal subjects. Anesthesia and Analgesia. 1997;**84**(5):1076-1080

[43] Borgeat A, Ekatodramis G, Schenker CA. Postoperative nausea and vomiting in regional anesthesia: A review. Anesthesiology. 2003;**98**(2):530-547

[44] Cassuto J, Sinclair R, Bonderovic M. Anti-inflammatory properties of local anesthetics and their present and potential clinical implications. Acta Anaesthesiologica Scandinavica. 2006;**50**(3):265-282

[45] Sasagawa S. Inhibitory effects of local anesthetics on migration, extracellular release of lysosomal enzyme, and superoxide anion production in human polymorphonuclear leukocytes. Immunopharmacology and Immunotoxicology. 1991;**13**(4):607-622

[46] Hodson M, Gajraj R, Scott NB. A comparison of the antibacterial activity of levobupivacaine vs. bupivacaine: An in vitro study with bacteria implicated in epidural infection. Anaesthesia. 1999;**54**(7):699-702. DOI: 10.1046/j.1365-2044.1999.00742.x

[47] Hocking G, Wildsmith JA. Intrathecal drug spread. British Journal of Anaesthesia. 2004;**93**(4):568-578. DOI: 10.1093/bja/aeh204

[48] Okutomi T, Nemoto M, Mishiba E, Goto F. Viscosity of diluent and sensory level of subarachnoid anaesthesia achieved with tetracaine. Canadian Journal of Anaesthesia. 1998;**45**(1): 84-86. DOI: 10.1007/BF03012001

[49] Hartwell BL, Aglio LS, Hauch MA, Datta S. Vertebral column length and spread of hyperbaric subarachnoid bupivacaine in the term parturient. Regional Anesthesia. 1991;**16**(1):17-19

[50] Danelli G, Zangrillo A, Nucera D, Giorgi E, Fanelli G, Senatore R, et al. The minimum effective dose of 0.5% hyperbaric spinal bupivacaine for cesarean section. Minerva Anestesiologica. 2001;**67**(7-8):573-577

[51] Veering BT, Burm AG, Spierdijk J. Spinal anaesthesia with hyperbaric bupivacaine. Effects of age on neural blockade and pharmacokinetics. British Journal of Anaesthesia. 1988;**60**(2):187-194. DOI: 10.1093/bja/60.2.187

[52] Richardson MG, Wissler RN. Density of lumbar cerebrospinal fluid in pregnant and nonpregnant humans. Anesthesiology.1996;**85**(2):326-330. DOI:10.1097/00000542-199608000-00014

[53] Nightingale PJ. Barbotage and spinal anaesthesia. The effect of barbotage on the spread of analgesia during isobaric spinal anaesthesia. Anaesthesia. 1983;**38**(1):7-9

[54] Janik R, Dick W, Stanton-Hicks MD. Influence of barbotage on block characteristics during spinal anesthesia with hyperbaric tetracaine and bupivacaine. Regional Anesthesia. 1989;**14**(1):26-30

[55] Schroder W, Schwagmeier R, Schmidt A, Nolte H. The effect of barbotage on the sensory spread in spinal anesthesia using isobaric and hyperbaric 0.5% bupivacaine. Regional-Anaesthesie. 1990;**13**(7): 168-171

[56] Singh SI, Morley-Forster PK, Shamsah M, Butler R. Influence of injection rate of hyperbaric bupivacaine on spinal block in parturients: A randomized trial. Canadian Journal of Anaesthesia. 2007;**54**(4):290-295. DOI: 10.1007/BF03022774

[57] James KS, Stott SM, McGrady EM, Pearsall FJ, Frame WT, Russell D. Spinal anaesthesia for caesarean section: Effect of Sprotte needle orientation. British Journal of Anaesthesia. 1996;**77**(2): 150-152. DOI: 10.1093/bja/77.2.150

[58] Urmey WF, Stanton J, Bassin P, Sharrock NE. The direction of the Whitacre needle aperture affects the extent and duration of isobaric spinal anesthesia. Anesthesia and Analgesia. 1997;**84**(2):337-341. DOI: 10.1097/00000539-199702000-00017

[59] Neigh JL, Kane PB, Smith TC. Effects of speed and direction of injection on the level and duration of spinal anesthesia. Anesthesia and Analgesia. 1970;**49**(6):912-918

[60] Masse E, Drolet P, Girard M. Direction of injection does not affect the spread of spinal bupivacaine in parturients. Canadian Journal of Anaesthesia. 1997;**44**(8):816-819. DOI: 10.1007/BF03013156

[61] Stienstra R, van Poorten F, Kroon JW. Needle direction affects the sensory level of spinal anesthesia. Anesthesia and Analgesia. 1989;**68**(4):497-500

[62] El-Boghdadly K, Chin KJ. Local anesthetic systemic toxicity: Continuing professional development. Canadian Journal of Anaesthesia. 2016;**63**(3):330-349. DOI: 10.1007/s12630-015-0564-z

[63] Christie LE, Picard J, Weinberg GL. Local anaesthetic systemic toxicity. BJA

Education. 2014;**15**(3):136-142. DOI: 10.1093/bjaceaccp/mku027

[64] Rosenblatt MA, Abel M, Fischer GW, Itzkovich CJ, Eisenkraft JB. Successful use of a 20% lipid emulsion to resuscitate a patient after a presumed bupivacaine-related cardiac arrest. Anesthesiology. 2006;**105** (1):217-218.DOI: 10.1097/00000542-200607000-00033

[65] Verlinde M, Hollmann MW, Stevens MF, Hermanns H, Werdehausen R, Lirk P. Local anesthetic-induced neurotoxicity. International Journal of Molecular Sciences. 2016;**17**(3):339. DOI: 10.3390/ijms17030339

[66] Pollock JE. Neurotoxicity of intrathecal local anaesthetics and transient neurological symptoms. Best Practice & Research. Clinical Anaesthesiology. 2003;**17**(3):471-484

[67] Brull R, McCartney CJ, Chan VW, El-Beheiry H. Neurological complications after regional anesthesia: Contemporary estimates of risk. Anesthesia and Analgesia. 2007;**104**(4):965-974. DOI: 10.1213/01.ane.0000258740.17193.ec

[68] Lofstrom JB. 1991 Labat lecture. The effect of local anesthetics on the peripheral vasculature. Regional Anesthesia. 1992;**17**(1):1-11

[69] Haller I, Hausott B, Tomaselli B, Keller C, Klimaschewski L, Gerner P, et al. Neurotoxicity of lidocaine involves specific activation of the p38 mitogen-activated protein kinase, but not extracellular signal-regulated or c-Jun N-terminal kinases, and is mediated by arachidonic acid metabolites. Anesthesiology.2006;**105** (5):1024-1033. DOI:10.1097/00000542-200611000-00025

[70] Kan H, Wang Y, Wang D, Sun H, Zhou S, Wang H, et al. Cordycepin rescues lidocaine-induced neurotoxicity in dorsal root ganglion by interacting with inflammatory signaling pathway MMP3. European Journal of Pharmacology. 2018;**827**:88-93. DOI: 10.1016/j.ejphar.2018.01.049

[71] Klohr S, Roth R, Hofmann T, Rossaint R, Heesen M. Definitions of hypotension after spinal anaesthesia for caesarean section: Literature search and application to parturients. Acta Anaesthesiologica Scandinavica. 2010; **54**(8):909-921. DOI: 10.1111/j.1399-6576.2010.02239.x

[72] Moore DC, Bridenbaugh LD. Spinal (subarachnoid) block. A review of 11,574 cases. Journal of the American Medical Association. 1966;**195**(11):907-912

[73] Horlocker TT, McGregor DG, Matsushige DK, Schroeder DR, Besse JA. A retrospective review of 4767 consecutive spinal anesthetics: Central nervous system complications. Perioperative Outcomes Group. Anesthesia & Analgesia. 1997;**84**(3):578-584. DOI: 10.1097/00000539-199703000-00021

[74] Green L, Machin SJ. Managing anticoagulated patients during neuraxial anaesthesia. British Journal of Haematology. 2010;**149**(2):195-208. DOI: 10.1111/j.1365-2141.2010.08094.x

[75] Lagerkranser M. Neuraxial blocks and spinal haematoma: Review of 166 case reports published 1994- 2015. Part 1: Demographics and risk-factors. Scandinavian Journal of Pain. 2017;**15**: 118-129. DOI: 10.1016/j. sjpain.2016.11.008

[76] Moen V, Dahlgren N, Irestedt L. Severe neurological complications after central neuraxial blockades in Sweden 1990-1999. Anesthesiology. 2004;**101**(4):950-959.DOI:10.1097/00000542-200410000-00021

[77] D'Angelo R, Smiley RM, Riley ET, Segal S. Serious complications related to obstetric anesthesia: The serious complication repository project of the Society for Obstetric Anesthesia and Perinatology. Anesthesiology. 2014;**120** (6):1505-1512. DOI: 10.1097/ALN.0000000000000253

[78] Cook TM, Counsell D, Wildsmith JA. Royal College of Anaesthetists Third National Audit Project. Major complications of central neuraxial block: Report on the Third National Audit Project of the Royal College of Anaesthetists. British Journal of Anaesthesia. 2009;**102**(2):179-190. DOI: 10.1093/bja/aen360

[79] Kurz A, Sessler DI, Schroeder M, Kurz M. Thermoregulatory response thresholds during spinal anesthesia. Anesthesia and Analgesia.1993;**77**(4): 721-726

[80] Joris J, Ozaki M, Sessler DI, Hardy AF, Lamy M, McGuire J, et al. Epidural anesthesia impairs both central and peripheral thermoregulatory control during general anesthesia. Anesthesiology. 1994;**80**(2):268-277. DOI: 10.1097/00000542-199402000-00006

[81] Saito T, Sessler DI, Fujita K, Ooi Y, Jeffrey R. Thermoregulatory effects of spinal and epidural anesthesia during cesarean delivery. Regional Anesthesia and Pain Medicine. 1998;**23**(4):418-423

[82] Kwak KH. Postdural puncture headache. Korean Journal of Anesthesiology. 2017;**70**(2):136-143. DOI: 10.4097/kjae.2017.70.2.136

[83] Sprung J, Bourke DL, Contreras MG, Warner ME, Findlay J. Perioperative hearing impairment. Anesthesiology. 2003;**98**(1):241-257

[84] Bromage PR. Epidural Analgesia. Philadelphia: Saunders; 1978

[85] Reina MA, Villanueva MC, Maches F, Carrera A, Lopez A, De Andres JA. The ultrastructure of the human spinal nerve root cuff in the lumbar spine. Anesthesia and Analgesia. 2008;**106**(1):339-344. DOI: 10.1213/01.ane.0000295803.31074.dc

[86] Tretjakoff D. Das epidurales Fettgewebe. Zeitschrift fur Anatomie und Entwicklungsgeschichte. 1926;**79**(1):101-111

[87] Ramsey HJ. Fat in the epidural space in young and adult cats. The American Journal of Anatomy. 1959;**104**:345-379

[88] Burm AG. Clinical pharmacokinetics of epidural and spinal anaesthesia. Clinical Pharmacokinetics. 1989;**16**(5): 283-311

[89] Hogan Q. Distribution of solution in the epidural space: Examination by cryomicrotome section. Regional Anesthesia and Pain Medicine. 2002;**27**(2):150-156

[90] Erdemir HA, Soper LE, Sweet RB. Studies of factors affecting peridural anesthesia. Anesthesia and Analgesia. 1965;**44**(4):400-404

[91] Moore PA, Hersh EV. Local anesthetics: Pharmacology and toxicity. Dental Clinics of North America. 2010;**54**(4):587-599. DOI: 10.1016/j.cden.2010.06.015

[92] Covino BG. The pharmacology of local anesthetic agents. In: Stanley TH, Petty WC, editors. Anesthesiology, Developments in Critical Care Medicine and Anesthesiology. Vol. 11. Dordrecht: Springer; 1986

[93] Oda Y, Furuichi K, Tanaka K, Hiroi T, Imaoka S, Asada A, et al. Metabolism of a new local anesthetic, ropivacaine, by human hepatic cytochrome P450. Anesthesiology.

1995;**82**(1):214-220. DOI: 10.1097/00000542-199501000-00026

[94] Bromage PR, Pettigrew RT, Crowell DE. Tachyphylaxis in epidural analgesia: I. Augmentation and decay of local anesthesia. The Journal of Clinical Pharmacology and the Journal of New Drugs. 1969;**9**(1):30-38

2

Local Anesthetics in Odontology

Enrique Hernández-Cortez, Cecilia G. Sandoval Larios and Juan Carlos Flores-Carrillo

Abstract

Pain has been a faithful companion of human beings and is a result of most of the dental procedures and illness; therefore a good control of dental pain is inevitable and feasible. The administration of local anesthetics has come to be the standard of care of dental profession. All local anesthetics are effective and high safety margin in all patients including childhood. The choice of using a local anesthetic depends on time of the surgical procedure, patient's medical history, and the interaction between local anesthetics and patient usual medications. The use of vasoconstrictors is priority in surgical/dental bleeding, but it must be used with caution in patients with cardiovascular disease to avoid a dental catastrophe. Dentists should be experts in dental-anesthetic techniques and in pharmacology of local anesthetics, since they are the most used medications in odontology. The accidental injection or a high absorption of local anesthetics in blood results in systemic toxicity. In such situation sedation, stunning, diplopia, sensory disturbances, disorientation, muscles spasm, respiratory depression, seizures, or cardiac arrest may be present; the dentist must immediately recognize this clinical complication to stablish an early treatment.

Keywords: local anesthetics, dental, local anesthesia, local analgesia, complications

1. Introduction

Local anesthetics (LAs) are the most used drugs by dentists. Actually, they are safer drugs. More than 40% or urgent dental procedures cause pain that needs and injection of LA. Therefore, dentists should be experts in dental-anesthetic techniques and in pharmacology of LA drugs. The safe administration of LA is the standard of care of dentists.

Pain has been a companion of human beings since their appearance on earth. Before local anesthetics, natural medicine was first used to relieve dental pain. Such medicine has evolved since ancient Egypt and Greek culture until the nineteenth century when LA developed. Actually, LAs are the most secure and effective drugs in medicine for pain prevention and treatment. There are no drugs more effective than LAs to avoid pain; no other drug prevents a nociceptive impulse from reach-ing the patient's brain, to finally be interpreted as pain. Whenever local anesthetics are administered near a sensitive nerve, it produces an adequate control pain for a limited time with the aids of been a reversible and temporary effect without harm of the anesthetized nervous structure.

The first registered dental anesthesia in history was in 1885 of the alveolar inferior nervous, applied by the medical surgeon William Stewart Halsted. The injected drug was a combination of cocaine and epinephrine [1]. In 1905, 2% procaine with epinephrine 1:50,000 was introduced, giving a quick access to dentists worldwide. Procaine, propoxycaine, and tetracaine were the most used LAs until the middle 1940s. Lidocaine was synthetized in Sweden in 1948 [2]. Articaine was synthetized in 1973 and introduced in dental clinic in 1976 and approved in Canada in 1984 and in the USA until 2000. Articaine has special characteristics of both amino amide and amino ester anesthetics. Its popularity has increased rapidly and is currently displacing the use of lidocaine in dental anesthesia [3].

Annually, a dentist in Canada applies 1800 LA cartridges, while in the USA, more than 300 million of cartridges are administered each year. Therefore, dentists should be experts in pharmacology, complications, and secondary effects of LA. In daily practice there are few complications related to LA, owing its security and the relative low doses that are applied. Nonetheless, it is necessary to consider possible complications, to detect it as soon as possible.

2. Pharmacology of LA

The synthetic LA has a common chemical structure, constituted by an aromatic ring, a hydrocarbon channel, and an amino group; the hydrocarbon channel and aromatic ring are joined by an ester or amide bond. Most of LAs are tertiary amines. The lipophilic portion is the biggest of the molecule. The aromatic portion proceeds from benzoic acid, aniline, or thiophene (articaine) and is the lipophilic portion. This portion is responsible for the affinity of nerve cells. The hydrophilic portion is an amino ethanol or acetic acid derivative and is responsible of water solubility and diffusion across tissues. LAs are amphipathic; that is, they have lipophilic and hydrophilic characteristics at their opposite ends of their molecules (**Figure 1**) [4]. Amides are the most common molecules; procaine is the prototype of this group and benzocaine for topic application. The minimal concentration of LA to block the conduction of a nociceptive impulse is named potency. The therapeutic value of the drug in terms of efficacy and tolerability is called toxicity. The ability of the drug to reach tissues far from the site of administration of LA is called diffusion. Time between the action of LA and the metabolism of its compounds is named time of action [5].

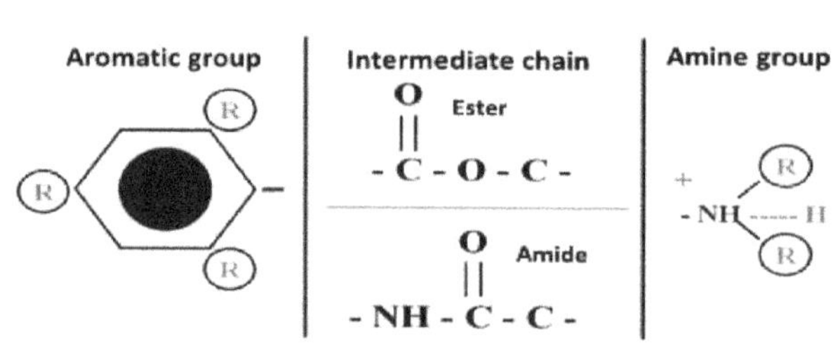

Figure 1.
Local anesthetic molecule.

3. Mechanism of action of LA

The type of nervous blockade produced by LA is named non-depolarizing nervous block. Local anesthetics block sodium channels permeability, they selectively inhibit the maximum permeability to sodium, whose values usually are five to six times greater than the necessary minimum to conduct the impulse, when this value fail, and the nerve block occurs. In other words, local anesthesia is induced when the spread of action potential is inhibited, so a painful sensation cannot be trans-mitted from the site of origin to the brain. Or, LA alter the mechanism to sodium ions to gain access to the axoplasm nerve. The nerve membrane stays in a polarized state due to the impossibility of ionic movement responsible of action potential. LA blocks the entrance of sodium ions into their channels in the nerve cellular mem-brane. The permeability to sodium is necessary to generate a new action potential to transmit nerve impulses to the brain [6]. The sequence of action mechanism proposed for LA is described in **Table 1**.

LAs are classified into two large groups depending on its chemical bond: amides or ester; the latter are almost disappearing in dentistry. The ester LAs are easily hydrolyzed in aqueous solution, while amide bond LAs are relatively resistant to hydrolysis. The most important factors that affect onset and duration of action of LA are tissue pH, drug pKa, diffusion time from the tip of the needle to nerve, nerve morphology, drug concentration, and drug solubility in lipids [7]. The most important of the abovementioned factors are tissue pH and drug pKa. The pH may be reduced in infection sites, so the result would be a delay in the LA onset. In clinics, the amides pK is similar, with the exception of bupivacaine that has a slightly greater pK and an onset time more prolonged. The proximity of the anesthetic to the nerve is another factor that influences the action time of LA; a very clear example is the Gow-Gates blockade, very slow in its installation. The nerve morphology is also an important factor, which thin fibers are quickly anesthetized compared to thicker ones. The duration of action depends on the depth at which the drug may be blocking the sodium channels in the nerve mem-brane. If the LA causes vasodilatation, it allows a more or less rapid diffusion in the site of action and therefore a short duration of action, especially if the drug is administered alone. This diffusion may be reduced with the aid of vasoconstric-tors like epinephrine, although bupivacaine is the only LA that has a prolonged action duration [8]. The two most important factors involved in the action of LA are the drug diffusion across the nerve sheath and the bind to the receptor in the ionic channel; a lipid-soluble free base and without electric charge is responsible of the diffusion across the nerve sheath.

The biotransformation of amides occurs mainly in the liver, although prilocaine is metabolized in plasma and eliminated in the kidney. One of its metabolites could be the origin of methemoglobinemia [9]. The ester LAs are biotransformed in plasma by enzymes called cholinesterase or pseudocholinesterase produced in the liver [10].

1. Displacement of sodium ions from the sodium channel receptor
2. Binding of the LA molecule to the receptor
3. Block of the sodium channel
4. Decreased sodium conduction
5. Depressed velocity of electric depolarization
6. Failed to teach the value of umbral potential
7. Absence of propagated action potentials
8. Conduction block

Table 1.
Sequence of mechanisms of LA to produce conduction block.

Important properties of LA
Specific action
Reversible action
Quickly onset action
Adequate duration of action
Active, injected, or topically administered
Non-irritating
Non-permanent harm
No systemic toxicity when properly used
High therapeutic ratio
Chemically stable
Long half-life
Ability to combine with other agents without losing their properties
Sterilizable without losing its properties
Slight allergenic

Table 2.
Important properties of LA.

Despite the great advances in the field or anesthetics in dentistry, the ideal agent do not exist; however, new ALs are increasingly safer. Some of its most important properties are listed in **Table 2**.

4. Most commonly used LA in dentistry

4.1 Lidocaine

This is the most common used LA in dentistry since its introduction in 1948 and now considered the gold standard for clinical use. It was the drug that displaced older anesthetics like procaine (Novocain). It has fast onset between 2 and 3 min-utes with a longer and profound anesthesia. It is available in various concentrations; the most used are 1 and 2% cartridges with 1:100,000 and 1:50,000 epinephrine. Using lidocaine without a vasoconstrictor is rare in dentistry because of rapid vasodilation and high plasma concentrations as well as higher adverse reaction. For patients who are sensitive to epinephrine, they should limit the amount to a maximum of two cartridges per procedure. Thus, it is true for hypertensive patients, patients with coronary heart disease, and the elderly. Lidocaine combined with 1:50,000 epinephrine is commonly used in active dental bleeding because of diminishing up to 50%. It gives a pulpal anesthesia for up to 90 minutes and some-times may be comparable to articaine (3–5 hours). Today, lidocaine is referred to local anesthetics toxicity. The maximum recommended dose in combination with epinephrine is 7 mg/kg for an adult or children over 15 kg, not exceeding 500 mg. Lidocaine alone is limited to 4.4 mg/kg, not exceeding 300 mg [11].

4.2 Mepivacaine

This is an amide type LA, available only in cartridge formed at concentration of 2 and 3%. Mepivacaine combined with a vasoconstrictor in 2% concentration. It is ideal for patients with an absolute contraindication to receive vasoconstrictor.

A maximum recommended dose in adult or children is 4.4 mg/kg without exceeding 300 mg a day. Simple mepivacaine at 3% gives anesthesia for about 20–40 minutes in gums, 40 minutes in nerve blocks, and a maximum of 3 hours in soft tissue. It is the most commonly used LA in pediatric patients because of its rapid onset and short dental procedures. It is available in 1:20,000 combination with levonordefrin which is a different profile compared to epinephrine. Their affinity to alpha and beta receptors is 75:25, a low effect on beta receptors. Levonordefrin is one-sixth of the potency of epinephrine. It has the lowest pKa of all LA used in dentistry, which explains the rapid onset [11]. Compared with lidocaine it has a potency of 2 and is metabolized thru oxidase in the liver, and renal elimination in 16% is unchanged.

4.3 Articaine

It is most recently introduced to dental practice. It is an amide type but possesses an ester group, making it the only hybrid LA, thus metabolizing in plasma as well as by the liver in which most of the process takes place, giving a result an inactive metabolite named articainic acid. It is equivalent to lidocaine in its vasodilation effect. It has a fast elimination time of approximately 27 minutes, compared to 40 minutes in amide anesthetics. It offers 90 minutes of pulpal anesthesia and 3 hours in soft tissue, being a reasonable choice in most dental procedures. This is available in dental cartridges at 4%, with epinephrine in 1:100,000 and 1:200,000 concentrations. The maximum dose is 7 mg/kg (72 mg per cartridge) for adults and 5 mg/kg for children under 15 kg [12]. It is the LA with higher risk of postoperative paresthesia in the jaw while rarely happening in other non-dental specialties such as orthopedic, spinal, or eye [13, 14].

4.4 Bupivacaine

It is a long-acting amide LA. Intrapulpal anesthesia as long as offers 6 hours and solf tissue up to 12 hours. It is also the most toxic drug, characterized by cardiovascular affection, inducing sudden collapse. In the same way it can induce longer duration of seizures which may be explained by its slower elimination (0.58 L/minute clearance) and a long half-life. It is four times more potent than lidocaine [15]. Although related to mepivacaine because of their molecular composition they differ chemically, it is 35 times more liposoluble, easily crossing the membrane in nerve cells, binding strongly at receptor sites with greater inactiva-tion of sodium channels which make slow recovery, hence the saying that it is not easily uncoupled from the receptor.

Nancarrow et al. studied fatal doses in several LA: for lidocaine 30.8 ± 5.8 mg/kg/h, ropivacaine 7.3 ± 1.0 mg/kg, and bupivacaine 3.7 ± 1.1 mg/kg. Due to this finding, the toxicity threshold of bupivacaine in dental procedures is low and, an unnoticed injection during infiltration is dangerous and not recommended or approved by the FDA in children [16].

Bupivacaine is available in dental cartridges in 0.5% with 1:200,000. Ropivacaine has demonstrated a 75% safer profile than bupivacaine. It is a long-acting LA with the highest pKa (8.1) and binding to plasmatic proteins in 95% compared to the rest of the drugs used in dentistry, which gives a slowest onset, although in dental procedures this is usually not an issue. With a fast onset of 4-8 minutes after injection, 99% of patients reported low sensitivity in the lips vs. 100% reported with lidocaine [17]. The majority of reports of bupivacaine used in third molar extractions and root canal has confirmed its efficiency and security.

It is four times more toxic than lidocaine, so the use in dentistry is in lower doses than other areas in anesthesiology. A low incidence in paresthesia near 0.5% with this LA in combination with epinephrine at 1:200000 in an inferior alveolar nerve block has been reported [18]. Chapman and Ganendran reported that patients blocked with bupivacaine and epinephrine for the third molar extractions did not need pain medication at 4 hours after surgery compared to the control group (lidocaine 2%) in which all of the patients were given pain medication at the same time. Seventy percent of the bupivacaine group received medication at 8 hours after surgery, versus 100% in the lidocaine 2% group [19].

4.5 Prilocaine

For dental anesthesia, it is available in 4% concentration with or without epinephrine 1:200,000. Prilocaine by itself induces more vasodilation than mepivacaine and less than lidocaine. It shares the same length of action, although a slower onset. Toxicity is lower than lidocaine. At doses above 600 mg, there is a higher risk of developing methemoglobinemia. In levels below 20%, clinical symptoms such as cyanosis, respiratory distress, and cardiovascular collapse are not seen. Mainstay treatment for methemoglobinemia is 1% methylene blue, 1–2 mg/kg intravenously slow 10-minute drip. Toxicity signs less severe than lidocaine. Prilocaine at 4% is contained in cream form commercially named EMLA (lidocaine-prilocaine) commonly used to produce skin numbness before any type of procedure such as phlebotomy; the downside is the time (30 minutes) to prepare the skin completely. The maximum recommended dose in adults is 600 mg and 400 mg in children. It may provide anesthesia up to 60 minutes in an inferior alveolar block or even 4 hours in soft tissue. It is important to remember that prilocaine is contraindicated in patients with congenital or idiopathic methemoglobinemia, heart failure, or chronic pulmonary disease.

5. Pharmacology of vasoconstrictors

The LAs commonly used in dental anesthesia are vasodilators, so they increase the blood flow in the injected site and perhaps enhance the concentration of the drug in blood and the probability of anesthetic overdose. The increase in blood flow also results in a short duration of action, although it depends on other factors, such as protein binding capacity.

Vasoconstrictors are adjuvant substances to LA that play an important role in dental anesthesia, producing deeper anesthesia and greater action duration, decreased systemic toxicity possibility, as well as bleeding reduction.

The most used vasoconstrictor in dental anesthesia is epinephrine, available in concentrations of 1:50,000; 1:100,000; and 1:200,000. It is rapidly metabolized by oxidation or conjugation, and its half-life is a few minutes, but its effects can last up to several hours. Malamed et al. showed in experimental animals that the application of 2% lidocaine with epinephrine 1:100,000 around the sciatic nerve reduces the blood flow in 79% (**Table 3**) [20]. Other vasoconstrictors used in this clinical setting are norepinephrine and levonordefrin [21]. Low plasmatic concentrations of adrenaline can raise heart rate, cardiac output, and systemic vasodilation because of its β1 adrenergic effect. The stimulation of adrenergic receptors alpha and beta occurs in 50/50 proportion; so that alpha-adrenergic stimulation causes peripheral vasoconstriction, while beta-adrenergic stimulation produces tachycardia. It is used to prolong the action time of LA, decrease dental bleeding, and improve the visibility of the surgical field. Its effect limits the diffusion of LA from the injection site and its systemic absorption reducing the possibility of systemic toxicity. Although, in general, vasoconstrictors are not contraindicated, the risk level depends on the characteristics of each patient; people with certain cardiac or endocrine diseases or

1:100,000 = 0.01 mg/mL or 10 μg/mL
1:200,000 = 0.05 mg/mL or 5 μg/mL
1:50,000 = 0.02 mg/mL or 20 μg/mL
1 epinephrine cartridge 1:200,000 = 9 μg/mL
1 epinephrine cartridge 1:100,000 = 18 μg/mL
1 epinephrine cartridge 1:50,000 = 36 μg/mL
1 levonordefrin cartridge 1:20,000 = 90 μg/mL

Table 3.
Vasoconstrictor concentrations in mg/mL.

taking medicines that affect the sympathetic nervous system have a greater risk of having deleterious side effects.

The LA with epinephrine for dental use are in the following proportions: 1:50,000 (0.02 mg/mL), 1:100,000 (0.01 mg/mL), or 1:200,000 (0.004 mg/mL) [22]. The administration of 2% lidocaine with epinephrine 1:100,000 (a cartridge) produces plasmatic concentration of 240 ± 69ρ g/mL. With the administration of three cartridges of epinephrine or 54 μg, the blood concentration is 302 ± 142 ρg/mL.

Usually, the administration of one cartridge of LA with epinephrine is not associated with cardiovascular changes, while the administration of three cartridges of LA with epinephrine at the same concentration is associated with five times the concentration of epinephrine in plasma, and with it there may be systemic cardiovascular alterations. However, it is not necessarily associated with the dose [23].

The umbral value of plasmatic epinephrine to develop hypertension is between 50 and 100 ρg/mL; the umbral value for systolic blood pressure is 75–125 ρg/mL, while the umbral value to rise the diastolic blood pressure is 150–200 ρg/mL. Barkin et al. found that 2% lidocaine 1:100,000 can produce non-serious cardiac arrhythmias in 16% of dental patients. The study does not specify with was the most frequent arrhythmia or if any treatment was administered [24].

Unfortunately, the vasoconstrictor effects are not always beneficial. In special situations vasoconstrictors can affect the patient; an example of this are the patients with limited cardiovascular systemic reserves, such angina pectoris, pr evious myocardial infarction, systemic hypertension, and non-controlled hypothyroid-ism. In such patients, epinephrine can produce indirectly central nervous system excitation, including systemic hypertension, tachycardia, tremors, headache, palpitations, cardiac arrhythmias, and stroke. Comorbidities recommendable to use lidocaine with epinephrine 1:100,000 to epinephrine dose of 0.04 mg = 40 μg as a total dose.

Procaine is a potent vasodilator and cannot produce adequate anesthesia if it is used without a vasoconstrictor. Lidocaine is also a vasodilator but has enough potency to be used alone. In contrast, mepivacaine has minor vasodilator properties and can be used with or without vasoconstrictors [25].

Norepinephrine as a vasoconstrictor is seldom used since fatalities due to hyper-tension have been reported. Another disadvantage at a local level is being a quarter less vasoconstrictor than epinephrine and having a shorter half-life.

6. Local and systemic complications of LA

Local anesthesia is the gold standard for surgical dental procedures; it has defined as a technique that produces loss of sensitivity, without losing consciousness. Although anesthetics are defined as safe medications, some complications have been described.

The incidence of complications related to dental anesthesia is 4.5%, and the most common are needle break, paresthesia, transient facial paralysis, hematoma, toxicity and rarely allergy, dizziness 1.3%, tachycardia 1.1%, agitation 1.1%, nausea 0.8%, chills 0.7%, syncope, seizures, and bronchospasm [26].

As the same way, it can be complications related to additional vasoconstrictors of LA. It has been shown that the increases in plasmatic catecholamines observed after the LA infiltration are mainly due to higher doses of vasoconstrictors. Vasoconstrictors increase heart rate in 4.1% of patients and increase 20% with respect to baseline. Coronary insufficiency, arterial hypertension, myocardial infarction (in the last 6 months), congestive heart failure, pheochromocytoma, hyperthyroidism, and diabetes mellitus are risk factors for the use of vasoconstrictors during dental anesthesia [27].

Patients receiving LA are not always healthy; they can have hypertension, history of myocardial infarction, sequelae of diabetic neuropathy, cardiac disease, serious dental infections, are patients in extremes of life. Some are taking aspirin for various reasons: this drug inhibits the secretion of thromboxane, adenosine diphos-phate, and serotonin, chemicals mediators necessary to the platelet plug formation. Therefore, all patients taking aspirin should be recommended to suppress it at least 6 or 7 days before the dental intervention. The aspirin binds to the platelet during its half-life of approximately 7 days, so by removing aspirin, the new platelets will function adequately. In arrhythmic patients the use of anesthetics with vasocon-strictors is not recommended.

More than 45% of dental patients have one or more concomitant disease in their medical history, and near 20% of patients will have some disease and drug or food allergy. The secondary effects of LA are mainly present in patients with risk factors; in such patients the secondary effects can raise to 5.7% [28], which may result in greater morbidity. Nowadays, although lidocaine is the most used LA in dentistry, there are other LAs such as articaine that could displace the use of lidocaine.

Complications of LA include local and systemic effects. Local complications include:

6.1 LA failure

The possibility that local dental anesthesia fails is remote. Timely identification of the reasons of regional anesthesia failure in dental or maxillofacial surgery is essential to adopt the measures required for its correction. Some factors of anesthetic failure involve bifid inferior alveolar nerve, retromolar foramen associated to accessory innervation, double or accessory mental foramen, the relation between the infiltration technique and bone density, accessory innervation in the case of the mylohyoid nerve and first cervical branches, cross innervation of the incisors, inactivity in the presence of tissue inflammation, inactive LA, incorrect technique, and subjective perception on the part of anxious patients [12]. **Table 4** lists other important factors.

6.2 Hematoma

Damage to blood vessels is usually caused by the tip needle, the blood accumulated inside the oral tissues, and the swelling located in any tissue which acts as an irritant of the tissue and causes pain and trismus. Accumulated blood can

1. Inadequate anatomical selection
2. Insufficient LA dose
3. Insufficient time for the LA diffusion
4. Administration of LA in swelling or infected tissue
5. Use of expired LA

Table 4.
LA failure in dental practice.

be a culture medium for oral bacteria, especially in diabetic patients or those with immune deficiency.

6.3 Nerve damage

The needle can damage a nerve which produces a partial or complete deficit with motor or sensory abnormalities that usually have a full recovery.

6.4 Transient facial nerve paralysis

This complication is caused by the introduction of LA into the parotid gland capsule, which is located at the back of the edge of the mandibular branch. If the LA is deposited on this site, a transient paralysis of muscles of the face occurs. The LA is applied next to the facial nerve, so the motor blockade would cause a temporary paralysis of the muscles of the face; clinically a modification in the face expression appears. The duration of motor paralysis lasts between 3 and 5 hours, and treatment is not required. An important clinical situation is that patient cannot close the affected eye and is necessary to avoid the dry eye during this period of involvement [29].

6.5 Needle rupture

Since the introduction of non-reusable needles in dental anesthesia, needle rupture has been an extremely rare complication. Progrel et al. estimated this risk at 1:14 million, more specifically in the case of inferior alveolar nerve block. In the analysis of broken needles, it was found that the majority were short or G30 ultra-short needles (20 and 10 mm). The inferior alveolar nerve block was the most frequent in 79% of the cases and the alveolar superior posterior nerve in the rest of the cases. Additional factors are pre-bending of the needle before injection, the unexpected and sudden movement of the patient at the time the needle is entering the soft tissue, and strong contact of the needle with the bone [30].

6.6 Systemic complications of LA

Local anesthetic-related systemic complications are associated with the nature of the drug and/or their composition. Systemic complications are as followed:

6.6.1 Systemic or local infection

Spreading the potentially dangerous infection within mouth soft tissue to neck or head may be caused by needle trauma. Dental abscess is a great danger to patient's health and a high risk for airway management by the anesthesiologist due to the possibility of rupturing it during the intubation. It is important to emphasize that LA should not be applied in infected soft tissue.

Bacterial endocarditis is not a complication related to the use of LA per se; however it can be related as a post procedure bacteremia after any type of injection to the mouth. Dental surgery that involves mucosa o contaminated tissue such as a molar extraction can produce a transient bacteremia and facilitate infections at a distance, especially in cardiac valves or endocardium. The most common bacteria is hemolytic streptococcus viridians. Patients with dentures can develop bacteremia from gum ulcers or gingivitis. Numerous studies have shown a possible odontology-related etiology of bacterial endocarditis in up to 20% of the patients. Although prophylactic antibiotics are a commonly accepted practice, the American Heart Association (AHA) in 1997 described multiple prophylactic strategies: (a) amoxicil-lin 2 g, 1 hour prior to the treatment, and (b) clindamycin 600 mg, 1 hour prior to treatment [31].

6.7 Cardiovascular manifestations

Heart complications related to dental procedures may increase up to a 5.7% in patients with identified risk factors. Patients with coronary heart disease, cardiac surgery, or heart failure show greater plasmatic lidocaine levels; therefore a 50% reduction in maximum dosage of LA is recommended. Potassium levels and acidosis may worsen the adverse effects in the myocardium. High-risk patients should be limited to 30-minute dental surgery; after that time complications may rise up to 15% [32].

Cardiovascular collapse is described as the most severe LA complication, associated with high mortality. It is produced by intravascular injection of AL and is manifested by arrhythmias, heart failure, and arterial hypotension that can end in death if not treated in a timely manner. Usually, the doses of LA used in dentistry rarely exceed the limits to cause cardiovascular problems, although in exceptional cases, small amounts of AL may be capable of cardiac arrest [33]. For more information, we refer the reader to the chapter on LA systemic toxicity included in this book.

6.8 Local anesthetic overdose

Most overdose reactions occur during LA injection or within the next 5–10 minutes. Clinical symptoms involving the CNS are, for example, generalized numbness, facial numbing, anxiety, restlessness, confusion, chills, seizures, or respiratory arrest [7]. A simple way to avoid LA injection into the blood vessels is to aspirate before and during the injection. Systemic toxicity depends on several factors such as speed of injection, site, and combination with vasoconstrictors. For example, maximum dose of LA in a pediatric patient may be mistaken with an adult and cause an overdose. High concentrations of LA articaine and prilocaine may exacerbate and overdose. Serum concentration of LA less than 5 μg/mL produce moderate sedation and analgesia, but at concentrations as high as 5–10 μg/mL, it can cause incoherent talk, dysphoria, diplopia, muscle contractions, or seizures [34].

6.9 Plasma cholinesterase deficiency

Esther-type LA should be avoided in patients that may carry this rare enzyme deficiency, due to the metabolism of this anesthetic. Methemoglobinemia is a rare complication associated with excessive metabolites of certain LA, mainly prilocaine, causing oxidation of the ferrous component in the blood to a ferric form, and poorly delivered oxygen to tissues commonly expressed as hypoxia. Unique features, such as a saturation gap and chocolate-brown-colored blood, can raise suspicion for methemoglobinemia. The use of articaine and benzocaine have also been associated with methemoglobinemia and manifests with cyanosis that does not respond with supplemental oxygen. When high methemoglobinemia levels are present, clinical symptoms such as nausea, sedation, seizures, and coma may appear. Treatment is with methylene blue. Thus, patients with congenital or acquired plasma cholinesterase deficiency should avoid exposure to these LAs [34].

6.10 Allergic reactions

These reactions are extremely rare in dentistry. The most common allergic reactions are allergies to latex, acrylates, and formaldehyde. While polymethylmethacrylate and latex trigger delayed hypersensitivity reactions, sodium metabisulphite and nickel cause immediate reactions. Most adverse reactions are caused by systemic complications or anxiety as a result of pain or needles, generating hyper-ventilation or syncope that may be confused with a faulty allergic reaction. True allergic reactions are caused mainly by ester LA. They are not dose related. Only 0.7–1% of all allergies are authentic hypersensitivity reactions and caused after administering LA [35]. It is fundamental to have previous contact with the allergen, and then a usual latency period occurs until a second exposure. Hypersensitivity reactions related to LA are classified into two types: type I reactions or humoral are immediate and severe such as anaphylactic shock, angioedema, fever, and photo sensibility. Type IV or cellular are delayed and manifested through moderate dermatologic reactions such as hives or cutaneous rash. Anaphylactic shock usually occurs within a short exposure to the antigen, and symptoms include cardiovascular collapse in 76.3%, bronchospasm in 44.2%, and skin in 69.9%. Cardiovascular collapse presents as abrupt drop in blood pressure, bradycardia, and desaturation followed by bronchospasm and redness in thoracic area and face are common. Initial management is epinephrine 1-5 mcg/kg [36]. Intramuscular application, fluid bolus, secured airway, and increase in oxygen concentration. There is a frequently reported contact dermatitis in healthcare workers that are exposed to parabens and bisulfates used as preservatives in local anesthetic preparations which can cause an allergic reaction [37, 38].

6.11 Drug interactions

There are some well-known interactions with LA, such as tricyclic antidepressants and beta blockers. The first act is by inhibiting the catecholamine reuptake, thus increasing the concentration at the presynaptic sympathetic binding site. In patients taking this kind of medication, it is recommended to limit the amount of epinephrine to a maximum of 0.05 mg/dose. Beta blockers, on the other hand, inhibit arteriolar vasodilation effect of drugs as epinephrine in combination with LA, which increase the predominant vasoconstrictor alpha adrenergic effect. The end result could be an increase of arterial blood pressure and sympathetic effects.

Another reported interaction is the diminished metabolism of amide LA. Sedatives, opioids, opioids, antihistamines, magnesium sulfate, and LA may increase CNS depression and respiratory drive which has to be titrated with caution. LA and some antiarrhythmic like quinidine may increase myocardial depression. Antimyasthenic agents such as neostigmine could antagonize the effect or muscle contraction. Anticholinesterase lowers the metabolism of ester LA. Ester LA such as procaine combined with sulfas could inhibit antimicrobial action [34].

7. Conclusions

Anxiety, stress, and pain are very frequent characteristics in dentistry. Dental anxiety can be considered as a universal phenomenon with a high prevalence, being one of the main causes of medical emergencies in the dental office, so its preven-tion is an essential part of patient safety and quality of care. The LA used in this clinical setting must be selective in nerve tissue; be powerful enough to produce complete anesthesia without tissue damage; have a reversible action within a predictable time; have minimal side effects and, also, reduced systemic toxicity, and few hypersensitivity reactions; have a short latency period with the duration of the effect adaptable to the desired; not cause pain during injection; be compatible with other components in the solution and not easily modified by sterilization processes; not be sensitive to variations in pH; be stable in the solution; and have sufficient penetration. Lidocaine and articaine with epinephrine are the most used, although mepivacaine and prilocaine are still options. It is mandatory to monitor side reac-tions, especially systemic toxicity.

Author details

Enrique Hernández-Cortez[1]*, Cecilia G. Sandoval Larios[2]
and Juan Carlos Flores-Carrillo[3]

1 Department of Anesthesia, Federación Mexicana de Colegios de Anestesiología, A.C., León, México

2 Anesthesia and Cardiovascular Anesthesia, Airway Committee Federación Mexicana de Colegios de Anestesiologia AC, Hospital Angeles León, México

3 Anesthesia and Critical Care Medicine, Hospital Angeles Tijuana, México

*Address all correspondence to: kikinhedz@gmail.com

References

[1] López-Valverde A, de Vicente J, Cutando A. The surgeons Halsted and Hall, cocaine and the discovery of dental anaesthesia by nerve blocking. British Dental Journal. 2011;**2011**:485-487

[2] Lofgren N. Studies on Local Anesthetics: Xylocaine, a New Synthetic Drug. Hoeggstroms: Stockhlm; 1948

[3] Vree TB, Gielen MJ. Clinical pharmacology and the use of articaine for local and regional anaesthesia. Best Practice and Research in Clinical Anaesthesiology. 2005;**19**(2):293-308

[4] Yagiela JA. Recent developments in local anesthesia and oral sedation. The Compendium of Continuing Education in Dentistry. 2004;**25**(9):697-706

[5] Suresh S, Ecoffey C, Bosenberg A, Lonnqvist PA, De Oliveira GS, De Leon CO, et al. Recommendations ESRA/ASRA on local anesthetics and adjuvants dosage in pediatric Regional anesthesia. The European Society of Regional Anaesthesia and Pain Therapy/American Society of Regional Anesthesia and Pain Medicine. 2018;**43**(2):211-216. Available from: https://doi.org/10.1097/AAP.0000000000000702

[6] De B, Reed KL. Local anesthetics: Review of pharmacological considerations. Anesthesia Progress. 2013;**59**:90-102

[7] Has DA. An update of local anesthetics in dentistry. Journal of the Canadian Dental Association. 2002;**68**(9):546-551

[8] Alcaina-Lorente MA, Cortes-Lillo O, German Cecilia C, Castejon-Navas I. Parestesia con el uso de anestésicos locales. A propósito de dos casos. Odontologia Pediátrica. 2010;**18**(3): 201-208

[9] Manani G, Charanda M, Benatti M, Narne S, Zanardi L, Rusca F, et al. Gow-gates block for beginners. Giornale di Anestesia Stomatologica. 1989;**18**(3):7-17

[10] Johnson TM, Badovinac R, Shaefer J. Teaching alternatives to the standard inferior alveolar nerve block in dental education: Outcomes in clinical practice. Journal of Dental Education. 2007; **71**(9):1145-1152

[11] Malamed SF, Reed KL, Okundeye A, Fonner A. Local and regional anesthesia in dental and oral surgery. Complications of Regional Anesthesia. 2017. DOI: 10.1007/978-3-319-49386-2_21

[12] Boronat López A, Peñarrocha DM. Failure of locoregional anesthesia in dental practice. Review of the literature. Medicina Oral, Patología Oral y Cirugía Bucal. 2006;**11**(6):E510-E513

[13] Malamed SF. Local anesthetics dentistry's most important drugs, clinical update 2006: CDA. Journal of the California Dental Association. 2006;**34**(12):971-976

[14] Batista da Silva C, Berto LA, Volpato MC, Ramacciato JC, Motta RH, Ranali J, et al. Anesthetic efficacy of articaine and lidocaine for incisive/mental nerve block. Journal of Endodontics. 2010;**36**(3):438-441

[15] Sambrook PJ, Smith W, Elijah J, Goss AN. Severe adverse reactions to dental local anaesthetics: Systemic reactions. Australian Dental Journal. 2011; **56**:148-153. DOI: 10.1111/j.1834-7819.2011.01316.x

[16] Liu W, Yang X, Li C, Mo A. Adverse drug reactions to local anesthetics: A systematic review. Oral Surgery, Oral Medicine, Oral Pathology, Oral Radiology. 2013;**115**(3):319-327. DOI: 10.1016/j.oooo

[17] Sancho-Puchades M, Vilchez-Perez MA, Valmaseda-Castellon E,

Paredes-Garcia J, Berini-Aytes L, Gay-Escoda C. Bupivacaine 0.5% versus articaine 4% for the removal of lower third molars. A crossover randomized controlled trial. Medicina Oral, Patología Oral y Cirugía Bucal. 2012;**17**(3):e4 62-e468

[18] Feldman G, Nordenram A. Bupivacaine in oral surgery. Acta Anaesthesiologica Scandinavica. 1983;**23**:409-413

[19] Sisk AL. Long-acting local anesthetics in dentistry. Anesthesia Progress. 1992;**39**:53-60

[20] Malamed SF, Gagnon S, Lebalanc D. Efficacy of articaine: A new amide local anesthetic. Journal of the American Dental Association (1939). 2000;**131**(5):635-642

[21] James O, Ladeinde AL, Ogunlewe MO, Ajuluchukwu JN, Adeyemo WL. Hemodynamic response after injection of local anesthetics with or without adrenaline in adult Nigerian subjects undergoing simple tooth extraction. Journal of Clinical Sciences. 2015; **12**:90-95

[22] Lawaty I, Drum M, Reader A, Nusstein J. A prospective, randomized, double-blind comparison of 2% mepivacaine with 1 : 20,000 levonordefrin versus 2% lidocaine with 1 : 100,000 epinephrine for maxillary infiltrations. Anesthesia Progress. 2010;**57**(4):139-144. DOI: 10.2344/0003-3006-57.4.139

[23] Sisk AL. Vasoconstrictors in local anesthesia for dentistry. Anesthesia Progress. 1992;**39**:187-193

[24] Becker DE, Reed KL. Essentials of local anesthetics pharmacology. Anesthesia Progress. 2006;**53**:98-109

[25] Hass DA. Drugs in dentistry. In: Compendium of Pharmaceuticals and Specialties. 37th ed. Canada: Canadian Pharmaceurical Association; 2002. pp. L26-L29

[26] Daublander M, Muller R, Lipp MDW. The incidence of complications associated with local anesthesia in dentistry. American Dental Society of Anesthesiology. 1997;**44**:132-141

[27] Seminario-Amez M,González-Navarro B, Velasco-Ortega E, Jane-Salas E, Lopéz-LopézJ.Use of local anesthetics associated with vasoconstrictors in dentistry. Is it a safe treatment? A literature update. EC Anesthesia. 2017;**3.2**:50-54

[28] Daublander M, Muller R, Lipp MDW. The incidence of complications associated with local anesthesia in dentistry. American Dental Society of Anesthesiology. 1999;**50**:102-106

[29] Malamed SF. Nerve injury caused by mandibular block analgesia. International Journal of Oral and Maxillofacial Surgery. 2006;**35**:876-877

[30] Progrel MA. Broken local anesthetic needle: A series of 16 patients, with recommendations. Journal of the American Dental Association. 2009;**140**:1517-1522

[31] Tomás-Carmona I, Diz-Dios P, Limeres-Posse J, Outumuro-Rial M, Caamaño-Durán F, Fernández-Feijoo J, et al. Pautas de profilaxis antibiótica de Endocarditis Bacteriana, recomendadas por los odontólogos en España. Medicina Oral. 2004;**9**:56-62

[32] Bahl R. Local anesthesia in dentistry. Anesthesia Progress. 2004;**51**: 138-142

[33] Becker DE, Reed KL. Local anesthetics: Review of pharmacological considerations. Anesthesia Progress. 2012;**59**:90-101

[34] Yagiela JA. Local anesthetics. Anesthesia Progress. 1991;**38**:128-141

[35] Speca SJ, Boynes SG, Cuddy MA. Allergic reactions to local anesthetic formulations. Dental Clinics of North America. 2010;**54**:655-664

[36] Truhlar A, Deakin CD, Soar J, Khalifa GE, Alfonzo A, Bierens JJ. European resuscitation council guidelines for resuscitation. Cardiac arrest in special circumstances. Resuscitation. 2015;**95**:148-201

[37] Gaitan-Padron MA, Hernández-Cortez E. Alergia al latex en el paciente pediátrico. Anestesia en México. 2013; **25**(S1):25-32

[38] Bina B, Hersh EV, Hilario M, Alvarez K, McLaughlin B. True allergy to amide local anesthetics: A review and case presentation. Anesthesia Progress. 2018;**65**(2):119-123. DOI: 10.2344/anpr-65-03-06

3

Pharmacokinetics and Pharmacodynamics of Local Anesthetics

Javier Marcos Michel-Levy

Abstract

Local anesthetics are basically weak bases whose structure consists of an aromatic half connected to a substituted amine through an ester amide linkage. The pKa values of local anesthetics are close to physiological pH, both protonated and unprotonated forms are present. The individual structures confer different physiochemical and clinical characteristics. Potency is correlated to lipid solubility in vitro, but less so in vivo. The duration of action is associated with the extent of protein binding. The onset of action is related to pKa. The intrinsic vasodilator activity varies between drugs and influences potency and duration of action. Local anesthetics block nerve conduction and interact directly with specific receptor on the Na^+ channel, inhibiting Na^+ ion influx and impairing Propagation of the action potential in axons. There are some characteristics in the blocking of nerve conduction and are related to size and function of the peripheral nerves, and to the fact that a specific concentration of local anesthetics may produce a different intensity of block. Some pathological states like decreased cardiac output, severe hepatic disease, renal disease, cholinesterase activity, fetal acidosis, sepsis, etc. altered the pharmacokinetics and pharmacodynamics of local anesthetics.

Keywords: esters, amides, pKa, Na^+ channel, pH, nerve fibers kinetics, block conduction

1. Introduction

When applied locally to nerve tissues in appropriate concentrations, local anesthetics (LAs) reversibly block the action potentials responsible for nerve conduction. They act anywhere in the nervous system and in any type of nerve fiber. Therefore, a LA in contact with a nerve trunk can produce both sensory and motor paralysis in the innervated region.

The practical advantage of LAs is that their action is reversible in concentrations of clinical importance; their administration is followed by complete recovery of nerve function [1] (**Figure 1**).

LAs are drugs primarily utilized in clinical settings to induce local anesthesia. The term local anesthesia, unlike general anesthesia, is defined as loss of sensation within a confined region without loss of the patient's consciousness. LAs are purposely used to relieve pain and induce numbness during surgical procedures and are normally applied by local injection [2].

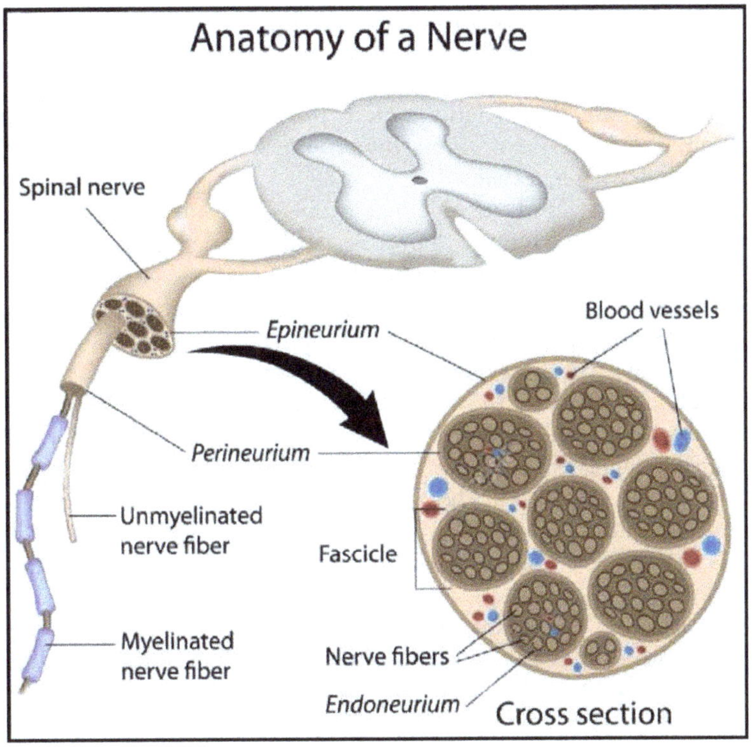

Figure 1.
Notes cards google.

2. Anatomy of the peripheral nerve

All peripheral nerves are similar in structure; neuron is the basic functional neuronal unit responsible for the conduction of nerve impulses. A typical neuron consists of a cell body (soma) that contains a large nucleus; the soma is attached to several branching processes called dendrites and a single axon. Axons vary in length and there is one only per neuron, they are a long and slender, and are also called nerve fibers; while dendrites receive incoming information and axons conduct outgoing information. Individual nerve fibers bind together, like wires in an electrical cable, and each axon is enveloped by the endoneurium (delicate layer of loose connective tissue around each axon). Groups of axons are closely associated within a bundle called a fascicle that is surrounded by perineurium (imparts mechanical strength and also acts as a diffusion barrier). Epineurium is a denser collagenous tissue that surrounds the entire nerve and holds it loosely to the connective tissue through which it travels. The paraneurium consists of loose connective tissue that keeps a stable relationship between adjacent structures filling the spaces in between them; this tissue promotes functional mobility of nerves during joint and muscular motion.

Nerves take in blood from the contiguous blood vessels along their course. These vessels that nourish larger nerves are macroscopic in bore and irregularly settled, conceive anastomoses to put on longitudinally common vessels that provision the nerve and emit subsidiary embranchments [3].

Each peripheral axon has its own cell membrane called axolemma, non-myelinated nerves such as nociceptive afferent type C fibers, and autonomous postganglionic efferent fibers contain axons coated by only one layer of cells. All large-caliber sensory and motor fibers are lined with multiple layers of myelin, which consist of the plasma membranes of Schawnn cells that wrap themselves around the axon during growth.

Myelin considerably increases the speed of nerve conduction as it achieves that action current generated by an action potential travels through the axoplasm to the nodes of Ranvier, these are periodic interruptions of the myelin sheath, where action potentials are regenerated.

In the nodes of Ranvier of the myelinated fibers, there is a high concentration of sodium channels Na^+, which serve to propagate the impulses, although they are also observed along the axons of unmyelinated fibers.

During the transmission of an impulse, the intra and extracellular ratios of Na^+ and K^+ ions are inverted. Na^+/K^+-ATPase is stopped during depolarization and Na^+ ion perviousness increases, leaving Na^+ ions to move inside the cell and the resting membrane potential be moved. An action potential is released when depolarization enough for the membrane potential to come a threshold value, it is concerning +15 mV. During repolarization, the electrical status of the cell is restored by K^+ diffusing out of the cell, and at the end the resting membrane potential has been restored; but the cell has effectively gained Na^+ and lost K^+. However, when Na^+/K $^+$-ATPase is reactivated, the normal intra and extracellular ratios of Na^+ and K^+ ions are restored.

In a depolarization stream, Na^+ channels they are activated, admitting extracellular Na^+ ions influx into the cell. After that (ms), Na^+ channels inactivate. The channels get back to the initial repolarization state. The course that involves sodium channels passing from an open or closed state is called a "gate." Gate is the result of the change of polarities after a potential. It is about explaining the mode of action of

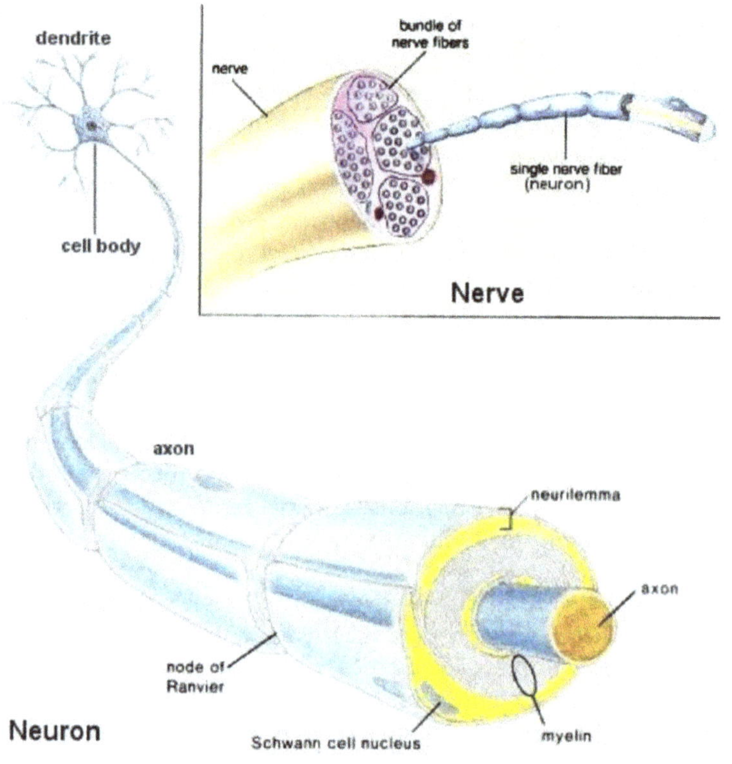

Figure 2.
Universo-review.ca free Google.

Fiber type	Function	Myelinated	Diameter (mm)	Conduction velocity (m/s)	Spike duration (ms)
Aα	Proprioception, somatic motor	Yes	12–20	70–120	0.4–0.5
Aβ	Touch, pressure	Yes	5–12	30–70	0.4–0.5
Aγ	Motor to muscle spindle	Yes	3–6	15–30	0.4–0.5
Aδ	Pain, cold, touch	Yes	2–5	12–30	0.4–0.5
C	Pain, temperature (dr) mechanoreception, reflex responses	No	0.4–1.2	0.5–2	2
B	Preganglionic autonomic	Yes	<3	3–15	1.2
C	Postganglionic sympathetic	No	0.3–1.3	0.7–2.3	2

Table 1.
Fiber type.

these channels, with the presence of voltage-dependent doors in the light of the same (**Figure 2**).

The currents of depolarization and repolarization move longitudinally along the nerve membrane and result in conduction of the nerve impulse. In unmyelinated nerves, the impulses spread at speeds of about 2 m/s. In myelinated nerves, the depolarization current jumps from node to node; this phenomenon, known as saltatory conduction, increases conduction velocity to around 120 m/s and is highly energy-efficient [4].

Neurons can usefully be classified according their diameter and speed of conduction (**Table 1**).

3. Local anesthetic molecule

The local anesthetic molecule consists of three components: (a) lipophilic aromatic ring, (b) intermediate ester or amide chain, and (c) terminal amine. Each of these contributes distinct properties to the molecule [5].

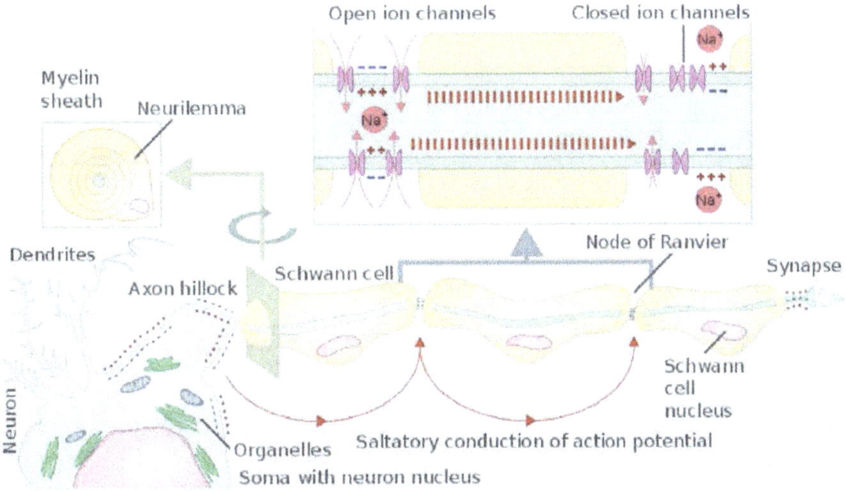

Figure 3.
Saltatory conduction. Wikiwand free Google.

In this way, local anesthetics can be classified into two groups: aminoesters and aminoamides. The aromatic ring provides a lipophilic character to the portion of the molecule in which it is found, while the tertiary amine end is hydrophilic, because it is protonated and has a positive charge in the physiological pH range [6] (**Figure 3**).

The ester-type LAs include benzocaine, procaine, cocaine, and tetracaine. The amide-type LAs include mepivacaine, lidocaine, ropivacaine, bupivacaine, and etidocaine. Lidocaine and bupivacaine are the most commonly used LAs, both are amide-type compounds, which are much more resistant than ester-type compounds to hydrolysis (**Table 2**).

In addition to the intrinsic binding affinities of LA drugs to the Na^+ channel, other variables also strongly influence the relative duration of local anesthesia; these include the volume, concentration, lipophilicity, pKa, pH, repeated injections, the presence of vasoconstrictors, and the precision of drug injection.

3.1 Hydrogen ion concentration

LAs in solution maintain a rapid chemical equilibrium between the basic uncharged form (B) and the charged cationic form (BH^+), the ratio of the two states is given by the Henderson-Hasselbach equation (it was originally derived to describe the pH changes resulting from the addition of H^+ or OH^- ions to any buffer system). At a certain concentration of hydrogen ion ($\log10^{-}_{1}$ [-pH]) specified for each drug, the concentration of LA in its basic form in a solution is equal to the

Structural groups of some commonly used local anesthetics (duration of action)
Amides
Bupivacaine (2–8 h)
Cinchocaine (2–3 h)
Etidocaine (2–6 h)
Levobupivacaine (2–8 h)
Lidocaine (1–2 h)
Mepivacaine (1.5–3 h)
Prilocaine (1–2 h)
Ropivacaine (4–6 h)
Ester of benzoic acid
Cocaine
Esters of meta-aminobenzoic acid
Proxymetacaine
Esters of para-aminobenzoic acid
Benzocaine
Chloroprocaine
Oxybuprocaine
Procaine (30–45 min)
Propoxycaine
Tetracaine

Table 2.
Groups of LA.

concentration of loaded cation. The logarithm of this concentration of hydrogen ion is called pKa.

$$pH = pKa + \log[HCO_3^-]/[H_2CO_3]$$
$$pKa = pH - \log[\text{base}]/[\text{conjugate acid}]$$
$$[\text{base}]/[\text{conjugate acid}] = 1.0$$

The dissociation constant of LA (pKa value) is the highly significant fact affecting the quickness of their beginning of action. The pKa values rule the ratio of the LA that is present in nonprotonated pattern at physiological pH values and hence disposable to spread through tissue walls to its spot of action.

Lower pKa values are conjoint with a prompt beginning of blockade, then more of the drug is present as the unprotonated base at pH 7.4. In contradistinction, bigger values are conjointed with a slower beginning, since fewer of the drug is present as the nonprotonated base at pH 7.4. For instance, lidocaine has a pKa value roughly 7.7. At pH 7.4, around one-third of these drugs is present in solution as the nonprotonated base B and is disposable to spread through the nerve scabbard. In contradistinction, bupivacaine and ropivacaine have a pKa value of 8.1, and at a pH 7.4 only 17% is present in solution as nonprotonated, diffusible base. These discrepancies are responsible for the more prompt beginning of action of lidocaine and slower beginning of action of ropivacaine and bupivacaine.

3.2 Alkalization of local anesthetics

Factors that increase the conversion of the free LA base (B) to the active form (BH^+) in the neuroplasm increase the diffusion gradient and the concentration of BH^+ in the Na^+ channel. This technique is of clinical interest because it is used to shorten the latency of onset of effective anesthesia, particularly useful in the context of extending an epidural block for urgent operative delivery.

The addition of bicarbonate will raise the pH of the weakly acidic solution nearer the pKa. Example: addition of 1.0 mL $NaHCO_3$ 8.4% to 10.0 mL of lidocaine 2% will raise its pH from 6.5 to 7.2; this means more drug will exist in the non-ionized form, so penetration will be more rapid [7].

Carbonation is a variation on alkalization, and is based on a similar principle but with a different site of action; when carbon dioxide diffuses across the neurilemma, it is rapidly buffered by intracellular proteins, so that changes in pH are minimal. Carbonated solutions are unstable, the LA may be precipitated and any added vasoconstrictor is more easily hydrolyzed [8].

3.3 Chirality

Chirality is derived from Greek, and means "having handedness," and is defined a particular type of stereoisomerism. Right and left hands are mirror images of each other but cannot be superimposed when the palms are facing in the same direction (**Figure 4**) [9]. These particular isomers are known as enantiomers and this form of stereoisomerism is dependent on the presence of one or more chiral centers, which typically comprise a carbon atom with four groups attached. These enantiomers have the capacity to rotate polarized light, and, so, are also known as optical isomers.

Enantiomers that rotate polarized light to the right are described as (+), and are the same as dextro or D isomers. Enantiomers that rotate polarized light to the left are described as (–),and are the same as levo or L isomers. The currently accepted convention is that which assigns a sequence of priority to the four atoms or group attached to the chiral center. The molecule is described as though it were being viewed from the front with the smallest group extending away from the viewer. If the arrangement of the largest to the smallest groups is clockwise, the enantiomer is designated "R" for rectus. If the arrangement is anticlockwise it is designated "S" for sinister. The optical direction is the added to complete the description. Most synthetic chiral drugs are racemic mixtures, less potent because the D-forms are much less active. The clinical behavior of the enantiomers, and in particular their toxicity, is related to the chiral form [10] (**Figure 5** and **Table 3**).

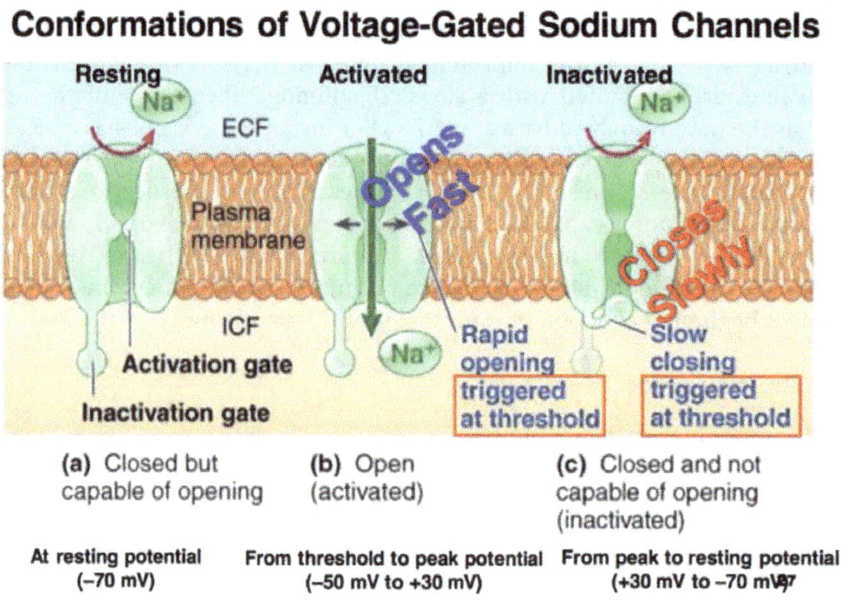

Figure 4.
Na receptor. Memorang.

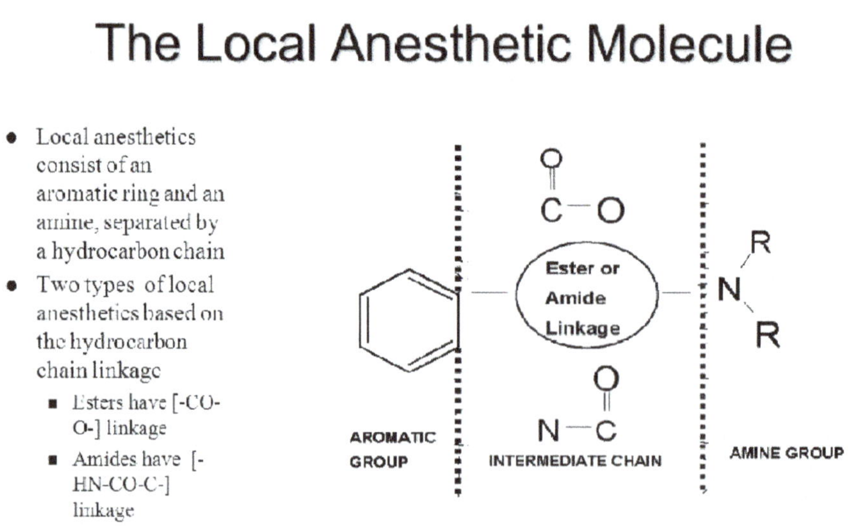

Figure 5.
LA molecule free Google.

Bupivacaine: S(−) enantiomer has less affinity for, and dissociates quicker from myocardial Na^+ channels. The cardio and central nervous system toxicity is reduced. S(−) exerts some vasoconstrictor activity.
Ropivacaine: S(−) enantiomer is a safer cardiovascular profile.
Prilocaine: S(+) enantiomer is a stronger vasoconstrictor, metabolized slowly than the R(−) form which therefore produces higher concentrations of 0-toluidine and a greater risk of methaemoglobinaemia.
Lidocaine: Achiral.

Table 3.
Quimical structure.

4. Pharmacodynamics

Most LA drugs are tertiary amine bases (B), which are dispensed as hydrochloride salts (B.HCL). In this way, their easily disband to pattern acidic solutions:

$$\mathrm{B.HCL} < > \mathrm{BH}^+ + \mathrm{CL}^-$$

After infiltrating the tissues, a ratio of the protonated basic pattern (BH^+) is turned to the unprotonated basic pattern (B) at the pH of the extracellular fluid:

$$\mathrm{BH}^+ + \mathrm{HCO_3}^- < > \mathrm{B} + \mathrm{H_2O} + \mathrm{CO_2}$$

Solely the unprotonated pattern B penetrates through the neurilemmal membrane, captures H^+ in the neuroplasm, and raises approach to its spot of action in the open Na^+ channel, inducing its blockade. The unprotonated pattern B may further straight permeate to the Na^+ channel across the neurilemma, and recruits H^+ into the Na^+ channel.

It is able to induce blockade by membrane expansion (ME), bring about puffiness of the lipoprotein matrix of the Na^+ channel (e.g., benzocaine). Tetrodotoxin and saxitoxin directly block the Na^+ channel from the exterior of the membrane, close to the external pore [11–13] (**Figure 6**).

The primary target of LAs is the voltage-gated Na^+ channel, which is responsible for the generation of action potentials in excitable membranes, there is an inverse relationship between action potentials and local anesthesia [13]. LAs also interact with many other types of ion channels, particularly K^+ and Ca^{2+} channels, notwithstanding they have a limited relationship at these sites. They do not mostly alter the neuronal resting potential, save in exceedingly raised concentrations. In the same way, they do not change the sill potential needed for impulse spread, even if the gear of depolarization and repolarization is diminished, and conduction velocity is reduced and may cause undesirable side effects, usually considered that the toxic effects of bupivacaine on the heart are partially related to its effects on K^+ and Ca^{2+} channels.

Mammalian voltage-gated Na^+ channels exist in different isoforms in various excitable tissues such as skeletal muscles, cardiac tissues, central nervous system (CNS), and peripheral nervous system (PNS) [14]. In addition, multiple major isoforms are present in CNS and PNS, some of these neuronal Na^+ channels are sensitive to tetrodotoxin (TTX) and some are resistant. Tetrodotoxin (TTX) is a potent naturally occurring neurotoxin isolated from puffer fish; it has been responsible for human intoxications and fatalities. Its usual route of toxicity is via the ingestion of contaminated puffer fish, which are a culinary delicacy, especially in

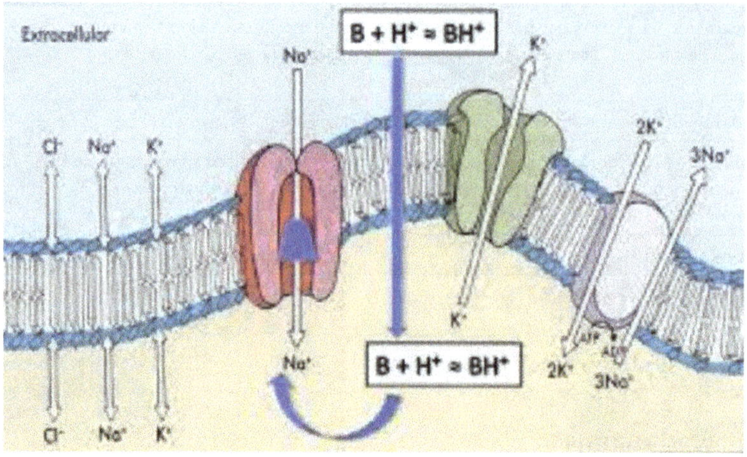

Figure 6.
Amino-base free Google.

Japan. TTX has been an invaluable tool for the identification of various neuronal Na^+ channel isoforms [11–13].

The concentration of LA in blood is determined by the amount injected, the rate of absorption from the injection site, the rate of distribution by tissues, the rate of biotransformation and drug elimination [14]. The patient's factors, such as age, cardiovascular situation, and hepatic function, influence the physiological disposition and the plasma concentration resulting from the LA injected [14, 15].

4.1 Mode and site of action of local anesthetics in Na^+ channels

Mammalian voltage-gated Na^+ channels are normally activated at a threshold of around −50 mV, and the probability of channels being open is maximal around+20 mV. At a single-channel level, the time course of Na channel activation is strongly voltage dependent. The probability of being open during depolarization rises slowly at the threshold and becomes rather fast at the more positive poten-tials. In contrast, the open Na^+ channels inactivate rapidly, with a dwell time that is generally 1 ms or less. Unlike the activation process, the time course of inacti-vation of the open Na^+ channel is not voltage dependent [16]. At the level of macroscopic currents, Na^+ currents rise (activate) and decay (inactivate) with overlapping time course, as would be expected from an ensemble of currents from single channels [17, 18].

Detailed kinetic analyses of macroscopic Na^+ currents in the presence of vari-ous LAs reveal complicated pharmacological profiles under voltage-clamp condi-tions. Voltage-sensitive Na^+ channels are integral proteins that cross neuronal membranes and surround an aqueous pore. Most Na^+ channels consist of three subunits (α1, β1, and β2), the largest subunit being α1, the site of ion conduction and LAs binding; the external surface of the α-subunit is heavily glycosylated, which serves to orient the channel properly within the plasma membrane. The α1 unit bears a molecular weight up of 260 kDa, and consists of an unique long peptide chain holding four hydrophobic regions (domains I–IV), which go across the membrane and symmetrically encircle the pore. The four domains are joined to each other by intracellular bridgeworks.

Every domain includes six membrane-spanning somites (S1–S6). The S4 somite is a potential sensor, and the brief curl among S5 and S6 forms portion of the sheathing of the external pore of the gutter. The intracellular bridgework among two of the domains (III and IV) is the speedy inactivation gateway. This gateway is liable for the speedy inactivation of Na^+ channels.

LAs reduce peak Na^+ currents during the test potential a few minutes after external perfusion of the drug solution at the holding potential (<−100 mV). This reduction in peak current is dose dependent, and the potency ranking of various LAs derived from their dose-response curves correlates well with the relative duration of local anesthesia they elicit in vivo. This LA block of the Na^+ channel at resting potential is termed "tonic block."

Most LAs are found to shift the apparent steady-state inactivation curve to the hyperpolarizing direction. Steady-state inactivation measures the availability of resting Na^+ channels at various prepulse voltages at which Na^+ channels normally do not open [7]. This closed-channel inactivation is strongly voltage dependent, unlike the open channel inactivation. A shift of the steady-state inactivation curve by LA toward the hyperpolarizing direction has significant physiological consequences. To begin with, if the steady-state inactivation curve is indeed shifted by LAs upon binding, a large fraction of Na^+ channels with LAs bound will be in their inactivated state at the resting potential and therefore will be unavailable to carry currents for the generation of action potentials. Another implication is that the inactivated state of the Na^+ channel binds more strongly than other channel states (generalized modulated receptor hypothesis envisioned by Hondeghem and Katzung [19]). They proposed that different states of Na^+ channels (open, resting, and inactivated) have different binding affinities for LAs, and that the affinity of the inactivated state is the highest.

Repetitive pulses produce an additional block of Na^+ currents in the presence of LA. This additional block of Na^+ currents is termed "use-dependent block" or "frequency-dependent block," with the two terms used interchangeably. The use-dependent block by LAs may be physiologically important for pain therapy, as many afferent fibers fire action potentials at a high frequency, particularly in the pathological states. In theory, LAs with a potent use-dependent attribute will be more effective than LAs without this attribute in blocking the high-frequency abnormal firings of sensory afferent fibers.

4.2 Potency of local anesthetic

The potency of a LA is regulated mainly by lipid solubility, the time of onset by the pKa of the substance, and the duration of action by protein binding. The more lipophilic the LA, the more potent it is [20, 21]. Nerve-blocking potency of LAs increases also with increasing molecular weight [22].

LA appears to have a ceiling effect. Above a partition coefficient of 4 there is no observed increase in potency [23]. Unfortunately, greater lipid solubility also increases toxicity, decreasing the therapeutic index for more hydrophobic drugs. Larger more lipophilic LAs permeate nerve membrane more readily and bind Na^+ channels with greater affinity (**Table 4**).

More lipid-soluble LAs are relatively water insoluble, high protein bound in blood, and less readily removed by bloodstream from nerve membranes, and this affinity of the drug to lipid membranes and therefore greater proximity to its site of action in the Na^+ channel.

4.3 Onset and duration of action of local anesthetics

The onset of nerve conduction blockade depends on the physicochemical properties of each LA. The latency also depends on the dose or concentration of the drug used. The duration of the effect of local anesthetics is very variable (**Table 5**).

Local anesthetic	Partition coefficient
Benzocaine	1.44
Procaine	2.51
Mepivacaine	2.69
Prilocaine	2.73
Lidocaine	3.40
Bupivacaine	4.05
Etidocaine	4.19
Tetracaine	4.32
Oxybuprocaine	4.38

Table 4.
Partition coefficients (n-octanol/water) of some local anesthetics.

Short effect	Procaine
	Cloroprocaine
Moderate effect	Lidocaine
	Mepivacaine
	Prilocaine
Long effect	Tetracaine
	Bupivacaine
	Ropivacaine
	Etidocaine

Table 5.
Onset and duration.

The peripheral vascular effects of the local anesthetic have significant effects; many anesthetics have a biphasic effect on vascular smooth muscle, at low concentrations they produce vasoconstriction and at higher concentrations they produce vasodilation. However, the vasodilator effect differs between the different drugs, the effects on vascular blood flow and its tone are complex, and vary among other factors, depending on the concentration, time, and vascular bed near the point of application.

5. Pharmacokinetics

Pharmacokinetics was originally described as the quantitative studio and mathematical review of drug and it's metabolite in the organism. The concept has been mostly obsequious to the prosecution of drug absorption, distribution, metabolism and excretion, and to their explanation in numerical terminus. Pharmacokinetics is once in a while portrayed as "what the body does to drugs." The two highly large pharmacokinetic uniforms are:

- Volume of distribution (V)
- Clearance (CL)

The volume of distribution depicts the seeming volume disposable in the organism for the allocation of the drug, whereas the clearance shows capacity of the organism to eliminate the drug. These two uniforms are kindred to the terminal or elimination half-life of the drug. In other words, after one half-life, the concentration of the drug in the body will be half of the starting dose. Half-life is defined as the time required for the plasma concentration to decrease by 50% during the terminal phase of decline, by the following expression:

$$t½ = 0.693 \times Vd/CL.$$

Accordingly, the terminal half-life is regularly heterogeneous, which depends on the early pharmacokinetics constant volume (V) and clearance (CL). A prolonged terminal half-life can throw back an enhanced volume of distribution, a narrow clearance, or together these changes, while a brief terminal half-life can reflect a decreased volume of distribution, an enhanced clearance or both together [8] (**Table 6**).

Clearance depicts the quantity of blood or plasma since that a drug would need to be thoroughly eliminated in unit time in order to guarantee its put-out from the body. It is a theoretic thought, inasmuch as in practice drugs are incompletely withdrawn from a nay larger quantity of plasma. Clearance values are generally expressed as a quantity cleared in unit time and are generally measured in $mL\ min^{-1}$ or $L\ h^{-1}$.

Also, clearance can be determined as the timing of drug elimination ($mg\ min^{-1}$) per unit of blood or plasma concentration ($mg\ mL^{-1}$).

$$\text{plasma clearance}\left(\text{mL min}^{-1}\right) = \frac{\text{timing of drug removal}\left(\text{mg min}^{-1}\right)}{\text{plasma centralization}\left(\text{mg mL}^{-1}\right)}$$

Plasma clearance is as a rule steadfast; the cadence of drug removal is right away proportional to plasma concentration. Total body clearance is the addition of various ways of drug elimination that are carried out by various organs in the body:

$$CL = CL_R + CL_H + CL_X$$

where CL is total clearance, CL_R is renal clearance, CL_H is hepatic clearance and CL_X is clearance by other routes (**Table 7**).

After absorption from the site of injection, the plasma concentration of LAs depends on their rate of distribution in tissues and their elimination from the body. Subsequent to an intravenous injection, the plasma concentration of all LAs in general falls in a biexponential ways. There is an incipient quick allocation time (half-life 1–3 min), conjoint with their rapid inlet by greatly perfused organs (e.g., lung, liver, kidney). Afterward, there is a slower reduction in plasma centralization, which depicts the put-out of LAs by metabolism and excretion. The final half-life of most ester anesthetics is comparatively brief (10 min) owing to their prompt

Drug	Volume of distribution (ml/kg)	Volume of distribution (L 70 kg)
Lidocaine	900 (500–1300)	63 (35–91)
Bupivacaine	1050 (650–1450)	74 (46–104)
Prilocaine	2700 (2100–3300)	189 (147–241)

Table 6.
Volume of distribution.

Drug	Hepatic clearance (mL min^{-1} kg^{-1})	Hepatic clearance (mL min^{-1} 70 kg^{-1})
Lidocaine	17.0 (12.6–21.4)	1190 (882–1498)

Table 7.
Hepatic clearance.

	Terminal half-life (min)	Clearance (mL min^{-1} kg^{-1})	Apparent volume of distribution	Metabolites (L kg^{-1})
Cocaine	48	31	2.0	Norcocaine
				Ecgonine
				Benzoylated
Procaine	8	60	0.7	Diethylaminoethanol
				p-aminobenzoate
Tetracaine	15	47	1.0	Butyl-aminobenzoate
				Dimethyl-aminoethanol
Lidocaine	100	15	1.3	Monoethylglycine-
				xylidide
				Ethylglycine
				2,6-xylidine
				4-hydroxy-2,6-xylidine
Prilocaine	100	34	2.7	N-propylamine
				o-toluidine
Bupivacaine	200	9	1.1	Pipecolic acid
				Pipecolyl-xylidide
Levobupivacaine	200	9	1.1	Pipecolic acid
				Pipecolyl-xylidide
Ropivacaine	110	7	0.7	3-Hydroxy-ropivacain
				4-Hydroxy-ropivacain

Table 8.
Pharmacokinetics and metabolism of local anesthetics.

hydrolysis by plasma cholinesterase, in hallmark, the terminal half-life of the amides oscillates from 100 min (lidocaine) to 200 min (bupivacaine).

Their volume of distribution is rather greater than total body water, while their plasma clearance is usually less than liver blood flow (**Table 8**).

Some clinical conditions can modify the pharmacokinetics of LAs, specially cardiovascular disorders and chronic hepatic diseases like cirrhosis can decline the clearance and volume of distribution of LAs, with changeable impact on the terminal half-life. In neonates, the clearance of LAs is diminished and their half-life is sustained.

6. Conclusions

LAs are drugs widely used in medicine and dentistry. These medications cause reversible neural block by their action in the sodium channels (**Figure 7**) located in

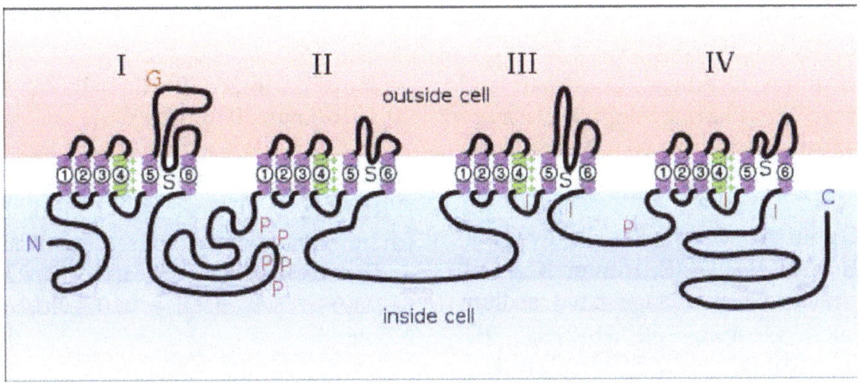

Figure 7.
Sodium channel. Wikipedia.

the nerve membranes. The unprotonated molecule configuration of the LA is introduced through the membrane from the outside and the protonated molecule acts with the sodium channel from the inside. The potency of a LA is given by liposolubility, the onset time by dissociation constant (pKa), and the duration of action by protein binding. Local anesthetics are weak bases whose structure consists of an aromatic moiety connected to a substituted amine through an ester or amide linkage. Consequently, LAs are classified as aminoester or aminoamide compounds. Amino acids are hydrolyzed by plasma cholinesterase, while aminoamides are metabolized in the liver. Aminoamides cause less allergic reactions.

Conflict of interest

The author declares no conflict of interests.

Author details

Javier Marcos Michel-Levy
Hospital Obrero N°8, Caja Nacional de Salud, Trinidad-Beni, Bolivia

*Address all correspondence to: jmichel_levy@hotmail.com

References

[1] Brunton L, editor. Goodman and Gilman. The Pharmacological Bases of Therapeutics. 12th ed. New York: McGraw Hill; 2011

[2] Goldin AL, Barchi RL, Caldwell JH, Hofmann F, Howe JR, Hunter JC, et al. Nomenclature of voltage-gated sodium channels. Neuron. 2000;**28**(2):365-368. DOI: 10.1016/s0896-6273(00)00116-1

[3] Hadzic A. Hadzic's Textbook of Regional Anesthesia and Acute Pain Management. The New York School of Regional Anesthesia. 2nd ed. NY: McGraw-Hill Education; 2017

[4] Bovill J, Fee H. Physiology for Anaesthesiologists. UK: Taylor and Francis Group; 2004

[5] Becker DE, Reed KL. Essentials of local anesthetic pharmacology. Anesthesia Progress. 2006;**53**(3):98-109. DOI: 10.2344/0003-3006(2006)53[98, EOLAP]2.0.CO;2

[6] Gropper MA, editor. Miller's Anesthesia. 9th ed. US: Elsevier; 2019

[7] Hodgkin AL, Huxley AF. A quantitative description of membrane current and its application to conduction and excitation in nerve. 1952. Bulletin of Mathematical Biology. 1990;**52**(1–2):25-71. DOI: 10.1007/bf02459568

[8] Calvey N, Williams N. Principles and Practice of Pharmacology for Anaesthetists. 5th ed. New Jersey: Wiley, John & Sons, Inc.; 2008

[9] Carrada PS. Carta al editor. Anestesia en México. 2006;**18**(2):181-182

[10] Weiskopf R, Nau C, Strichartz G. Drug chirality in anesthesia. Anesthesiology. 2002;**97**:497-502

[11] Lorentz MN, Stokes AN, Rößler DC, Lötters S. Tetrodotoxin. Current Biology. 2016;**26**(19):R870-R872. DOI: 10.1016/j.cub.2016.05.067

[12] Bane V, Lehane M, Dikshit M, O'Riordan A, Furey A. Tetrodotoxin: Chemistry, toxicity, source, distribution and detection. Toxins (Basel). 2014; **6**(2):693-755. DOI: 10.3390/toxins 6020693

[13] Thottumkara AP, Parsons WH, Du Bois J. Saxitoxin. Angewandte Chemie (International Ed. in English). 2014; **53**(23):5760-5784. DOI: 10.1002/anie.201308235

[14] Tucker GT. Pharmacokinetics of local anaesthetics. British Journal of Anaesthesia. 1986;**58**(7):717-731. DOI: 10.1093/bja/58.7.717

[15] Rosenberg PH, Veering BT, Urmey WF. Maximum recommended doses of local anesthetics: A multifactorial concept. Regional Anesthesia and Pain Medicine. 2004; **29**(6):564-575. DOI: 10.1016/j. rapm.2004.08.003

[16] Skou JC. Local anaesthetics. VI. Relation between blocking potency and penetration of a monomolecular layer of lipoids from nerves. Acta Pharmacologica et Toxicologica (Copenh). 1954;**10**(4):325-337. DOI: 10.1111/j.1600-0773.1954. tb01349.x

[17] Aldrich RW, Corey DP, Stevens CF. A reinterpretation of mammalian sodium channel gating based on single channel recording. Nature. 1983; **306**(5942):436-441. DOI: 10.1038/306436a0

[18] Hille B. Gating mechanisms. In: Ionic Channels of Excitable Membranes. Sunderland, Massachusetts: Sinauer; 1992. pp. 472-503

[19] Hondeghem LM, Katzung BG. Time - and voltage-dependent

interactions of antiarrhythmic drugs with cardiac sodium channels. Biochimica et Biophysica Acta. 1977;**472** (3–4):373-398. DOI: 10.1016/0304-4157 (77)90003-x

[20] Grouls RJ, Ackerman EW, Korsten HH, Hellebrekers LJ,Breimer DD. Partition coefficients(n-octanol/water) of N-butyl-p-aminobenzoate and other local anesthetics measured by reversed-phase high-performance liquid chromatography. Journal of Chromatography. B, Biomedical Sciences and Applications. 1997;**694**(2): 421-425. DOI: 10.1016/s0378-4347(97) 00207-7

[21] Dullenkopf A, Borgeat A. Local anesthetics. Differences and similarities in the "-cains". Anaesthesist. 2003; **52**(4):329-340. DOI: 10.1007/s00101-003-0463-5

[22] Sanchez V, Arthur GR, Strichartz GR. Fundamental properties of local anesthetics. I. The dependence of lidocaine's ionization and octanol: buffer partitioning on solvent and temperature. Anesthesia and Analgesia. 1987;**66**(2):159-165

[23] Bricker S. The Anaesthesia Science Viva Book. 3rd ed. New York, NY: Cambridge University Press; 2017

4

Complications Associated with Local Anesthesia in Oral and Maxillofacial Surgery

Basak Keskin Yalcin

Abstract

One of the important attempts in clinical oral surgery practice is to maintain safe and effective local anesthesia. Dental procedures are frequently performed under local anesthesia; thus, drug-related complications are often encountered. It is mandatory to have a preoperative evaluation of the patient and choosing the proper local anesthetic agent. Various complications including hypersensitivity, allergy, overdosage, toxicity, hematoma, trismus, paresthesia, or neuralgia can be observed during practice. Therefore, the practitioner should be aware of the possible compli-cations and management methods. The aim of this chapter is to review the preop-erative and postoperative complications associated with the local anesthetic in oral and maxillofacial surgery practice. The prevention of measures and treatment of the complications is also emphasized.

Keywords: local anesthesia, complication, local complications, systemic complications, treatment

1. Introduction

Local anesthetic agents have been used in clinical dentistry to allay or eliminate pain associated with invasive operations as early as the nineteenth century [1]. Local anesthetics are used routinely also in oral and maxillofacial surgery. Despite that local anesthetics are reliable and efficient drugs, the risks that practitioners need to be aware of were also reported [2].

Complications associated with local anesthetics can be evaluated systemically and locally. Common systemic reactions due to local anesthesia are reported as psy-chogenic reactions, systemic toxicity, allergy, and methemoglobinemia. Common local complications associated with local anesthesia are reported as pain at injec-tion, needle fracture, prolongation of anesthesia and various sensory disorders, lack of effect, trismus, infection, edema, hematoma, gingival lesions, soft tissue injury, and ophthalmologic complications [2, 3].

This chapter is presenting the local and systemic complications associated with the local anesthetics used in oral and maxillofacial surgery. The prevention of complications and management methods are also emphasized.

2. Classification and chemical structure of local anesthetics

Local anesthetics can be classified according to their chemical structure, a rate of onset, potency, and duration of action. Chemically, they are either amino esters or amino amides (i.e., an aromatic, lipophilic ring connected to a hydrophilic amine group by an intermediate chain containing either an ester or amide linkage). Ester local anesthetics are hydrolyzed in the plasma by pseudocholinesterase into para-aminobenzoic acid (PABA) and other derivatives, whereas amide-type local anesthetics are metabolized by the liver. The rate of hydrolysis has an effect on the potential toxicity of a local anesthetic. Allergic reactions that occur in response to ester local anesthetics usually are related to para-aminobenzoic acid, which is a major metabolic product of many ester local anesthetics. The rates of biotransformation of amide group lidocaine, mepivacaine, etidocaine, and bupivacaine are similar. Articaine, which contains both amide and ester, metabolizes both in the liver and blood. The ester group (cenzoic acid esters) includes cocaine, procaine, chloroprocaine, tetracaine, and benzocaine. The amide group includes lidocaine, mepivacaine (Carbocaine), prilocaine (Citanest), bupivacaine (Marcaine), etidocaine (curanest), dibucaine (nupercaine), and ropivacaine (Naropin).

Ester local anesthetics are not available in dental cartridges essentially because of several reasons such as the lack of efficacy, the potential for allergenicity, and the advantages of amino amides [4–7].

3. Systemic reactions due to local anesthesia

3.1 Psychogenic reactions

This psychogenic answer is associated with either the patient's body counterbalance to an anxiety-inducing situation or due to adrenaline secreted by the vasoconstrictor agent. As a result of mood changes, heart rate, respiratory rate, and blood pressure are altered. Patients often have a blush or erythema which mimics allergic reactions, hyperventilation, nausea, and vomiting [3]. It is important to understand the patient and make them relax. In more severe cases, these reactions should be maintained as syncope and hyperventilation. For preventing psychogenic reactions, the patient should be relaxed before administering local anesthetic injections. Using oral sedatives is an efficacious method to manage dental fears. Initial dosage should be dependent on patient health, age, weight, and duration of the operation. For healthy adult patients in short-term operations antihistamine-diphenhydramine (Benadryl) 50 mg 1 hour prior to the operation, moderate length (1–2 hours) operation benzodiazepine, triazolam (Halcion) 0.125–0.5 mg 1 hour before the operation triazolam, for longer duration (2–4 hours) benzodiazepine such as lorazepam (Ativan) 1–4 mg may be given 1–2 hours prior to the operation or 30–60 minutes prior for the sublingual prepa-ration may be described and given. Pharmacologically, mildly and moderately anxious dental patients can be managed using sedation or extremely anxious or phobic patients using general anesthesia [8, 9].

3.2 Systemic toxicity

Local anesthetic systemic toxicity develops when a sufficient (toxic) concentra-tion of anesthetic drug in the blood level reaches to the central nervous system and cardiovascular systems.

Initial symptoms are characterized by central nervous system signs such as excitation, convulsions, followed by loss of consciousness and respiratory arrest. These symptoms are often accompanied by cardiovascular signs such as hypertension, tachycardia, and premature ventricular contractions. The clinical signs and symptoms usually show objective symptoms such as quick talking, flicker, and tremor in the extremities [10, 11].

Predisposing factors are associated with age, weight, other drugs, gender, the presence of disease, genetics, vasoactivity, concentration, dose, route of administration, the rate of injection, vascularity of the injection site, and the presence of vasoconstrictors [7].

In order to prevent systemic toxicity, the patient should be evaluated. The volume of local anesthesia should be decreased, young or lightweight patients should not be treated all four quadrants at one visit using local anesthetic alone; accurate and slow injection technique, adjustment of dosage divided administra-tion and aspirating technique, using agents with low toxicity such as ropivacaine and levobupivacaine, and performing an aspiration test are recommended [11]. Preventing from a toxic dose complication, it should be evoked that for healthy adults, the suggested maximum safe dose of 2% lignocaine in 1:80,000 adrenaline is four-and-a-half 2 or 2.2 mL cartridges (180–198 mg lignocaine); for 3% prilo-caine and felypressin 0.03 i.u./mL, the maximum safe dose is 400 mg (six 2 mL cartridges) [12]. Another strategy to reduce toxicity is using the guideline of 1/10th cartridge per kilo as a rough guide to the maximum dose [13].

Dentists should be aware that excessive doses of topical anesthetics while these agents are more concentrated to facilitate infiltration may lead to toxic effects, particularly in children.

Treatment at the office includes airway support, administration of 100% oxygen, supine positioning, and protection from injury in the event of seizure activity, treating convulsions (benzodiazepines or thiopental; propofol cannot be used in patients with unstable blood pressure, heartbeat) [14]. If severe hypotension arrhythmia occurs, administration of the infusion of a 1.5 mL/kg 20% lipid emulsion over approximately 1 minute and then starting with continuous application at 0.25 mL/kg/min = 1000 mL/h. Studies have reported a resuscitation effect at a total dose of ≤10 mL/kg; therefore, 12 mL/kg can be used as an approximate estimate for the maximum dose. The adrenaline dose should be based on resuscitation guidelines such as those of the American Heart Association. The American Society of Regional Anesthesia and Pain Medicine standard of <1 μg/kg does not need to be strictly adhered to [11].

3.3 Allergy

Allergy is also known as hypersensitive reactions, initiated by immunological mechanisms acquired through exposure to a specific allergen; re-exposure to which produces a heightened capacity to react. The prevalence of allergic reactions to amide group local anesthetics is rare. It is predicted that less than 1% of all complications are caused by an allergy. Many of the complications doubt to be allergic are actually anxiety-induced reactions [15].

Ester-type local anesthetics are more allergenic than amide-type local anesthetics. Therefore, amide-type anesthetics are broadly used, among which lidocaine is the most commonly used for dental anesthesia epinephrine involving form. Adverse reactions to local anesthesia are caused by preservatives (e.g., methyl-p-hydroxybenzoate), antioxidants (e.g., bisulfate), antiseptics (e.g., chlorhexidine), vasoconstrictor (e.g., sulfites), and other antigens such as latex, as well as local anesthetic drugs themselves [5].

Allergic reactions may include mild symptoms, such as urticaria, erythema, and intense itching, as well as severe reactions in the form of angioedema and/or respiratory distress. Even more severe life-threatening anaphylactic responses include symptoms of apnea, hypotension, and loss of consciousness [15].

In order to diagnose allergies, the skin prick test is the most endorsed. When skin prick test results are determined to be negative, intradermal testing should be performed for patients who have a history of allergy to local anesthetics intradermal tests become obligatory [15, 16].

The following treatments a local anesthetic patient had tested negative in the allergy tests, should be used.

The initial treatment for an allergic reaction in office at the first step should be the removal of the causative agent. For the management of mild symptoms, oral or intramuscular antihistamine-diphenhydramine (Benadryl), 25 or 50 mg, should be given. Additionally, hydrocortisone cream may be prescribed to relieve skin itching or erythema. In life-threatening cases basic life support, intramus-cular or subcutaneous epinephrine 0.3–0.5 mg, and hospitalization services should be given.

Anaphylaxis is an acute potentially life-threatening hypersensitivity reaction. The clinical symptoms of anaphylaxis are depending on the organ systems involved. Uncontrolled co-existing asthma, mast cell disorders, and patients with specific allergens such as peanut and tree nut allergy are the risk factors for anaphylaxis. In emergency management of anaphylaxis in the office, due to guidelines of the Australasian Society of Clinical Immunology and Allergy should be in these steps, the patient should lie flat, but also in the case of breathing difficulty, the patient is allowed to sit. Adrenaline 1:1000 dilution (0.01 mg/kg up to 0.5 mg per dose) should be administered intramuscular with 1-mL syringes, 21 gauge needles, and should be repeated every 5 minutes as needed. Another recommendation for epinephrine is or children and adults who weigh 30 kg or over is 0.3 mg. For those weighing 15 to 30 kg, the epinephrine dose is 0.15 mg. The use of adrenaline auto-injector can also be chosen, which is carried mostly by heavy allergic patients themselves.

Adrenaline should be administered for anaphylaxis by intravenous (IV) route only in the case of profoundly hypotensive patients or patients who develop a cardiopulmonary arrest or those who fail to respond to multiple doses of IM adrenaline because of the potential cardiovascular adverse effects of IV administration of adrenaline [17, 18].

Estelle and Simons evaluated evidence-based pharmacologic treatment of anaphylaxis. They agreed using epinephrine at the first step intramuscular in the treatment of anaphylaxis. But the use of antihistamines and glucocorticoids is controversial. Some authors claim using antihistamines is not effective because they are not effective on upper or lower airway obstruction, hypotension, or shock, while others advocate that these drugs decrease the side effects urticaria, flushing, headache, hypotension, and rhinorrhea. In the World Allergy Organization survey, glucocorticoids were reported to be the second most widely available medications (after epinephrine) for anaphylaxis treatment globally, even though some claim glucocorticoids have no proven benefit in anaphylaxis [19].

As a result first step of treatment must be epinephrine additionally glucocorticoids and antihistamines may use to treat severe systemic reactions.

3.4 Methemoglobinemia

Methemoglobinemia is a unique dose-dependent reaction where the iron in hemoglobin is stabilized in the ferric ($Fe3+$) form, unable to attach oxygen, leading to tissue hypoxia and causing a varying degree of cyanosis. Methemoglobinemia can be either inherited or acquired [20].

The risk of methemoglobinemia increased in infants and the elderly. Patients with underlying health problems; liver cirrhosis, with underdeveloped hepatic and renal function; heart disease; and pulmonary disease (chronic obstructive pulmonary disease, pneumonia) are under the risk of methemoglobinemia. When administered in excessive doses, the local anesthetics mostly prilocaine and benzocaine (90% of reported cases) and barely lidocaine and articaine may also lead to methemoglobinemia [21].

Symptoms of cyanosis will be observed in nail beds and mucous membranes. In more severe cases, headache, dizziness, fatigue, dyspnea, and tachycardia are seen. For diagnosis in the dental clinic, pulse oximetry and in-hospital arterial blood analysis play an essential role [21].

Management of methemoglobinemia begins with supplemental oxygen (100%) immediately. As a guideline, methylene blue, which is a heterocyclic aromatic chemi-cal compound increasing the rate of conversion of methemoglobin to hemoglobin, may be given to a symptomatic patient. For severe cases, hyperbaric oxygenation may also be used if available. Methylene blue should be administrated in 1 to 2 mg/kg doses, given as 0.1 mL/kg of a 1% solution (10 mg/mL) intravenously over 5–10 min-utes every hour up to a 7 mg/kg maximum. Repeated doses may be necessary within 30–60 minutes of the initial dose [22, 23]. Guay summarizes 242 cases of methemo-globinemia complications related to dental local anesthetics lidocaine, bupivacaine, cocaine, mepivacaine, prilocaine, and tetracaine in children and adults. He concluded that benzocaine should be out of usage. In a specific patient group, in children younger than 6 months, in pregnant women, or in patients taking other oxidizing drugs, prilocaine should not be used. The dose should be limited to 2.5 mg/kg [21].

4. Local complications associated with local anesthesia

4.1 Pain on injection

Pain on injection can be due to specific circumstances such a temperate of the solution, velocity of injection, dull needles, needles with barbs, or aggressive insertion of the needle, damaging soft tissues, blood vessels, nerves, or the periosteum and causing more pain and other complications.

The burning is dependent on the rate of injection and the acidity of the solution. Lidocaine causes an intense burning sensation when injected locally. When the needle penetrates a nerve, the patient may also feel a sudden "electric" shock, suddenly moving the head, with the risk of self-inflicted damage [24].

In order to prevent discomfort, topical anesthetic application, warming anesthetics to body temperature, using a smaller-gauge needle (27 gauge), switching to a fresh needle when you have to inject multiple times in the same lesion or when you have multiple injection sites, and injecting slowly and with low pressure which reduces pain are done. A rate of 30 seconds per mL of solution is recommended. An inadequate injection site can lead to an intramuscular or intraneural injection blunt-ing of the needle, side of injection anatomic structure (palate) it is unacceptable to feel a little pain during injection [13, 24, 25].

4.2 Needle fracture

Needle breakage in the oral cavity after local anesthesia is a rare complication, since the establishment of non-reusable, stainless steel dental local anesthetic needles. In most cases, needle fracture happened with 30-gauge needles and during inferior alveolar nerve block, as a result of either incorrect injection technique, improper choice of hypodermic needle magnitude, or unexpected motion of the patient or assistants [26].

In order to prevent needle fracture, first the injection needles should be checked; 30-gauge and short needles should not be used for inferior alveolar nerve block in adults or children (25–27 should be chosen). Needles should not bend while insert-ing them into soft tissue [26, 27].

In the case of a broken needle, if visible, it should be removed immediately with a hemostat. If this is inaccessible, computed tomographic (CT) scanning should be taken to ensure the location of the needle, and under general anesthesia, the patient should be operated. In the literature for the removal of the fragment, mostly superficial mucosal incision perpendicular to the trajectory of the needle followed by blunt supra-periosteal dissection to spare vital structures is recommended [28, 29].

Acham et al. in 2018 made an analysis of the literature complication of needle fracture following dental local anesthesia on 36 reports and 59 needle breakage events; they concluded that three-dimensional imaging techniques should be taken to see the broken fragment and also surrounding structures like vessels and the the parotid gland. It is important because 27 out of 57 cannula fragments were located in the pterygomandibular space, and the choice of the removal of the fragment, whether general or local anesthesia, should be dependent on the patient's systemic condition [30].

4.3 Prolongation of anesthesia and various sensory disorders

Prolonged anesthesia, paresthesia, or neuralgia may occur following dental local anesthetic blocks. This may be temporary, where after a few days, weeks, or months, sensation returns or it may be permanent [31]. This mostly involves nervus lingualis or nervus mandibularis or both [32]. The nerve may be damaged during injection by direct injury, or the needle may damage the intraneural blood supply, resulting in a hematoma, or the needle may traumatize the medial pterygoid muscle which results in trismus. Neurotoxicity of the local anesthetic is another theory for nerve damage [33]. Procaine and tetracaine cause more damage than bupivacaine or lidocaine [34]. Paresthesia or neuralgia complication is mostly transient but may also be permanent if the anesthetic solution is injected directly into the nerve. Due to a numb feeling, the patient may have discomfort such as tongue biting, drool-ing, loss of taste, and speech impediment. Sullivan et al. conducted a randomized, double-blind, placebo-controlled trial on 496 patients with Bell's palsy. They main-tain treatment with steroids within 3 days after onset quite advances the chance for full recovery at 3 or 9 months [35]. Piccinni et al. conducted an analysis of reports to the FDA Adverse Event Reporting System; about 573 cases of paresthesia and dysesthesia after local anesthetics between 2004 and 2011 were performed. They concluded that the use of prilocaine, articaine, or both drugs has a higher risk of paresthesia [36].

If a nerve is damaged due to dental local anesthesia, the first treatment should be managing the pain. In order to decrease local anesthesia-dependent nerve injury, avoiding high concentration of anesthetic agent for inferior alveolar nerve blocks (use 2% lidocaine as standard), preventing iterative injections, and avoiding infe-rior alveolar nerve blocks are done by using high concentration agents (articaine) infiltrations only. The use of a low daily dose of multivitamin B, to regaining nerve healing and function, has been recommended [37, 38].

4.4 Lack of effect

Reasons for unsuccess in obtaining local anesthesia can be dependent on anatomical variants, pathological and psychological factors, choice of technique and solution, and poor technique [24].

Anatomical factors comprise accessory nerve supply, alteration in foramen location, atypical development of the nerves (bifid mandibular canals), and bone density [39, 40].

Pathological reasons for the failure of anesthesia are trismus, infection, inflammation, and previous surgery or trauma. Inflammatory diseases altering the pharmacokinetics and pharmacodynamics of local anesthetics cause a response to decrease and unfavorable effects to increase [41].

Local anesthetic failure or difficulty to obtain satisfactory analgesia commonly occurs in the situations with inflammations such as pulpitis and apical periodontitis acute periodontal abscess or pericoronitis [42]. Psychological determinants such as angst and anxiety can also cause local anesthesia failure [39].

Poor technique failure mostly occurs to obtain mandibular anesthesia. If the needle is inserted and advanced too deeply and too far dorsally, the terminal branches of the facial nerve within the deep lobe of the parotid gland are affected. Direct anesthesia to the facial nerve can force a rapid onset that occurs while the anesthetic agent is being injected; reflex vasospasms of the external carotid artery can lead to ischemia of the facial nerve, so facial nerve palsy occurs. The patient is unable to wrinkle the forehead, raise the eyebrow, close the upper eyelid, retract the commissure of the lips to smile, and turn down the lower lip on the affected side. The removal of contact lenses and closing of the eye on the affected side in Bell's palsy prevent corneal abrasion or drying [43, 44].

In most cases, paralysis occurs immediately after mandibular anesthesia injection, but there are also some cases in which paralysis starts lately. Cakarer et al. have a case report for late paralyses. They extracted simple teeth, without any complication, and 1 day after the patient returned with complaints of a weakness of the muscles of the left side of his face. On the examination, they observed Bell's palsy sign on the left side and unilateral expressionless, and there was no pathologic sign in the wound or any herpetic lesions. They consulted the patient with the Department of Ophthalmology and the Department of Physical Therapy and Rehabilitation. For the treatment lubricant eye drop (4 × 1), tobramycin ophthalmic solution (4 × 1) and lanolin eye ointment (during night) supported by eye patch were used. For 4 weeks, galvanic stimulation of the affected side of the facial nerve was performed, and mime therapy was recommended. In 2 weeks all of the symp-toms disappeared [45].

If the needle is inserted too high and deep, N. auriculotemporalis will be affected, and the feeling of "numbness" will occur. There has been a report of sudden unilateral deafness following inferior dental nerve anesthesia.

4.5 Trismus

Trismus is defined as a painful circumstance with inability to open the mouth normally. Several factors cause trismus such as multiple injections in a short period of time in the same area, intramuscular injections inside the muscle or trauma to muscles (either the lateral pterygoid muscle or the temporal muscle) which cause hematoma formation and fibrosis, needle fracture in the muscles inserting to styloid process, inaccurate positioning of the needle when giving the inferior nerve block or maxillary posterior injections or inflammation of the masseter and other masticatory muscles, a low-grade infection, and excessive volumes of local anes-thetic solution deposited into a bounded region which cause expansion of tissues. In the acute phase, pain from hemorrhage leads to muscle contraction and limitation of motion.

Once trismus develops, some cases will resolve spontaneously. Progression of trismus to chronic hypomobility and fibrous ankylosis may be prevented by the early institution of treatment consisting of heat therapy; soft diet; prescription of analgesics, anti-inflammatory drugs, antibiotics, muscle relaxants; or physiotherapy. Trismus caused by an infection needs to be treated by antibiotics. Usually, trismus will resolve in 6 weeks, with a range of 4 to 20 weeks.

Awareness of the anatomical landmarks and muscles: palpation of bony anterior ramus for temporalis muscle, pterygomandibular fold for pterygoid muscle, and appropriate angulation of the needle and bone contact before injecting are good methods for avoiding trismus via local anesthesia.

Intraorally the Vazirani-Akinosi technique, the closed-mouth mandibular nerve block technique, or extraoral techniques can provide anesthesia to trismus patients [43, 46].

4.6 Infection

Infection complication is rare since the usage of disposable needles and glass cartridges. Infection may extend to tissues by penetration of the needle through a contaminated tissue, because of the needle being contaminated before an operation or improper preparation of local anesthetic diluted solutions. On the other hand, a latent viral infection may be reactivated due to the trauma of the procedure which may be responsible for neural sheath inflammation.

The area to be penetrated should be cleaned with a topical antiseptic prior to insertion of the needle. Antiseptic mouthwash solutions such as chlorhexidine gluconate should be considered for all regional techniques. The local anesthesia should not be injected through the infected area.

Injecting local anesthesia during the presence of infection is important to increase the pH of anesthetic agent in order to increase efficiency because the infected tissue is more acidic. This process is called anesthetic buffering and leads to patient com-fort during injection, fast onset of anesthesia, and lower postinjection tissue injury. Recommendation for treatment of infection is antibiotics (penicillin V 500 mg every 6 hour for 7–10 days), analgesics, heat, drainage, and physiotherapy [2, 31, 47].

4.7 Edema

Swelling of tissues can be due to trauma during injection, infection, allergy, hemorrhage, and injection of irritating solutions.

The management of edema is dependent on the cause. Allergy-induced edema treatment consists of intramuscular epinephrine injection as mentioned above and, additionally, antihistamine and corticosteroid administration and consultation with an allergist to determine the precise cause of the edema. Trauma-induced edema should be managed as a hematoma. For the treatment of edema produced by infec-tion, antibiotics should be prescribed [27].

4.8 Hematoma

Hematoma formation as a complication of local anesthesia is the result of a venous or arterial laceration; intra-arterial blood pressure increase causes effusion of blood into the surrounding soft tissues. While injecting, if there is a high pres-sure, it may be a warning injecting against the bloodstream. The size of a hematoma depends on the density and compactness of the affected tissue; when a vein rupture is concerned, hematoma does not necessarily occur. Discoloration on the area, a bruise may accompany hematoma [48].

From the anatomical point of view, different nerve effects cause hematoma on specific regions such as anterior superior alveolar (infraorbital) nerve block below the lower eyelid, incisive (mental) nerve block at the chin area, buccal nerve block or any palatal injection within the mouth, and posterior superior alveolar nerve block extraoral in the lower buccal region of the mandible, intraoral distal to maxil-lary tuberosity.

Hematoma formation can be prevented by aspirating before injecting the anesthetic solution, by using a short needle and a minimum number of needle penetrations into tissues. When swelling forms immediately after injection, localized pressure should be applied with a minimum of 2 minutes. This will stop the hemorrhage.

Both swelling and discoloration usually subside in 10 to 15 days. Ice packs should be held for the first 24 hours after surgery following which intermittent hot moist packs can be used to resolve the condition and massage therapy using a heparin cream. Antibiotics should be prescribed if the hematoma is large in order to prevent the development of a wound infection [14, 49].

4.9 Gingival lesions

Gingival lesions consist of recurrent aphthous stomatitis, and herpes simplex can occur intraorally after a local anesthetic injection or after any trauma to the intraoral tissues. The exact mechanism is unknown, but any trauma to tissues by a needle may activate the latent form of the disease process that was present in the tissues with previous injection.

No management is necessary until there is severe pain. In order to relieve pain, topical anesthetic solutions (e.g., viscous lidocaine) may be used on affected areas. A concoction of identical amounts of diphenhydramine and milk of magnesia rinsed in the mouth effectively covers the ulcerations and provides relief from pain. Triamcinolone acetonide without corticosteroid can remedy pain [14, 27].

4.10 Soft tissue injury

Lip or tongue biting or chewing can occur on children with special needs or disabled patients, following dental local anesthesia with the unfamiliar sensation of being numb [50]. Shorter-acting local anesthetics such as plain mepivacaine should be chosen, and the patient or the guardian should be warned about eating, drinking hot fluids, and biting on the lips or tongue to test for anesthesia; cotton rolls can be placed between the teeth and soft tissues to prevent chewing. In order to accelerate recovery time for sensation, an alpha-adrenergic receptor, phentolamine mesylate (OraVerse), may be injected. For adults, the proposed dosage is 1 to 2 cartridges of phentolamine mesylate (a dose of 0.4 to 0.8 mg), while for children the proposed dosage is 0.5 to 1 cartridge (0.2 to 0.4 mg) [50, 51] Malamed [52].

Swelling may decay after 2 to 3 days. The lesion will heal over the next 10 to 14 days. For pain complains, analgesics may be prescribed and topical local anesthetic gel may be applied to the area.

4.11 Ophthalmologic complications

The most common complications include diplopia (dual vision), ophthalmoplegia (paralysis or weakening of eye muscles), ptosis, and mydriasis (dilatation of pupil). In extremely rare instances, amaurosis (partial/total blindness) can be seen. All these complications are transient and disappear on interruption of the anesthetic effects [53].

Intraarterial injection or perforation of the vascular wall would stimulate the sympathetic fibers running alongside the internal maxillary artery until reaching the orbit. The intravenous injection could reach the cavernous sinus via the pterygoid plexus and anesthetize the oculomotor, trochlear, or abducens nerves.

Horner's syndrome may occur after an inferior dental nerve block anesthesia because of penetration of the local anesthetic through the lateral pharyngeal and prevertebral spaces, causing barrier of the stellate ganglion [54, 55].

Alamanos et al. conducted a systematic review in 2016 on ophthalmologic complications following dental local anesthesia with 66 reports and 89 cases. They found that the Gow-Gates technique for mandibular block anesthesia is only associ-ated with diplopia, vision impairment is more associated with inferior alveolar nerve blocks than with posterior superior alveolar nerve blocks, and the latter technique has rarely been reported as a cause of amaurosis. Ocular complications in the literature are mostly with an injection of lidocaine [56].

In order to minimize the possible complications, visualization of the regional anatomy, numerous aspirations while injection, and aspiration on at least two planes before administration local anesthetic are performed.

5. Conclusion

Administration of a local anesthetic can be associated with complications of adverse events. In order to prevent local anesthetic complications, the medical history of the patients should routinely be evaluated in details, and effective anxiety management should be performed. Doses of local anesthetics should be always strictly assessed with body weight, and the maximum recommended dosages should be considered. While administrating anesthesia, the painless injection should be performed, avoiding intravascular or intramuscular or direct trauma to the nerve. New developments should be followed by the practitioners to reduce possible complications associated with the local anesthesia.

Author details

Basak Keskin Yalcin
Cerrahpasa Vocational School of Health Services, Istanbul University, Turkey

*Address all correspondence to: dr.basakkeskin@gmail.com

References

[1] Christopher A. Local anesthesia—An insight. International Journal of Oral Health and Medical Research. 2016;**3**(3):83-86

[2] Cummings DR, Yamashita DD, McAndrews JP. Complications of local anesthesia used in oral and maxillofacial surgery. Oral and Maxillofacial Surgery Clinics of North America. 2011;**23**(3):369-377

[3] Haas DA. An update on local anesthetics in dentistry. Journal of the Canadian Dental Association. 2002;**68**(9):546-551. DOI: 10.1111/ors.12252

[4] MacKenzie TA, Young ER. Local anesthetic update. Anesthesia Progress. 1993;**40**(2):29-34

[5] Kocak Berberoglu H, Gurkan Koseoglu B, Kasapoglu C. Dis Hekimliginde lokal anestezi. Istanbul: Quintessence; 2007. pp. 142-160. ISBN:9944 564137

[6] Giovannitti JAJR, Rosenberg MB, Phero JC. Pharmacology of local anesthetics used in oral surgery. Oral and Maxillofacial Surgery Clinics of North America. 2013;**25**(3):453-465

[7] Becker DE, Reed KL. Essentials of local anesthetic pharmacology. Anesthesia Progress. 2006;**53**(3):98-108

[8] Donaldson M, Gizzarelli G, Chanpong B. Oral sedation: A primer on anxiolysis for the adult patient. Anesthesia Progress. 2007;**54**(3):1 18-128

[9] Appukuttan DP. Strategies to manage patients with dental anxiety and dental phobia: Literature review. Clinical, Cosmetic and Investigational Dentistry. 2016;**8**:35-50. DOI: 10.2147/CCIDE. S63626

[10] Sekimoto K, Tobe M, Saito S. Local anesthetic toxicity: Acute and chronic management. Acute Medicine & Surgery. 2017;**4**(2):152-160

[11] Safety Committee of Japanese Society of Anesthesiologists. Practical guide for the management of systemic toxicity caused by local anesthetics. Journal of Anesthesia. 2019;**33**:1-8. DOI: 10.1007/s00540-018-2542-4

[12] Singh P. An emphasis on the wide usage and important role of local anesthesia in dentistry: A strategic review. Dental Research Journal (Isfahan). 2012;**9**(2):127-132

[13] Meechan JG. Local anaesthesia: Risks and controversies. Dental Update. 2009;**36**(5):278-280

[14] Bosack RC, Lieblich S. Anesthesia Complications in the Dental Office. 1st ed. Wiley-Blackwell; 2014. pp. 211-218

[15] Batinac T, Sotosek Tokmadzic V, Peharda V, Brajac I. Adverse reactions and alleged allergy to local anesthetics: Analysis of 331 patients. The Journal of Dermatology. 2013;**40**(7):522-527

[16] Lee J, Lee JY, Kim HJ, Seo KS. Dental anesthesia for patients with allergic reactions to lidocaine: Two case reports. Journal of Dental Anesthesia and Pain Medicine. 2016;**16**(3):209-212

[17] Muraro A, Roberts G, Worm M, Bilo MB, Brockow K, Fern andez Rivas M, et al. Anaphylaxis: Guidelines from the European academy of allergy and clinical immunology. Allergy. 2014; **69**:1026- 1045. DOI: 10.1111/all.12437

[18] Australasian Society of Clinical Immunology and Allergy guidelines. 2017. Available from: www.allergy.org. au/health-professionals/papers/acute-management-of-anaphylaxis-guidelines

[19] Simons FER. Pharmacologic treatment of anaphylaxis: Can the

evidence base be strengthened? Current Opinion in Allergy and Clinical Immunology. 2010;**10**(4):384-393. DOI: 10.1097/ACI.0b013e32833c2038

[20] Barash M, Reich KA, Rademaker D. Lidocaine-induced methemoglobinemia: A clinical reminder. The Journal of the American Osteopathic Association. 2015;**115**(2):94-98

[21] Guay J. Methemoglobinemia related to local anesthetics: A summary of 242 episodes. Anesthesia and Analgesia. 2009;**108**(3):837-845. DOI: 10.1213/ane.0b013e318187c4b1

[22] Chowdhary S, Bukoye B, Bhansali AM, Carbo AR, Adra M, Barnett S, et al. Risk of topical anesthetic–induced methemoglobinemia: A 10-year retrospective case-control study. JAMA Internal Medicine. 2013;**173**(9): 771-776

[23] Hegedus F, Herb K. Benzocaine-induced methemoglobinemia. Anesthesia Progress. 2005;**52**(4):136-139

[24] Säkkinen J, Huppunen M, Suuronen R. Complications following local anaesthesia. Den Norske Tannlaegeforenings Tidende. 2005;**115**: 48-52

[25] Kudo M. Initial injection pressure for dental local anesthesia: Effects on pain and anxiety. Anesthesia Progress. 2005;**52**(3):95-101

[26] Augello M, Jackowski J, Grätz KW, Jacobsen C. Needle breakage during local anesthesia in the oral cavity—A retrospective of the last 50 years with guidelines for treatment and prevention. Clinical Oral Investigations. 20 11;**15**(1): 3-8. DOI: 10.1007/s00784-010-0442-6

[27] Malamed SF, Reed K, Poorsattar S. Needle breakage: Incidence and prevention. Dental Clinics of North America. 2010;**54**(4):745-756. DOI: 10.1016/j.cden.2010.06.013

[28] Brand HS, Bekker W, Baart JA. Complications of local anaesthesia. An observational study. International Journal of Dental Hygiene. 2009;**7**(4):270-272

[29] Zeltser R, Cohen C, Casap N. The implications of a broken needle in the pterygomandibular space: Clinical guidelines for prevention and retrieval. Pediatric Dentistry. 2002;**24**(2):153-156

[30] Acham S, Truschnegg A, Rugani P, Kirnbauer B, Reinbacher KE, Zemann W, et al. Needle fracture as a complication of dental local anesthesia: Recommendations for prevention and a comprehensive treatment algorithm based on literature from the past four decades. Clinical Oral Investigations. 2019;**23**(3):1109-1119. DOI: 10.1007/s00784-018-2525-8

[31] Crean SJ, Powis A. Neurological complications of local anaesthetics in dentistry. Dental Update. 1999;**26**(8): 344-349

[32] Pogrel MA. Permanent nerve damage from inferior alveolar nerve blocks-an update to include articaine. Journal of the California Dental Association. 2007;**35**(4):271-273

[33] Smith MH, Lung KE. Nerve injuries after dental injection: A review of the literature. Journal of the Canadian Dental Association. 2006;**72**(6):559-564

[34] Renton T. Oral surgery: Part 4. Minimizing and managing nerve injuries and other complications. British Dental Journal. 2013;**215**(8):393-399

[35] Sullivan FM, Swan IR, Donnan PT, Morrison JM, Smith BH, McKinstry B, et al. Early treatment with prednisolone or acyclovir in Bell's palsy. The New England Journal of Medicine. 2007;**357**(16):1598-1607

[36] Piccinni C, Gissi DB, Gabusi A, Montebugnoli L, Poluzzi E. Paraesthesia

after local anaesthetics: An analysis of reports to the FDA adverse event reporting system. Basic & Clinical Pharmacology & Toxicology. 2015;**117**(1):52-56. DOI: 10.1111/bcpt.12357. PMID:25420896

[37] Sambrook PJ, Goss AN. Severe adverse reactions to dental local anaesthetics: Prolonged mandibular and lingual nerve anaesthesia. Australian Dental Journal. 2011;**56**(2):154-159. DOI: 10.1111/j.1834-7819.2011.01317.x

[38] Vasconcelos BC, Bessa Nogueira RV, Maurette PE, Carneiro SC. Facial nerve paralysis after impacted lower third molar surgery: A literature review and case report. Medicina Oral, Patología Oral y Cirugía Bucal. 2006;**11**(2):175 178

[39] Meyer FU. Complications of local dental anesthesia and anatomical causes. Annals of Anatomy. 1999;**181**(1):105- 106. PMID:10081571

[40] Wolf KT, Brokaw EJ, Bell A, Joy A. Variant inferior alveolar nerves and implications for local anesthesia. Anesthesia Progress. 2016;**63**(2):84-90. DOI: 10.2344/0003-3006-63.2.84

[41] Siddiqui A, Shenoi R, Sharma HU, Harankhedkar N, Shrivastava A, Vats V, et al. Causes of failure of dental local anaesthesia—A review. International Journal of Contemporary Medical Research. 2015;**2**(2):415-419

[42] Wong MK, Jacobsen PL. Reasons for local anesthesia failures. Journal of the American Dental Association (1939). 1992;**123**(1):69-73. DOI: 10.14219/jada. archive.1992.0004

[43] Blanton PL, Jeske AH, ADA Council on Scientific Affairs, ADA Division of Science. Avoiding complications in local anesthesia induction anatomical considerations. The Journal of the American Dental Association. 2003;**134**(7):888-893

[44] Ogle OE, Mahjoubi G. Local anesthesia: Agents, techniques, and complications. Dental Clinics of North America. 2012;**56**(1):133-148. DOI: 10.1016/j.cden.2011.08.003

[45] Cakarer S, Can T, Cankaya B, Erdem MA, Yazici S, Ayintap E, et al. Peripheral facial nerve paralysis after upper third molar extraction. The Journal of Craniofacial Surgery. 2010;**21**(6):1825-1827. DOI: 10.1097/SCS.0b013e3181f43dcf

[46] Stone J, Kaban LB. Trismus after injection of local anesthetic. Oral Surgery. 1979;**48**:29-32

[47] Fonseca RJ, Frost DE, Hersh EV, Levin LM. Oral and Maxillofacial Surgery. Philadelphia, PA: Saunders; 2009

[48] Baiju A, Krishnakumar K, Panayappan L. Anaesthesia complications: An overview. Journal of Bio Innovation. 2018;**7**(4):526-534

[49] Biočić J, Brajdić D, Perić B, Đanić P, Salarić I, Macan D. A large cheek hematoma as a complication of local anesthesia: Case report. Acta Stomatologica Croatica. 2018;**52**(2):156-159. DOI: 10.15644/asc52/2/9

[50] Bendgude V, Akkareddy B, Jawale BA, Chaudhary S. An unusual pattern of self-inflicted injury after dental local anesthesia: A report of 2 cases. The Journal of Contemporary Dental Practice. 2011;**12**(5):404-407. DOI: 10.5005/jp-journals-[10024-1067]

[51] Jung RM, Rybak M, Milner P, Lewkowicz N. Local anesthetics and advances in their administration-an overview. Journal of Pre-Clinical and Clinical Research. 2017;**11**:94-101

[52] Malamed SF. Handbook of Local Anesthesia. 5th ed. St Louis, Missouri: Elsevier Mosby; 2004. pp. 621-655

[53] Pandey R, Dixit N, Dixit KK, Roy S, Gaba C. Amaurosis, an unusual complication secondary to inferior alveolar nerve anesthesia: A case report and literature review. Journal of Endodontia. 2018;**44**(9):1442-1444. DOI: 10.1016/j.joen.2018.05.005

[54] Peñarrocha-Diago M, Sanchis-Bielsa JM. Ophthalmologic complications after intraoral local anesthesia with articaine. Oral Surgery, Oral Medicine, Oral Pathology, Oral Radiology, and Endodontics. 2000;**90**(1): 21-24

[55] von Arx T, Lozanoff S, Zinkernagel M. Ophthalmologic complications after intraoral local anesthesia an analysis of 65 published case reports. Research and Science Swiss Dental Journal. 2014;**124**:784-795

[56] Alamanos C, Raab P, Gamulescu A, Behr M. Ophthalmologic complications after administration of local anesthesia in dentistry: A systematic review. Oral Surgery, Oral Medicine, Oral Pathology, Oral Radiology. 2016;**121**(3):39-50

5

Bupivacaine Pharmacokinetics in Pregnant Women

Yazmín Guillén-Dolores

Abstract

Pregnancy, labor, and delivery are accompanied by physiological changes that impact on the use of the drugs to which they are exposed. The anesthesiologist needs to understand the principal differences in management of this particular population. The study of the main pharmacokinetic changes associated with pregnancy is relevant for the proper management of drugs to avoid adverse effects. The objective of this chapter is to review the physiological changes that impact on the pharmacokinetics of the pregnant woman with a focus on local anesthetics of the amide type, specifically bupivacaine, and the main studies that have led to a deeper understanding.

Keywords: pharmacokinetics, pregnant, bupivacaine

1. Introduction

Pregnancy and labor are accompanied by important physiological and anatomical changes. There is a modification in the metabolism of drugs and changes in their pharmacokinetics as well as their interaction with organs and systems. Anesthesia in the obstetric patient is influenced by physiological changes, concomitant dis-eases, and preferences for a specific drug. Local anesthetics are a special topic due to the frequent use of them during labor, the performance of cesarean section, or another non-obstetric procedure in the pregnant patient. It is necessary to know the pharmacokinetics of the local anesthetic most frequently used in our practice, bupivacaine, plain or hyperbaric, or one of its enantiomers. The objective of this review is to know the main studies that have evaluated pharmacokinetics and their interaction with systems and organs in the mother and placental passage.

2. Cardiovascular changes of pregnancy

During pregnancy many hemodynamic and hormonal changes occur like cardiovascular adaptations such as increased heart rate, plasmatic volume, cardiac output and sympathetic tone, or a reduction in peripheral resistances. The heart moves to the left and up during pregnancy, since the diaphragm progressively rises through the gravid uterus. These changes may be more important in post-term periods that are defined as pregnancies greater than 294 days (≥42 weeks of gestation periods) [1]. The increase in cardiac output and blood volume may increase the distribution of some drugs; the water-soluble ones will increase in their absorption as well as the liposoluble by the augmentation of the maternal fat, and there is an increase of the glomerular filtration and the renal sanguineous irrigation, which will produce an increase in the clearance of the drug [2].

The blood volume increases by 30–50%, and this rise begins in the first trimester and continues rising until week 30 of gestation and returns to its normal volume after pregnancy. A phenomenon is a dilutional anemia since the proportion of plasma volumes in relation to blood volume increases proportionally greater than red cells, and the hemoglobin concentrations will vary between 11 and 12 g/100 mL at the end of pregnancy. The increase in plasma volume is related to the size of the fetus; one theory is that the adrenal glands of the fetus can initiate an increase in blood volume by providing dehydroepiandrosterone (precursor of estrogen) to the placenta, stimulating the liver to produce angiotensin, which increases aldosterone production and fluid retention [3].

Increased blood volume and increased cardiac output may respond to an initial vasodilation caused by a vasodilating substance that may be prostacyclin or the endothelial-derived relaxing factor. This increase in blood volume is necessary to meet the needs of the fetus and compensate for the loss of maternal blood at delivery; the mother can lose up to 20% of their blood volume without a significant change in his hematocrit [3]. Cardiac output increases to 30–50% during preg-nancy, peaks at weeks 28–32, and then decreases a little during the last weeks. The values increase to 4.5–6.5 L/min and decrease as the term of pregnancy approaches but are considerably lower in the lateral position than in the supine position. The supine position during labor is associated with an 8% incidence of hypotension, and 15–20% of patients will have aortoiliac and vena cava compression. The reduced cardiac output lowers uterine blood flow, and this adversely affects the fetus. The cardiac return is diverted from the vena cava through the vertebral and azygos systems to the superior vena cava, and this enlarges the epidural veins and provides an explanation for the reduced amount of local anesthetic needed for spinal or epidural analgesia in pregnancy, and there is an increase in sympathetic activity that results in vasoconstriction that reduced the degree of hypotension observed [4].

Uterine blood flow increases to 200 mL/min by week 28 and 500 mL/min by the end of pregnancy, the uterine musculature receives approximately 20% of the total uterine blood flow, while the area of the placenta receives 80% by what to the placenta, that is to say, 400 mL of blood per minute or approximately 80 mL of blood per 100 g of tissue per minute [4].

3. Pharmacokinetics of bupivacaine and main studies

Bupivacaine is a local anesthetic amide type, synthesized in 1957 by Ekenstam in Switzerland, and has a mechanism of action through the obstruction of sodium channels to the nerve membrane, preventing the generation of an action potential. It is used for intraoperative local anesthesia, postoperative analgesia, and chronic pain treatment. It is widely used in pregnant patients and provides excellent sensory anesthesia with reported concentrations at 0.5% [5].

The effectiveness of bupivacaine was evaluated by the toxicity, the latency, and the degree of motor block, the sympathetic block, and the sensory block, as well as the elimination time. The absorption and distribution are influenced by the vascularity of the injection site, the mode of injection, and the degree of ionization of the drug. After IV administration, its half-life is 45 min correspond-ing to redistribution and 2.5 h due to elimination. It is metabolized by the liver by N-dealkylation and glucuronide conjugation. Elimination is urinary. Although some metabolites are eliminated via the pulmonary and bile fluid, the portion bound to proteins is the active part, and the unbound is responsible for the toxic effects [5].

The pharmacokinetics in the mother-fetus binomial changes, the fetus and the placenta function as deposits, the placenta has the capacity to metabolize drugs, and it is possible to modulate the elimination of the drug by producing metabolites and retaining large quantities for its release back to the fetus [6].

The apparent volume of distribution increases during pregnancy with the increase in plasma volume, approximately 40–50% from the beginning of pregnancy to a maximum of 32 weeks. During the placental growth phase, the peripheral hairy surface increases from 3.7 m^2 in week 25 to 11 m^2 during the last month of gestation, and the fetal-mother exchange surface decreases from 92 to 767 m^2 due to a decrease in density of the microvilli [6].

Since the drugs that cross the placenta reach the fetus via the umbilical venous blood and 50% of it enters the liver circulation and the rest goes through the venous duct, then half of the transported drug is susceptible to hepatic metabolism and the other half enters the fetal circulation directly. The distribution of a drug in the fetus is regulated by variations in pH and protein binding [6].

The drugs once inside the organism move between the compartments, and to analyze it the changes in the concentration of the drug in a compartment as a function of time are studied, according to the following formula [7]:

$$\frac{dC}{dt} = -kCn \tag{1}$$

where dC/dt equals the change in concentration in relation to time and −kCn refers to the decrease in the concentration of a drug which is an exponential type function [7].

When the rate of change is independent of the concentration of the drug, it is called a zero-order process, and when the process and the rate of change are proportional to the concentration of the drug, it is called a first-order process, the mother-fetus, which behaves like a model of two compartments with bidirectional distribution [7].

Bupivacaine has an asymmetric carbon atom and can take the form of two enantiomers (R + dextrobupivacaine and S-levobupivacaine), form different three-dimensional relationships in the asymmetric medium of receptors and enzymes, and result in differences in toxicity, distribution, cardiotoxicity, and neurotoxicity [8]. Levobupivacaine is soluble in water with a molecular weight of 325, a partition coefficient of 1624, and a pKa of 8.09. Both the partition coefficient and the pKa are very similar to those of bupivacaine. Its pH is 4.0–6.5. Its maximum plasma concentration reaches 30 min, and its volume of distribution is 67 L [8]. Liposomal bupivacaine is composed of multivesicular liposomes with 10–30 micrometers in diameter and has a duration of analgesia of up to 72 h [9].

Bupivacaine has a pKa of 8.1, ionized fraction of 15% at a pH of 7.4, fat/buffer coefficient of 115, protein binding 95%, molecular weight of 288 Daltons, and an effective anesthetic concentration in the rat sciatic nerve of 0.25. The main determinant of adverse systemic effects is the free fraction, which is not bound to proteins [10].

4. Studies of bupivacaine in QT interval

Spinal anesthesia involves changes in the mother's hemodynamic, including decreased venous return, decreased systemic vascular resistance, and a compensatory increase in cardiac output. These changes increase the risk of intraoperative arrhythmias in patients [1].

Local anesthetics routinely used include bupivacaine and its enantiomer levobupivacaine, the latter having a clinical profile close to bupivacaine, but it is less toxic to both the nervous system and the cardiovascular system, which makes it useful in obstetric anesthesia, where large volumes of local anesthetics may be required. It has been reported that bupivacaine and levobupivacaine cause a concentration-dependent inhibition of the amplitude of gravid myometrial contractions in rats [11].

Local anesthetics are amphiphilic and can enter a variety of cellular compartments and potentially interact with many different cell membranes, organelles (including the inhibition of mitochondrial adenosine production), and a variety of membrane junctions and charged cytosol molecules. Other mechanisms, which can contribute to myometrial inhibition, include the blocking of ionotropic signaling pathways (sodium, potassium, or calcium) and interference with protein modulation of calcium and potassium channels [11].

The practice of using low concentrations (0.125–0.25%) makes it less likely that the inhibitory concentrations in the plasma reach the clinical practice [11]. The toxic effect of local anesthetics on myocardial contractility and cardiac conduction is due to the alteration of the calcium channel [12]. In a study by Mahmut et al., 40 healthy pregnant patients were included; they evaluated QT interval, which increased significantly in the post-term group, which makes them susceptible to the development of arrhythmias; and they concluded that care must be taken during the induction of spinal anesthesia in term pregnancies as well as cardiovascular monitoring should be prolonged in this type of patients [13].

The Dogan et al. study used 12 mg of 0.5% hyperbaric bupivacaine or 0.5% of levobupivacaine for the spinal levobupivacaine group and calculated the QTc with the Bazzett formula and the QT dispersion (difference between the maximum and minimum QTc). They studied 60 patients. The mean maximum QTc was longer in levobupivacaine, and the minimum mean QTc was also longer. In the bupivacaine group, the maximum QTc was longer than levobupivacaine [14].

5. Pharmacokinetic studies in rats

It is known that the placenta does not limit the fetal transfer of local anesthetics administered to the mother; using a human placental model in rats, it is suggested that bupivacaine accumulates in the placenta [15]. The study of Morishima et al., a study in the University of Columbia with a model of rats, administered 1 mg/kg of bupivacaine followed by an infusion of 0.33 mg/kg/min, over a total period of 15 min. The maximum dose of bupivacaine was 1200–1400 ng/mL, which is similar to the concentration of plasma bupivacaine in pregnant women under cesarean section with epidural anesthesia [1].

The pharmacokinetic analysis of bupivacaine was assumed as an open two-compartment model. A transient reduction in heart rate occurred during the infusion of bupivacaine [1].

5.1 Pharmacokinetic parameters

The mean peak concentration of bupivacaine in maternal plasma was 3123 ± 370 ng/mL, the concentration decreased to 26 ± 12 ng/mL at 180 min, and after 240 min, it became undetectable. In plasma 4′-hydroxybupivacaine and 2,6-pipecoloxylidine were not detected. The half-life of distribution was 37.7 ± 2.4 min, the volume of distribution in stable state 3.86 ± 0.29 l/kg, and the total clearance 93.3 ± 8.6 $mL/min^{-1}.kg^{-1}$; other parameters were K_{12} 0.462 ± 0.066; K_{21} 0.081 ± 0.008 and K_{10} 0.166 ± 0.021. In fetal plasma, a bupivacaine peak of

320 ± 38 ng/mL was detected rapidly, and the drug became undetectable at 4 h. A bupivacaine concentration of 4817 ± 976 ng/g in the amnion at the end of the infusion was the highest sample of those obtained at any time [1].

While the dose of bupivacaine decreases, 3-hydroxybupivacaine remains virtually constant in the amnion and myometrium, and the 3-hydroxybupivacaine also kept increasing. Despite a high concentration of 3-hydroxybupivacaine in these tissues, the amniotic fluid concentration was not as high as expected. The 4-hydroxybupivacaine and the 2.6 pipecoloxylidide were only detected in traces in samples obtained in 2 h. The largest metabolite detected in rats was 3-hydroxybupivacaine [1].

In the fetus, the 3-hydroxybupivacaine remains detectable in the liver up to 4 h, while it virtually disappears from other tissues, because most of the umbilical venous blood perfused in fetal liver, and bupivacaine transmitted to the fetus, can directly enter the fetal liver; this may suggest that the fetal liver is capable of metabolizing bupivacaine. However, because polar metabolites do not cross the placental membrane bidirectionally, 3-hydroxybupivacaine probably accumulates in the fetus [1].

6. Studies about bupivacaine in multimodal analgesia

6.1 Blockage of the transverse abdominal muscle

In the study by Eslamian et al., a randomized, double-blind, placebo-controlled study of 50 pregnant women under elective cesarean section, transverse abdominis plane (TAP) block was used. The preparation was performed with 40 mL of 0.25% hyperbaric bupivacaine plus 2 mL of normal saline for the placebo group of 400 mL of 0.25% hyperbaric bupivacaine plus 2 mL of sufentanil for the study group. The block was guided with ultrasound; the patients who received 40 mL of hyperbaric bupivacaine 0.25% plus 10 μg of sufentanil consumed less morphine during 24 h after surgery compared to the control group ($p = 0.002$); the mean difference in morphine consumption was 15.6 mg in the first 24 h of the postoperative period. There were no differences in the EVA scale between one group and another with>0.05 [15].

In the Trabelsi et al. study, a group of 17 pregnant patients were administered with spinal anesthesia with hyperbaric bupivacaine with 5 μg of sufentanil, and abdominal ultrasound-guided TAP block was placed with 20 mL 0.25% bupivacaine bilaterally. They found an accumulated average of bupivacaine of 1.4 ± 0.2 mg/kg (range of 1.05–1.79 mg/kg); the C_{MAX} was 802.36 ng/mL (231.8–3504.5 ng/mL) and was reached at 30 min (T_{MAX}). The mean area under the curve (AUC) (0–24 h) was 4505.4 ng/mL, and the elimination half-life was 8.75 h for bupivacaine, demonstrating that bilateral blockade increases the total concentration of bupivacaine in the plasma after administering spinal anesthesia with bupivacaine. Plasma concentrations occurred at 30 min after injection, all peak concentrations were reached between 10 and 90 min and a second delayed peak of 90 min [10].

In the Lacassie study, in 12 pregnant women and 11 healthy volunteers, the transverse muscle was blocked with levobupivacaine 0.25%, 20 mL with epinephrine 5 μg/ml^{-1}, venous concentrations were 2.62 mg/L^{-1}, below the level toxic, the volume of distribution of levobupivacaine was 172 L (70 kg) (IC 95% 137–207) higher than in healthy volunteers [16].

6.2 Use of patient-controlled analgesia (PCA pumps) in different combinations

The Stourac study worked with pregnant women under epidural analgesia; they used 12.5 mg of bupivacaine and 5 μg of sufentanil in 10 mL of normal saline, and boluses of half the dose every 60–90 min were administered. Another group using

PCA pumps with remifentanil connecting a 50 mL syringe with remifentanil at a concentration of 20 μg/mL studied a total of 24 patients, and there was no significant difference between the groups. The level of satisfaction of the patients was 88% with epidural analgesia and 85% with PCA pump. Among the complications, only one had hypotension, with remifentanil, and experienced drowsiness and dizziness as well as temporary anxiolysis [8].

In the Chen et al. study, they determined the lowest effective concentration of levobupivacaine and levobupivacaine with fentanyl, and one group received 1.2 mg/mL of levobupivacaine and 2 μg/mL of fentanyl. They determined that the concentrations of 0.6 mg/mL of levobupivacaine plus 2 μg/mL of fentanyl and 1 mg/mL of levobupiva-caine were the lowest concentrations of the drugs required for effective analgesia, and they analyzed a total of 83 pregnant women and showed that levobupivacaine alone produces a comparable analgesia with levobupivacaine with narcotic; in addition, those who received narcotics had more adverse effects [17].

6.3 Studies in the capacity of blocking muscle fibers

In the Fanning et al. study, pregnant patients received spinal anesthesia with 10–12 mg at 0.5% hyperbaric bupivacaine with 20–25 μg of intrathecal fentanyl and 100–150 μg of intrathecal morphine. After the placental extraction, a small segment of the myometrium was removed from the incisional surface of the lower uterine segment. Each sample was dissected in four longitudinal muscles. The muscle was exposed to bupivacaine or levobupivacaine and chemical contractions were induced. Eight muscle samples were included. Bupivacaine and levobupivacaine caused a concentration-dependent decrease in the amplitude of the contractions reaching a statistical significance of $p = 0.002$ for bupivacaine and $p = 0.001$ for levobupivacaine compared to the control period before the administration of any drug [18]. There was no significant difference between bupivacaine and levobu-pivacaine in its effects on contraction of the myometrium, in the amplitude of the contractions, and in the interval between contractions for bupivacaine and levobu-pivacaine; there was no difference between the EC_{50} (effective concentration 50) and the effect of both drugs in contractility which was reversible. No increase in contractile amplitude was observed. The maximum concentrations in plasma were 1053 μg/mL (3.24×10^{-6} m) for bupivacaine and 1017 μg/mL (3.13×10^{-6} m) for levobupivacaine. They concluded that bupivacaine and its enantiomer levobupiva-caine cause a similar decrease in concentration-dependent contractions. The con-centrations required for their inhibitory effect on the amplitude of the contractions were much higher (33 times) than the clinically relevant plasma concentrations of these drugs after epidural administration and are unlikely to be significant in the low epidural dose scenario to analgesia in labor periods [18].

The combination with clonidine, a partial agonist of alpha 2 adrenergic receptors, interacts with the local anesthetic in the neural axis. The analgesic effect is due to its action in spinal and supraspinal α-adrenergic receptors, including the activation of postsynaptic α-2 receptors, since the noradrenergic descending pathways of cholinergic neurons and the release of nitric oxide and substances such as enkephalin reduce the absorption of local anesthetics by a vasoconstrictor effect, improving quality and increasing the duration of anesthetic blockade. It is recommended at doses of 1 μg/kg combined with bupivacaine [12]. In a Brazilian study, 66 pregnant patients were divided into two groups: a group with 8 mg of bupiva-caine +75 μg of clonidine and 100 μg of morphine +0.9% saline and another group with 10 mg of bupivacaine +75 μg of clonidine +100 μg of morphine + saline 0.9%; the total volume administered was 4 ml in both groups, and there was no difference in hemodynamic parameters, adverse effects, and level of consciousness, only the regression time of the motor block, in group 1, of 198.48 ± 47.63 min, and in group 2 of 232.84 ± 63.66 min; p = 0.00073. They concluded that morphine and clonidine at low doses produce adequate postoperative analgesia in pregnant patients [12].

In the study Zhan et al., 70 pregnant or obstetric patients were studied; 0.5% spinal isobaric bupivacaine was 4 mg; the ED50 of intrathecal bupivacaine for motor block was 3.96 mg (IC 95% 3.83–4.98) for pregnant women versus 4.51 mg (95% CI 4.27–4.76) for nonpregnant women. The potency of bupivacaine for motor block in pregnant versus non-pregnant women was 1.14 times higher (95% CI 1.05–1.24). This is because the supine position can increase the dissemination of the injected drugs due to the increase in intra-abdominal pressure, in addition to the increase in blood flow in the vasculature in the epidural veins, which distends and compresses the intraspinal space decreasing the volume of the spinal fluid cerebral [19].

7. Bupivacaine and placental transfer to fetus

The analysis of the placental intervillous space shows to be an appropriate place of investigation because this space is initially filled with blood coming from the maternal spiral arteries that interchange with the fetal venous blood, when the blood of the mother flows toward the branched villi. Although it is an important interchange interface, the intervillous space has been studied as the transport of substances between the mother, the placenta, and the fetus; obtaining blood from this compartment has provided a unique opportunity to study the maternal-fetal physiological relationship in a more physiological way [20]. The importance of this is that the reduced ability of the fetus to eliminate drugs can cause prolonged effects on the fetus, since half of the fetal circulation reaches the umbilical vein and directly reaches the fetal heart and brain by passing to the fetus. Liver immaturity contributes to the presentation of adverse effects, the fetus eliminates the drug by diffusion into the maternal compartment, although the majority of the metabolites are more polar and it is unlikely that the placental membrane crosses the placental membrane back to the compartment maternal, possibly resulting in the accumulation of metabolites in various fetal tissues [20].

In the study by Barros et al., a Brazilian study, the concentrations of bupivacaine and lidocaine as well as its metabolite (MEGX) and its placental transfer were analyzed in 10 healthy pregnant patients, under elective cesarean and epidural anesthesia. The administration of the medication was epidural of 0.1 mg of fentanyl citrate, 112.5 mg of 0.5% bupivacaine with 2:200000 epinephrine, and 200 mg of lidocaine 2% without vasoconstrictor injected into the epidural space [11]. The concentrations of bupivacaine enantiomers were high in the maternal plasma and placental intervillous space than in the umbilical vein and the umbilical artery. The concentrations of S-bupivacaine in the maternal plasma were higher than the R-bupivacaine concentrations, and the values were 195 .2 and 186.0 ng/mL. There were no significant differences ($P < 0.05$) between their concentrations in umbilical fetal vessels [11]. The placental transfer was 33% for R-bupivacaine and 31% for the S-bupivacaine. The concentrations of the enantiomer S-bupivacaine were 3.5 and 3.82 times higher in the placental intervillous space than that of the umbilical vein and the umbilical artery, respectively [11].

The R-bupivacaine concentrations were 2.9 times higher in the placental intervillous space than the fetal umbilical vein concentrations and 3.16 times higher than the concentrations in the fetal umbilical artery. There were no cardiocirculatory changes, neonatal repercussions in the APGAR, or respiratory depression. There was no significant difference in the ratio of enantiomer concentrations between the different compartments, maternal or fetal. This study showed that the intervillous space acts as a drug reservoir [11].

8. Conclusion

In conclusion, local anesthetics, including bupivacaine, are among the drugs most commonly used in clinical practice for the management of pregnant patients for obstetric or non-obstetric procedures. It is essential to know the pharmacokinet-ics of the drug in order to understand the concentrations of the drugs which we can obtain adequate analgesic and anesthetic effects, trying to diminish the toxic effects.

Acknowledgements

I thank the Instituto Nacional de Cardiología Ignacio Chávez for allowing me to carry out my work, promoting research and dissemination of knowledge.

Conflict of interest

I declared that I do not have any conflict of interests.

Author details

Yazmín Guillén-Dolores
Instituto Nacional de Cardiología Ignacio Chávez, México City, México

*Address all correspondence to: gudyyazy@hotmail.com

References

[1] Morishima HO, Ishizaki A, Zhang Y, Whittington RA, Suckow RF, Cooper TB. Disposition of bupivacaine and its metabolites in the maternal, placental, and fetal compartments in rats. Anesthesiology. 2000;**93**(4):1069-1074

[2] Babst CR, Gilling BN. Bupivacaine: A review. Anesthesia Progress. 1978;**25**(3):87-91

[3] Elkayam U. Pregnancy and cardiovascular disease. In: Braunwald E, editor. Heart Disease. A Textbook of Cardiovascular Medicine. 8th ed. Philadelphia: WB Saunders; 2007. pp. 1843-1844

[4] González I, Armada E, Díaz J, Gallego P, García-Moll M, González A, et al. Guías de práctica clínica de la Sociedad Española de Cardiología en la gestante con cardiopatía. Revista Española de Cardiología. 2006;**53**:1 474-1495

[5] Rudolph AM. Pharmacodynamics in the maternal-fetal-placental unit. NIDA Research Monograph. 1995;**154**: 163-174

[6] Briggs GG, Freeman RK, Yaffe SS. Drugs in Pregnancy and Lactation. 4th ed. Baltimore: Williams and Wilkins; 1994

[7] Foster RH, Markham A. Levobupivacaine: A review of its pharmacology and use as a local anaesthetic. Drugs. 2000;**59**(3):5 51-579

[8] Stourac P, Suchomelova H, Stodulkova M, Huser M, Krikava I, Janku P, et al. Comparison of parturient - controlled remifentanil with epidural bupivacain and sufentanil for labour analgesia: Randomised controlled trial. Biomedical Papers of the Medical Faculty of the University Palacky, Olomouc, Czech Republic. 2014;**158**(2):227-232. DOI: 10.5507/bp.2012.073

[9] Lirk P, Picardi S, Hollmann MW. Local anaesthetics: 10 essentials. European Journal of Anaesthesiology. 2014;**31**(11):575-585. DOI: 10.1097/EJA.0000000000000137

[10] Trabelsi B, Charfi R, Bennasr L, Marzouk SB, Eljebari H, Jebabli N, et al. Pharmacokinetics of bupivacaine after bilateral ultrasound-guided transversus abdominis planeblock following cesarean delivery under spinal anesthesia. International Journal of Obstetric Anesthesia. 2017;**32**:17-20. DOI: 10.1016/j.ijoa.2017.04.007

[11] de Barros Duarte L, Dantas Móises EC, Cavalli RC, Lanchote VL, Duarte G, da Cunha SP. Distribution of bupivacaine enantiomers and lidocaine and its metabolite in the placental intervillous space and in the different maternal and fetal compartments in term pregnant women. Journal of Clinical Pharmacology. 2011; **51**(2):212-217. DOI: 10.1177/0091270010365551

[12] Braga Ade F, Frias JA, Braga FS, Pereira RI, Titotto SM. Spinal anesthesia for elective ceasarean section: Use of different doses of hyperbaric bupivacaine associated with morphine and clonidine. Acta Cirúrgica Brasileira. 2013;**28**(1):26-32

[13] Mahmut Alp K, Adnan I, Evren B, Nuray A, Orhan B, Besli F. Effect of spinal anesthesia on the QT interval in term and post-term pregnancies scheduled for elective cesarean section, a prospective study. The Journal of Maternal Fetal and Neonatal Medicine. 27 Jan 2019:1-5. DOI: 10.1080/14767058.2019.1569620. [Epub ahead of print]

[14] Dogan Z, Yildiz H, Akcay A, Coskuner I, Arikan DC, Silay E, et al. The effect of intraspinal bupivacaine versus levobupivacaine on the QTc intervals during caesarean section:

A randomized, double-blind, prospective study. Basic and Clinical Pharmacology and Toxicology. 2014;**114**(3):248-253. DOI: 10.1111/bcpt.12146

[15] Eslamian L, Kabiri-Nasab M, Agha-Husseini M, Azimaraghi O, Barzin G, Movafegh A. Adding sufentanil to TAP block hyperbaric bupivacaine decreases post-cesarean delivery morphine consumption. Acta Medica Iranica. 2016;**54**(3):185-190

[16] Lacassie HJ, Rolle A, Cortínez LI, Solari S, Corvetto MA, Altermatt FR. Pharmacokinetics of levobupivacaine with epinephrine in transversus abdominis plane block for postoperative analgesia after caesarean section. British Journal of Anaesthesia. 2018;**121**(2): 469-475. DOI: 10.1016/j.bja.2018.02.070

[17] Chen SY, Liu FL, Cherng YG, Fan SZ, Leighton BL, Chang HC, et al. Patient-controlled epidural levobupivacaine with or without fentanyl for post-cesarean section pain relief. BioMed Research International. 2014;**2014**:965152. DOI: 10.1155/2014/965152

[18] Fanning RA, Campion DP, Collins CB, Keely S, Briggs LP, O'Connor JJ, et al. A comparison of the inhibitory effects of bupivacaine and levobupivacaine on isolated human pregnant myometrium contractility. Anesthesia and Analgesia. 2008;**107**(4):1303-1307. DOI: 10.1213/ane.0b013e3181804245

[19] Zhan Q, Huang S, Geng G, Xie Y. Comparison of relative potency of intrathecal bupivacaine for motor block in pregnant versus non-pregnant women. International Journal of Obstetric Anesthesia. 2011;**20**(3): 219-223. DOI: 10.1016/j.ijoa.2011.01.001

[20] Pacifici GM, Nottoli R. Placental transfer of drugs administered to the mother. Clinical Pharmacokinetics. 1995;**28**(3):235-269. DOI: 10.2165/00003088-199528030-00005

6

Local Anesthetics Infiltration and Wound Healing Process

João Abrão, Marcelo Antunes and Luis Vicente Garcia

Abstract

It is a good practice, nowadays, to infiltrate local anesthetics along the incision to prevent postoperative pain. This can reduce the use of opioids and the side effects they cause. It is known clearly that the surgical trauma causes inflammatory reaction, and this can be the beginning of a bad cicatrization or even a scar. The use of local anesthetics preventing the acute pain is a very simple technique and has proved to be useful. Nevertheless, the reaction that various anesthetics have over the tissues and the cicatrization process is yet controversial and deserves to be investigated deeply. The use of different formulations of these drugs has been stimulated. The duration and secureness have been the goals of many researches. Levobupivacaine, ropivacaine, and bupivacaine for their long action; lidocaine for less toxicity; and liposomal formulation for the longest duration ever seen, all of them have been indicated in the postoperative pain management. The aim of this chapter is to evaluate the role of long duration local anesthetics on the inflammatory reaction and consequently the collagen production and resistance of the tissue to traction.

Keywords: local anesthetics, pharmacology, ropivacaine, bupivacaine, tensile strength, wound healing, drug effects

1. Introduction (local anesthetics, general comments, classification regarding structure and duration)

Local anesthetics (LA) are widely used in clinical practice in anesthesiology. They possess the common property of transient interruption in the neural conduction, and in the fibers C and Aδ, they cause interruption of pain transmission. Pharmacologically, there is a selective blockade of Na^+ channels [1, 2]. The mechanism of action of LA is not related only to binding to the Na^+ channels. LA have an important role in other targets (channels and receptors); for example, in K^+ and Ca^{++} channels, they have an anti-inflammatory effect by bounding to G protein (inhibiting the adhesion of polymorphonuclear leukocytes, macrophages, and monocytes), increase the release of glutamate, as well as interfering in the activity of some intracellular signaling pathways [3, 4].

There are at least five applications for the use of LA in anesthesiology: local infiltration, regional intravenous anesthesia (Bier block), peripheral nerve block, central nervous system (CNS) blockade (spinal anesthesia, epidural, and caudal), and topical deposit (EMLA, eye drops in ophthalmology) [3]. In this chapter, we will discuss its application in the infiltration of the operative wound and its effects in the inflammatory process, after a brief discussion about the pharmacological structure of LA.

2. Na^+ channel structure: the main target of conventional LA

The Na^+ channel is composed of one alpha subunit and one or two beta subunits, which can be present in three different states: resting, open, and inactivated (**Figure 1**). The AL binds to the Na^+ channel after crossing the plasma membrane, that is, they bind to an internal portion of the alpha subunit preventing its activation and conse-quent depolarization of the membrane (**Figure 2**). Thus, the impulse is not propagated through the neurons, which prevents the perception of nociceptive pain [5, 6].

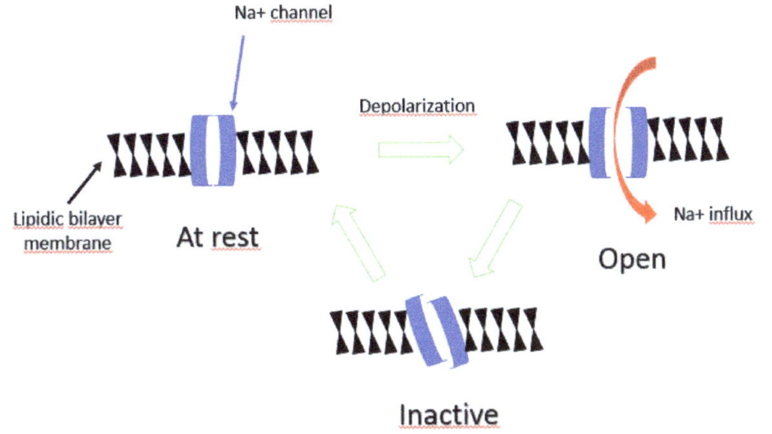

Figure 1.
Na^+ channels—it opens with the voltage changes (depolarization) propagated by the electrical impulse.

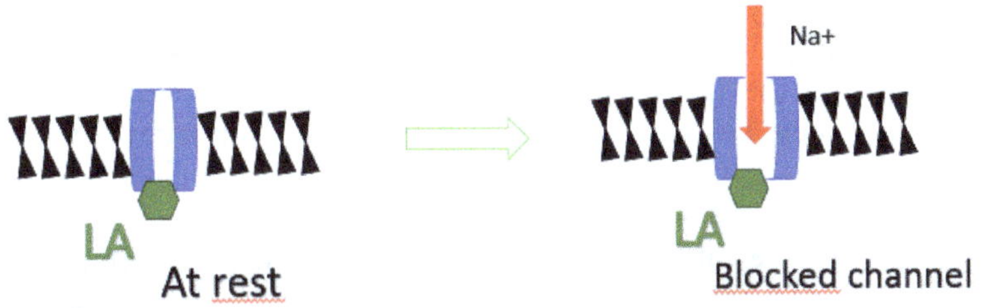

Figure 2.
The electric stimuli are not able to open the Na^+ channel because it is blocked by the LA.

3. Classification of AL (esters and amides and justify the use of each)

In its chemical structure, the LA are weak bases that possess in its molecule a lipophilic portion (aromatic ring) and another hydrophilic (tertiary amine) separated by an intermediate chain (hydrocarbon chain containing an ester or an amide group) (**Figure 3**) [7, 8].

The latter allows the classification of LA in amino-esters or amino-amides. These two groups differ in relation to its biotransformation site (the ester forms are metabolized by plasmatic esterases, while amide forms are degraded by hepatic enzymes) [9, 10].

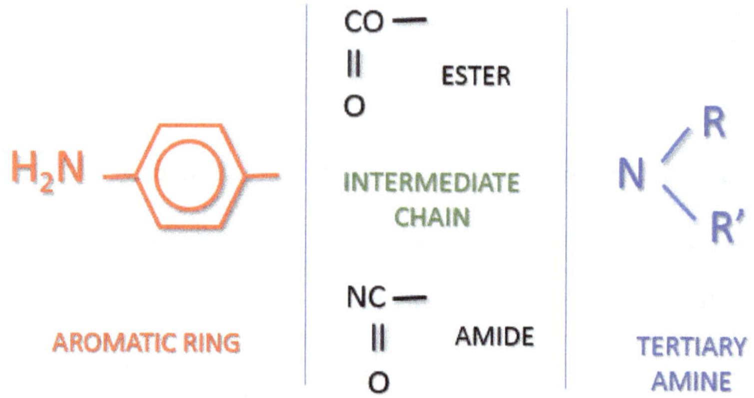

Figure 3.
LA generic structural formula.

Regarding the allergenic potential—the para amino benzoic acid (PABA) is an allergenic metabolite of the amino esters. Caution must be observed with some LA formulations, because methylparaben and metabisulfite are allergenic used as a preservative [11].

The size of the alkyl chain, in the amino group or aromatic ring, confers the LA molecule its hydrophobic character and its permeability in the lipid bilayer. So, the larger the nitrogenated radicals will be their potency and duration of LA blockades [12].

4. LA toxicity

Followed by the application of AL in the patient, a fraction will be absorbed by the bloodstream (plasma). Depending on the dose administered, the LA may reach higher or lesser degree the noble organs (e.g., brain and heart) producing physiological alterations in these tissues as well. The total dose used should comply with a maximum limit to try to avoid these undesirable effects, known as systemic LA toxicity [13]. Usually, in clinical practice, we must respect the maximum dose of each LA. Note that the CNS effects of lidocaine vary according to its plasma concen-tration (**Table 1**)—the higher the plasma concentration, the greater the risk to the patient, even develop a cardio-respiratory arrest. Thus, it is mandatory to observe the maximum allowable doses for each LA.

LA may also induce cardiac toxicity depending on the dose employed, acting directly in the heart (specialized conduction tissues) and decreasing the contractility of ventricular myocytes. Bupivacaine is more cardio depressor than lidocaine [14–16].

Plasma concentration (mcg/mL)	Effect
1–5	Analgesia
5–10	Numbness of tongue, tinnitus
10–15	Seizures
15–25	Coma, respiratory failure
>25	CV depression

Table 1.
CNS toxicity—lidocaine plasma concentrations and its effects [17].

5. Long-term local anesthetics: ropivacaine, bupivacaine, and levobupivacaine. (Pharmacological characteristics: concentration used in practice, toxic dose and care). Liposome formulations

The duration of action of LA is influenced by its effect on the vascular smooth muscle tone (vasoconstriction/vasodilatation) adjacent to the place where it is deposited. Other factors that determine its duration include the volume and concentration used, the approach itself (infiltrative versus regional peripheral nerve versus CNS blocks), the target tissue (fiber's diameter and myelin sheath), and the plasma protein binding (drug-specific affinity).

Long-term LA are the most used in clinical practice in anesthesiology at the following maximal allowed doses—bupivacaine (2 mg/kg), levobupivacaine (2 mg/kg), and ropivacaine (3 mg/kg).

5.1 Bupivacaine

Bupivacaine is presented as a racemic mixture of enantiomers R^+ and S^-. The optical isometry due to the presence of a chiral carbon (asymmetric) confers several possibilities in the formulation of the LA.

Bupivacaine promotes differential conduction blockade. As it produces more sensory than motor blockade, it plays an important role in the postoperative pain control. The use of epinephrine (5 μg/mL) gives a small increase in its duration of action (as opposed to lidocaine, which takes great advantage over this association). The use of large volumes for infiltration should be taken with cautious and done gradually and intermittently (3–5 mL at 5 min intervals). The patient should always be monitored to detect any unintentional intravascular injection of LA. Bupivacaine presents a higher risk of cardiac toxicity, when compared to levobupivacaine and ropivacaine. Every injection of this anesthetic should be done with the utmost care, always checking the positioning of the needle (by aspirating the syringe ensuring that the needle bevel is not intravascular).

5.2 Levobupivacaine

This anesthetic is the S-isomer of the bupivacaine, having the advantage of less neuro-cardio-toxicity due to lower affinity for these tissues. From a cardiac point of view, it causes a shorter prolongation of the QT interval and lower negative inotropism than racemic or R+ bupivacaine [18]. Its analgesic profile is similar to bupivacaine, because its duration of action is also long-lasting. Like ropivacaine, it has an intrinsic vasoconstrictor effect.

5.3 Ropivacaine

It is an anesthetic formulated by the pure enantiomer S of 1-propyl 2′-6′ pipecoloxylide [19]. As levobupivacaine, it has a safer profile than bupivacaine, because it has a lower toxicity in the CNS and heart. Its duration of action is long-lasting, like that of bupivacaine and levobupivacaine. It is widely used in infiltrative anesthesia and peripheral nerve blocks in anesthesiology. The same precautions should be taken with the use (intermittent and monitored injections). It is worth remembering that ropivacaine possesses intrinsic vasoconstrictor effect, which confers lower vascular absorption and increases its duration of action (levobupivacaine also owns this property).

6. Liposomal formulations

New methods of releasing the LA have been used in order to prolong the analgesia conferred by these anesthetic drugs. One of them is to produce liposomes spheres loaded with LA. This system allows LA deposit in the center of the liposomes, being involved by a double lipid layer. This setting allows a slower, controlled, and gradual release of LA, (72–96 h), consequently providing extended analgesic duration [20–23]. Liposomal bupivacaine (LB) has a decreased spread when compared with conventional bupivacaine. Therefore, several injections are needed and next to each other to obtain better results. In the infiltrative technique, it should be injected continuously from the fascia to the dermis. Unlike conventional formulations, which use bupivacaine HCl, the LB is produced only with its unprotonated basic form.

7. Infiltrative or transdermal techniques: practical recommendations

When the LA is used to infiltrate the operative wound, the anesthesiologist should seek a balance between the dose employed considering the size of the area to be anesthetized. In other words, it is sought to dilute the total dose used to cover most of the tissues operated. Thus, the same amount of LA used for infiltration on one side (e.g., right breast) needs to be diluted (doubling the volume) and to be employed bilaterally (e.g., right and left breast), always keep in mind that we must respect the maximum safety doses.

This approach allows an alternative to single dose injection of LA, namely the implantation of catheters for complementary use of the medication (continuous and/or in bolus, known as Patient Controlled Analgesia PCA) in order to prolong its therapeutic effect. In clinical practice, these resources increase costs because they need to be supervised, in addition to the increased risk of infection at the catheter implant site. New approaches are being investigated to optimize postoperative analgesia—use of newer drugs, innovative delivery systems (liposomal bupivacaine and ropivacaine), and the use of adjuvants along with LA.

8. Non-anesthetic drugs (adjuvants) injected together with LA (magnesium, epinephrine, clonidine, morphine, dexmedetomidine, and steroids). Is it worth?

With the advent of several approaches in the treatment of postoperative pain, the anesthesiologist can associate the use of various drugs and techniques aiming at greater efficacy in their control. The simultaneous use of several drugs (with pharmacological synergism) allows the anesthesiologist to decrease the total dose employed, when compared to the isolated use of each of them. This is one of the reasons for the use of adjuvants with the LA [24–26]. Another reason is to reduce opioid consumption in the post-operative period and associated collateral effects.

Usually, there is a consensus about the use of adjuvants in anesthesia, that is, the anesthesiologist must balance risks versus benefits and mainly the common sense. It is his/her responsibility to do the best choice in each case.

8.1 Magnesium

Magnesium sulfate antagonizes ionotropic N-methyl-D-aspartate (NMDA) glutamatergic receptor interfering in calcium homeostasis (membrane potential).

When injected together with LA in regional anesthesia, some evidence suggest that its use is beneficial [27]. Conversely, the use of magnesium sulfate intravenously is controversial [28, 29].

8.2 Dexmedetomidine

Dexmedetomidine (DMD) is a strong and highly selective α2-adrenoceptor agonist. When added to local anesthetics can enhance the analgesic efficacy of the peripheral regional nerve block [30]. DMD is eight times more selective than cloni-dine. It has analgesic, sedative, and antihypertensive effects, when used in systemic route. This substance has been associated with bupivacaine and lidocaine aiming prolonging the analgesic effect [31].

8.3 Epinephrine

Epinephrine has been used mixed to local anesthetics since a long time ago, and its recommended concentration is 5–10 µg/mL. It has, besides vasoconstrictive action that prolongates the local anesthesia, an analgesic effect mediated by alpha-2 adrenoceptor activation [32]. The vasoconstrictor effect of epinephrine can prevent inadvertent intravascular administration of local anesthetic solutions. Nowadays, the use of ultrasonography made such use largely redundant [33].

The onset time of local anesthesia after single injection was considered clinically significantly reduced when epinephrine was added to lidocaine or bupivacaine, when performing peripheral nerve blocks [34]. Current recommendations, however, allow the use of epinephrine in peripheral blocks only when ultrasonography is not available [35].

8.4 Clonidine

Clonidine applied at perineural sites, in doses up to 1.5 mcg/kg, acts as an adjuvant to local anesthetics prolonging analgesia and sensory/motor blocks [36]. It has intrinsic analgesic properties, inhibiting action potentials of C and Aδ fibers, as well as modulates the redistribution of local anesthetics through alpha1-receptors activation [37].

Side effects of this drug are dose dependent and include sedation, by decreasing sympathetic outflow (suppressing the release of norepinephrine in locus ceruleus (CNS) and substantia gelatinosa), hypotension, bradycardia, dry mouth, constipation, dizziness, and drowsiness [38].

Clonidine represents a good addition for the armamentarium of anesthesiologists because it prolongs the duration of analgesia, provides a faster onset of action, and improves the quality of nerve blocks (decreasing opioid consumption) [39, 40].

8.5 Morphine

Morphine is used by several routes and dosages (intrathecal: 100–200 mcg, epidural: 1–5 mg, peripheral nerve block: 75–100 mcg/kg, intravenous and intramuscular) [41]. Despite its use to prolong the analgesia, it is important to the anesthesiologist to pay attention at recommended doses to avoid the undesirable side effects (pruritus, nausea, vomiting, urinary retention, and respiratory failure). Always double check the vials before the administration of this medication because there are several vials currently in use (2, 4, 5, 8, and 10 mg/ml). All vital signals must be monitored at post-anesthetic care unit after the morphine use to early detect any cardiovascular or respiratory complications: bradycardia, hypotension, hypoxemia, and respiratory failure [42].

8.6 Steroids

Dexamethasone, a potent anti-inflammatory agent, has been investigated for its role as an adjuvant to local anesthetics in neuraxial as well as peripheral nerve blocks. This steroid has been used in intrathecal anesthesia (8 mg preservative free), in epidural analgesia (4–8 mg) and as an adjuvant in a variety of peripheral blocks, like brachial plexus, ankle block, and TAP block. A meta-analysis has found it to significantly prolong the duration of brachial plexus block when using conventional local anesthetics solutions [43]. Besides all the researches about the role of dexamethasone in neural block, one question has not been answered yet: is the better and prolonged analgesia caused by systemic effects of the steroid?

9. The four stages of wound healing

The wound healing is a continuous process, but for didactic understanding, it can be divided into four phases [44, 45]. The first phase occurs just after the incision or lesion of the skin, as soon as the blood leaks out of the body. There is a vasoconstriction, and the platelets stick together to initiate the coagulation. This phase is called the hemostasis phase. The platelet plug is reinforced by threads of fibrin. The hemostasis phase occurs very rapidly, in a question of seconds. As the fibrin mesh is formed, the blood is transformed from liquid to a gel state, that is, the pro-coagulant effect of prothrombin. This clot keeps the platelets and blood cells trapped in the wound area. Just after the injury of the skin, the epidermal tissue and the keratinocytes release the interleukin-1 (IL-1) pre-stored in these sites. The coagulation process activates the clotting cascade which is responsible to give the matrix for the influx of inflammatory cells. The degranulation of the platelets releases alpha granules, which secrete growth factors, like epidermal growth factor (EGF), platelet derived growth factor (PDGF), and transforming growth factor-beta (TGF-β). The PDGF and the IL-1 are responsible for attracting neutrophils to the wound site to remove bacteria [44]. The monocytes cells are converted to macrophages by influence of TGF-β, what has an important role in the initiation of the granula-tion tissue and a many proinflammatory cytokines (IL-1 and IL-6), besides other growth factors, like fibroblast growth factor (FGF), EGF, TGF-β, and PDGF. All these growth factors and the added endothelial cell proliferation ensues the angio-genesis beginning. During this hemostasis phase, the injured blood vessels leak transudate causing localized swelling and cell migrations to the site of wound. The damaged cells, pathogens, and bacteria are removed. White cells, growth factors, nutrients, and enzymes create the swelling, heat, pain, and redness, normally seen in the wound healing. This phase where all these signs appear is called the inflam-matory phase. This phase is not a problem unless it is prolonged and excessive. After all the bacteria and debris are removed, the wound is rebuilt with a new tissue made up of collagen and extracellular matrix. This is the proliferative phase. In this phase, new blood vessels are formed, so that the granulation tissue can receive enough oxygen and nutrients. The myofibroblasts are responsible for the contraction of the wound, making the granulation tissue to take the ideal dimensions to the lesion. The granulation in this phase is pink or red. If there is a dark color is a sign of infection, ischemia or poor perfusion. At the end of this process the epitelial cells resurface the wound extension, what is called the maturation or remodelling phase. In this stage, it is wise to maintain the wound moist and hydrated to optimize the epithelialization [46]. Some authors consider that the wound healing has only three phases, and this is comprehensible as long as the hemostasis phase and the inflammatory phase are so concomitant, dynamic, and interactive, that they consider it just as an inflammation phase. In fact, the phases do not have a predetermined duration, as Witte and Barbul showed in their article (**Figures 4** and **5**), the migration of cells to the wound site and the matrix formation [47].

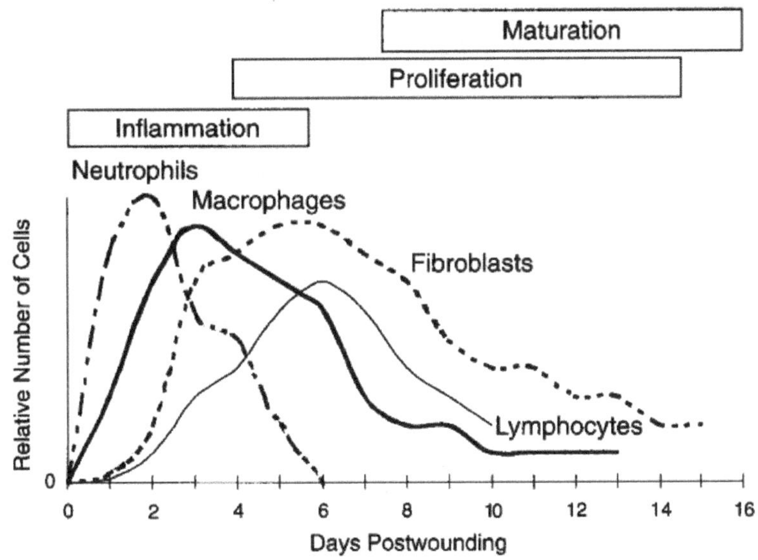

Figure 4.
The time course of different cells during healing process. Macrophages and neutrophils are predominant in inflammation phase, whereas lymphocytes peak somewhat later. In the proliferative phase, fibroblasts are more frequent [47].

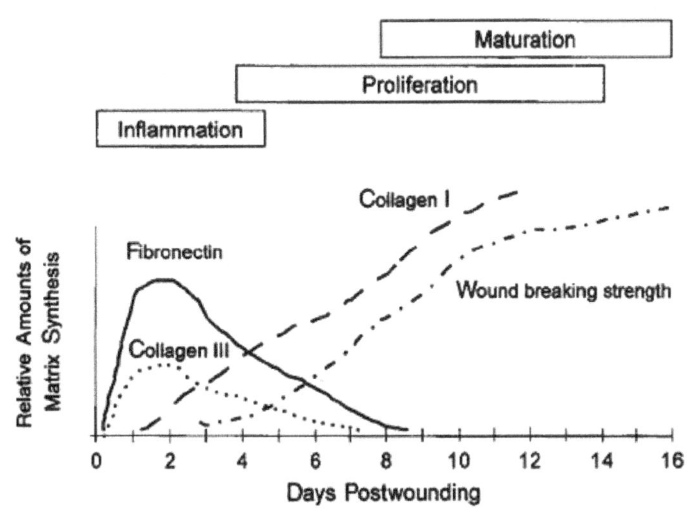

Figure 5.
Deposition of wound matrix components over time [47].

10. Local anesthetics can influence the process of wound healing?

When there is a rupture of vessels, there is an exposure of the subendothelial collagen to the platelets. This contact results in the aggregation and activation of the intrinsic factor of coagulation cascade. In the presence of thrombin, fibronectin, and their fragments, there is the release of cytokines and growth factors from platelets

(PDGF), transforming growth factor-β (TGF-β), platelet-activating factor (PAF), fibronectin, and serotonin. All this form the local fibrin clot that is the scaffolding for invading cells such as neutrophils, monocytes, fibroblasts, and endothelial cells. The neutrophils are the first cells to invade the wound, increasing the vascular permeability due to inflammation and release of prostaglandins. In the same time, chemotactic substances like complement factors, interleukin, tumor necrosis factor-α (TNF-α), TGF-β, platelet factor 4, and stimulate neutrophil migration [47–49]. The factors associated with wound healing can be seen in **Table 2**.

When analyzing the possible action of the LAs in the wound healing process, many aspects can take role. Injecting any substance in the surgery site, it is expected that it can have at least a pH influence, as the anesthetic has a pH different of the physiologic one. Many times, epinephrine is used to prolong the duration and lower the toxicity of the drug used [50, 51]. The influence of pain in the wound healing has been studied too [52–54]. The wound healing in the fetus has also been the object of research [55, 56]. And last, the LA probably can have a direct action in the eicosanoids or in the fibroblast formation and so in the cicatricial process [56].

These all are hypothesis that are discussed deeply, and many researches in human have to be done, unfortunately the majority of the manuscripts are in rats and they have a different immunologic system than humans.

The tissue injury caused by surgery produces directly and indirectly activa-tion of nociceptors and higher expression of proinflammatory cytokines and cyclooxygenase-2 (COX-2), leading to peripheral and central sensitization with subsequent hyperalgesia. The pain and inflammation are maintained by abundant eicosanoids, like prostaglandin E_2, released after surgical trauma. The long-acting local anesthetics such as bupivacaine and ropivacaine are used to provide prolonged perioperative pain relief and to diminish the occurrence of postoperative sensitization that manifests with hyperalgesia after the anesthetic effect has dissipated. The occurrence of hyperalgesia is very common when high doses of anesthetic are used [57, 58]. The routine of infiltrating the surgical site reduces the postoperative pain

	Function
Hemostatic factors	
Fibrin, plasma fibronectin	Coagulation, chemo attraction Structure for cell migration
Factor XIII (fibrin-stabilizing factor) Circulatory growth factors	Chemo attraction and adhesion Modulation of chemo attraction, mitogenesis, fibroplasia
Complement	Antimicrobial activity, chemo attraction
Platelet-derived factors	
Cytokines, growth factors	Regulation of chemo attraction, mitogenesis, fibroplasia
Fibronectin	Early matrix, ligand for platelet aggregation
Platelet-activating factor (PAF) Thromboxane A_2	Platelet aggregation Vasoconstriction, platelet aggregation, chemotaxis
Platelet factor IV	Chemotactic for fibroblasts and monocytes, neutralizes activity of heparin, inhibits collagenase
Serotonin	Induces vascular permeability, chemoattractant for neutrophils
Adenosine dinucleotide	Stimulates cell proliferation and migration, induces platelet aggregation

Table 2.
Hemostatic and platelet-derived factors associated with wound healing [47].

and morbidity and accelerates the recovery. This can be explained by reducing the production of cytokines. Although LA action is to block the nerve conduction, they have other cellular targets that modulate the inflammation, suggesting that the LAs have an anti-inflammatory effect [59, 60]. Several studies have shown that LA dose-dependently inhibits leukocyte adhesion to synthetic material and to blood vessel walls. LA can induce the release of prostacyclin, and this causes the release of leukocytes previously firmly adherent to vascular endothelium. It is shown that the LA can in low concentration stimulate the phospholipase A_2 (PLA_2) while in higher concentrations inhibited this enzyme [61].

All these considerations are important, but what is important in clinical aspects are the fibroblast formation and the quality of the wound healing. The first question the patient formulates is when he will return to normal life activity. To answer this question, it is important to have not only histological analyzes of the wound but also mechanical testing to be sure that the tissue is ready to normal work. Vasseur and cols in 1984 studied the effects of local anesthetics on abdominal wounds of rabbits [62]; using mechanical testing device, they could demonstrate that the breaking strength in the groups infiltrated with lidocaine or bupivacaine, do not vary con-sistently from the tissues infiltrated with saline solution, and so they conclude that the local infiltration with lidocaine and bupivacaine does not alter substantially the healing of midline abdominal incisions in rabbits. Abrão and cols in 2014 made a similar work using rats and long-lasting anesthetics, bupivacaine, and ropivacaine [63]. They used a computerized universal testing machine, and they concluded that there were no significant differences among the groups with respect to tensile strength after 14 days. These results, however, are not the same than Hanci and cols in 2012, who found that lidocaine and bupivacaine reduce the collagen production and the wound breaking strength in Wistar rats [64]. To further augment the argu-ment, Kesici and cols in 2018 studied the effect of bupivacaine, levobupivacaine, and procaine in the Sprague Dawley rats [65]. They found that bupivacaine and levobupivacaine affect negatively the wound healing, especially at the late period (21 days). The differences in these studies increase the uncertainty and discussion regarding the effects of local anesthetics. Many aspects must be considered like the animal gender, the use of other analgesic like paracetamol, the infiltration method, and the time of evaluation. Interestingly, there is no work done on humans, who certainly have a different response to pain. Probably, the reason is the difficulty to use the same methodology. All the researches in humans have only clinic evaluation, it is almost impossible to make mechanical tests. Uncertainties in this field only will be clarified with new studies. The clinical studies in human beings have a very sub-jective way to follow the wound healing. They constitute another subject that must be studied separately. The analogic scale of pain as the consume of opioids has been used as parameters to analyze the efficacy of the method. These studies conclude that ropivacaine (0.3%) can be used alone or with the addition of DMD (1 μg/kg), and there is no effect on wound healing [31, 66]. We must bear in mind that some authors only used a clinic evaluation, what can vary a lot from one researcher to another.

11. Conclusion

Nowadays, all the anesthesiologists are engaged in avoiding the excessive use of opioids for their side effects in the postoperative pain treatment. In fact, the μ-opioid receptors are impaired by the unrestricted use of morphine like drugs, besides there is an inhibition of the beta-endorphin release. Considering that the infiltration of LA in the surgical site does not produce, clinically any significant harm to the tissue cicatrization, and has the property of sparing opioid use, this technique is an important tool in the control of the postoperative pain and must be recommended.

Conflict of interest

We declare that we do not have any conflict of interest.

Author details

João Abrão[1*], Marcelo Antunes[2] and Luis Vicente Garcia[1]

1 Medical School of Ribeirão Preto, University of São Paulo, Ribeirão Preto, SP, Brazil

2 Educational Hospital of the Medical School of Ribeirão Preto, University of São Paulo, Ribeirão Preto, SP, Brazil

*Address all correspondence to: joaoabrao@fmrp.usp.br

References

[1] Catterall WA, Mackie K. Local anesthetics. In: Brunton L, Chabner B, Knollman B, editors. Goodman & Gilman's the Pharmacological Basis of Therapeutics. 12th ed. New York: The McGraw Hill Companies; 2011. pp. 565-582

[2] Cousins MJ, Bridenbaugh PO, Carr DB, Horlocker TT. Neural Blockade in Clinical Anesthesia and Management of Pain. 4th ed. Philadelphia: Lippincott-Williams & Wilkins; 2009. p. 1308

[3] Berde CB, Strichartz GR. Local anesthetics. In: Miller RD, editor. Miller's Anesthesia. 8th ed. Philadelphia: Elsevier Saunders; 2015. pp. 1028-1054

[4] Hollmann MW, Wieczorek KS, Berger A, Durieux ME. Local anesthetic inhibition of G protein-coupled receptor signaling by interference with Galpha(q) protein function. Molecular Pharmacology. 2001;**59**:294-301. DOI: 10.1124/mol.59.2.294

[5] Strichartz GR, Ritchie JM. The action of local anesthetics on ion channels of excitable tissues. In: Strichartz GR, editor. Local Anesthetics—Handbook of Experimental Pharmacology. Vol. 81. Berlin: Springer-Verlag; 1987. pp. 21-52. DOI: 10.1007/978-3-642-71110-7

[6] Catterall WA. From ionic currents to molecular mechanisms: The structure and function of voltage-gated sodium channels. Neuron. 2000;**26**:13-25. DOI: 10.1016/S0896-6273(00)81133-2

[7] Suzuki S, Koköfer A, Gerner P. Local anesthetics. In: Hemmings HC Jr, Egan TD, editors. Pharmacology and Physiology for Anesthesia—Foundations and Clinical Application. 1st ed. Philadelphia: Elsevier Saunders; 2013. pp. 291-308

[8] Lin Y, Liu SS. Local anesthetics. In: Barash PG, Cullen BF, Stoelting RK, Cahalan MK, Stock MC, Ortega R, et al. editors. Clinical Anesthesia. 8th ed. Philadelphia: Lippincott-Williams & Wilkins; 2017. pp. 564-584

[9] Kuhnert BR, Kuhnert RM, Philipson EH, Syracuse CD, Kaine CJ, Yun CH. The half-life of 2-chloroprocaine. Anesthesia and Analgesia. 1986;**65**: 273-278

[10] Scott DB, Jebson PJR, Boyes RN. Pharmacokinetic study of the local anaesthetics bupivacaine (Marcaine) and etidocaine (Duranest) in man. British Journal of Anaesthesia. 1973;**45**:1010-1012

[11] Boren E, Teuber SS, Naguwa SM, Gershwin ME. A critical review of local anesthetic sensitivity. Clinical Reviews in Allergy and Immunology. 2007;**32**: 119-128

[12] Strichartz GR, Sanchez V, Arthur GR, ChafetzR, Martin D. Fundamental properties of local anesthetics. II. Measured octanol: Buffer partition coefficients and pKa values of clinically used drugs. Anesthesia and Analgesia. 1990;**71**:158-170

[13] Groban L. Central nervous system and cardiac effects from long-acting amide local anesthetic toxicity in the intact animal model. Regional Anesthesia and Pain Medicine. 2003;**28**:3-11. DOI: 10.1053/rapm.2003.50014

[14] Chamberlain BK, Volpe P, Fleischer S. Inhibition of calcium-induced calcium release from purified cardiac sarcoplasmic reticulum vesicles. The Journal of Biological Chemistry. 1984;**259**:7547-7553

[15] Clarkson CW, Hondeghem LM. Mechanism for bupivacaine depression of cardiac conduction: Fast block of sodium

channels during the action potential with slow recovery from block during diastole. Anesthesiology. 1985;**62**:396-405

[16] Heavner JH. Cardiac toxicity of local anesthetics in the intact isolated heart model: A review. Regional Anesthesia and Pain Medicine. 2002;**27**:545-555

[17] Maheshwari K, Naguib MA. Local anesthetics. In: Flood P, Rathmell JP, Sahfer S, editors. Stoelting's Pharmacology & Physiology in Anesthetic Practice. 5th ed. Philadelphia: Lippincott-Williams & Wilkins; 2015. pp. 282-313

[18] Foster RH, Markham A. Levobupivacaine: A review of its pharmacology and use as a local anaesthetic. Drugs. 2000;**59**:551-579. DOI: 10.2165/00003495-200059030-00013

[19] McClure JH. Ropivacaine. British Journal of Anaesthesia. 1996;**76**:300-307. DOI: 10.1093/bja/76.2.300

[20] Tong YC, Kaye AD, Urman RD. Liposomal bupivacaine and clinical outcomes. Best Practice & Research. Clinical Anaesthesiology. 2014;**28**:15-27. DOI: 10.1016/j.bpa.2014.02.001

[21] Mantripragada S. A lipid based depot (DepoFoam® technology) for sustained release drug delivery. Progress in Lipid Research. 2002;**41**:392-406

[22] Kirkness CS, Asche CV, Ren J, Gordon K, Maurer P, Maurer B, et al. Assessment of liposome bupivacaine infiltration versus continuous femoral nerve block for postsurgical analgesia following total knee arthroplasty: A retrospective cohort study. Current Medical Research and Opinion. 2016;**32**:1727-1733. DOI: 10.1080/03007995.2016.1205007

[23] Hamilton TW, Athanassoglou V, Trivella M, Strickland LH, Mellon S, Murray D, et al. Liposomal bupivacaine peripheral nerve block for the management of postoperative pain. Cochrane Database of Systematic Reviews. 2016;**8**:CD011476. DOI: 10.1002/14651858.CD011476.pub2

[24] Bailard NS, Ortiz J, Flores RA. Additives to local anesthetics for peripheral nerve blocks: Evidence, limitations, and recommendations. American Journal of Health-System Pharmacy. 2014;**71**:373-385. DOI: 10.2146/ajhp130336

[25] Emelife PI, Eng MR, Menard BL, Myers AS, Cornett EM, Urman RD, et al. Adjunct medications for peripheral and neuraxial anesthesia. Best Practice & Research. Clinical Anaesthesiology. 2018;**32**:83-99. DOI: 10.1016/j.bpa.2018.06.011

[26] Thornton PC, Grant SA, Breslin DS. Adjuncts to local anesthetics in peripheral nerve blockade. International Anesthesiology Clinics. 2010;**48**(4):59-70. DOI: 10.1097/AIA.0b013e3181f89af1

[27] Koinig H, Wallner T, Marhofer P, Andel H, Hörauf K, Mayer N. Magnesium sulfate reduces intra and postoperative analgesic requirements. Anesthesia and Analgesia. 1998;**87**:206-210. DOI: 10.1097/00000539-199807000-00042

[28] Kara H, Sahin N, Ulusan V, Aydogdu T. Magnesium infusion reduces perioperative pain. European Journal of Anaesthesiology. 2002;**19**:52-56

[29] Ko SH, Lim HR, Kim DC, Han YJ, Choe H, Song HS. Magnesium sulfate does not reduce postoperative analgesic requirements. Anesthesiology. 2001;**95**:640-646. DOI: 10.1097/00000542-200109000-00016.

[30] Mandal D, Das A, Chhaule S, Halder PS, Joydip Paul J, Roy Basunia S, et al. The effect of dexmedetomidine added to preemptive (2% lignocaine with epinephrine) infiltration on

intraoperative hemodynamics and postoperative pain after ambulatory maxillofacial surgeries under general anesthesia. Anesthesia, Essays and Researches. 2016;**10**:324-331. DOI: 10.4103/0259-1162.167837

[31] Vallapu S, Panda NB, Samagh N, Bharti N. Efficacy of dexmedetomidine as an adjuvant to local anesthetic agent in scalp block and scalp infiltration to control postcraniotomy pain: A double-blind randomized trial. Journal of Neurosciences in Rural Practice. 2018; **9**:73-79. DOI: 10.4103/jnrp. jnrp_310_17

[32] Collins JG, Kitahata LM, Matsumoto M, Homma E, Suzukawa M. Spinally administered epinephrine suppresses noxiously evokeactivity of WDR neurons in the dorsal horn of the spinal cord. Anesthesiology. 1984;**60**:269-275. DOI: 10.1097/00000542-198404000-0 0001

[33] Swain A, Nag DS, Sahu S, Samaddar DP. Adjuvants to local anesthetics: Current understanding and future trends. World Journal of Clinical Cases. 2017;**5**(8):307-323. DOI: 10.12998/wjcc.v5.i8.307

[34] Córdoba-Fernández A, Gonzá lez-Benítez J, Lobo-Martín A. Onset time of local anesthesia after single injection in toe nerve blocks: A randomized double-blind trial. Journal of Perianesthesia Nursing. 2019;**34** (4):820-828. DOI: 10.1016/j. jopan.20 18.09.014

[35] Brummett CM, Williams BA. Additives to local anesthetics for peripheral nerve blockade. International Anesthesiology Clinics. 2011; **49**(4):104-116. DOI: 10.1097/ AIA.0b013e31820e4a49.

[36] Murphy DB, McCartney CJ, Chan VW. Novel analgesic adjuncts for brachial plexus block: A systematic review. Anesthesia and Analgesia. 2000;**90**:1122-1128. DOI: 10.1097/00000539-200005000-00023

[37] Butterworth JF 5th, Strichartz GR. The alpha 2-adrenergic agonists clonidine and guanfacine produce tonic and phasic block of conduction in rat sciatic nerve fibers. Anesthesia and Analgesia. 1993;**76**:295-301

[38] Kaye AD, Cornett EM, Helander E, Menard B, Hsu E, Hart B, et al. An update on nonopioids: Intravenous or oral analgesics for perioperative pain management. Anesthesiology Clinics. 2017;**35**(2):e55-e71. DOI: 10.1016/j. anclin.2017.01.006

[39] Jellinge ME, Petersen RH. Clonidine can reduce opioid medication during post-operative pain. Ugeskrift for Laeger. 2015;**177**(49):V05150415

[40] Blaudszun G, Lysakowski C, Elia N, Tramèr MR. Effect of perioperative systemic α2 agonists on postoperative morphine consumption and pain intensity: Systematic review and meta-analysis of randomized controlled trials. Anesthesiology. 2012;**116**(6):1312-1322. DOI: 10.1097/ALN.0b013e31825681cb

[41] Cummings K III, Naguib MA. Opioid agonists and antagonists. In: Flood P, Rathmell JP, Shafer S, editors. Stoelting's Pharmacology & Physiology in Anesthetic Practice. 5th ed. Philadelphia: Lippincott-Williams & Wilkins; 2015. pp. 217-256

[42] Dahan A, Niesters M, Smith T, Overdyk F. Opioids. In: Barash PG, Cullen BF, Stoelting RK, Cahalan MK, Stock MC, Ortega R, Sharar SR, Holt NF, editors. Clinical Anesthesia. 8th ed. Philadelphia: Lippincott-Williams & Wilkins; 2017. pp. 505-526

[43] Choi S, Rodseth R, McCartney CJ. Effects of dexamethasone as a local anaesthetic adjuvant for brachial plexus block: A systematic review and

meta-analysis of randomized trials. British Journal of Anaesthesia. 2014; **112**(3): 427- 439. DOI: 10.1093/bja/aet417

[44] Hantash BM, Zhao L, Knowles JA, Lorenz HP. Adult and fetal wound healing. Frontiers in Bioscience. 2008;**13**: 51-61

[45] Gilmore MA. Phases of wound healing. Dimensions in Oncology Nursing. 1991;**5**(3):32-34

[46] Wound Healing Phases [Internet]. 2019. Available from: https://www.ncbi.nlm.nih.gov/books/NBK470443/ [Accessed on: 24 June 2019]

[47] Witte MB, Barbul A. General principles of wound healing. Surgical Clinics of North America. 1997;**77**(3):5 09-528

[48] Broughton G 2nd, Janis JE, Attinger CE. The basic science of wound healing. Plastic and Reconstructive Surgery. 2006;**117** (7Suppl):12S-34S. D OI: 10.1097/01. prs.0000225430.425 31.c2

[49] Pakyari M, Farrokhi A, Maharlooei MK, Ghahary A. Critical role of transforming growth factor beta in different phases of wound healing. Advances in Wound Care. 2013;**2**(5):215-224. DOI: 10.1089/wound.2012.0406

[50] Robson MC, Steed DL, Franz MG. Wound healing: Biologic features and approaches to maximize healing trajectories. Current Problems in Surgery. 2001;**38**(2):72-140. DOI: 10.1067/msg.2001.111167

[51] Velnar T, Bailey T, Smrkolj V. The wound healing process: An overview of the cellular and molecular mechanisms. Journal of International Medical Research. 2009;**37**(5):1528-1542. DOI: 10.1177/147323000903700531

[52] McGuire L, Heffner K, Glaser R, et al. Pain and wound healing in surgical patients. Annals of Behavioral Medicine. 2006;**31**(2):165-172. DOI: 10.1207/s15324796abm3102_8

[53] Kasaj A, Heib A, Willershausen B. Effectiveness of a topical salve (Dynexan) on pain sensitivity and early wound healing following nonsurgical periodontal therapy. European Journal of Medical Research. 2007;**12**(5):19 6-199

[54] Gao Z, Cui F, Cao X, Wang D, Li X, Li T. Local infiltration of the surgical wounds with levobupivacaine, dexibuprofen, and norepinephrine to reduce postoperative pain: A randomized, vehicle-controlled, and preclinical study. Biomedicine & Pharmacotherapy. 2017; **92**:459-467. DOI: 10.1016/j.biopha.2017. 05.038

[55] Cowin AJ, Brosnan MP, Holmes TM, Ferguson MW. Endogenous inflammatory response to dermal wound healing in the fetal and adult mouse. Developmental Dynamics. 1998;**212**(3):385-393

[56] Samad TA, Moore KA, Saierstein A, et al. Interleukin-1b-mediated induction of cox-2 in the CNS contributes to inflammatory pain hypersensitivity. Nature. 2001;**410**:471-475. DOI: 10.10 38/35068566

[57] Hay JL, White JM, Bochner F, Somogyi AA, Semple TJ, Rounsefell B. Hyperalgesia in opioid-managed chronic pain and opioid-dependent patients. Pain. 2009;**10**(3):316-322. DOI: 10.10 16/j.jpain.2008.10.003

[58] Krishnan S, Salter A, Sullivan T, Gentgall M, White J, Rolan P. Comparison of pain models to detect opioid-induced hyperalgesia. Journal of Pain Research. 2012;**5**:99-106. DOI: 10.2147/JPR.S27738

[59] Gordon SM, Chuang BP, Wang XM, et al. The differential effects of bupivacaine and lidocaine

on prostaglandin E2 release, cyclooxygenase gene expression and pain in a clinical pain model. Anest-hesia and Analgesia. 2008;**106**(1):321-327. DOI: 10.1213/01. ane.0000296474.79437.23

[60] Cassuto J, Sinclair R, Bonderovic M. Anti-inflammatory properties of local anesthetics and their present and potential clinical implications. Acta Anaesthesiologica Scandinavica. 2006; **50**(3):265-282. DOI: 10.1111/j.1399-65 76.2006.00936.x

[61] Kunze H, Nahas N, Traynor JR, Wurl M. Effects of local anaesthetics on phospholipases. Biochimica et Biophysica Acta. 1976;**441**(1):93-102

[62] Vasseur PB, Paul HA, Dybdal N, Crumley L. Effects of local anesthetics on healing of abdominal wounds in rabbits. American Journal of Vete-rinary Research. 1984;**45**(11):2385-2 388

[63] Abrão J, Fernandes CR, White PF, et al. Effect of local anaesthetic infilt-ration with bupivacaine and ropivacaine on wound healing: A placebo-controlled study. International Wound Journal. 2014;**11**(4):379-385. DOI: 10.1111/ j.1742-481X.2012.01101

[64] Hancı V, Hakimoğlu S, Özaçmak H, et al. Comparison of the effects of bupivacaine, lidocaine, and tramadol infiltration on wound healing in rats. Revista Brasileira de Anestesiologia. 2012;**62**(6):799-810. DOI: 10.1016/ S0034-7094(12)70180-0

[65] Kesici S, Kesici U, Ulusoy H, Erturkuner P, Turkmen A, Arda O. Effects of local anesthetics on wound healing. Revista Brasileira de Anestesiologia. 2018;**68**(4):375-382. DOI: 10.1016/j.bjan.2018.01.016

[66] Luan H, Zhu P, Zhang X, et al. Effect of dexmedetomidine as an adjuvant to ropivacaine for wound infiltration in patients undergoing open gastrectomy: A prospective randomized controlled trial. Medicine. 2017;**96**(38):e7950. DOI: 10.1097/ MD.0000000000007950

7

Local Anesthetic Systemic Toxicity

Divya Garg, Shikha Soni and Rakesh Karnawat

Abstract

Local anesthetics are used very often in medicine and dentistry. They have few adverse effects, but the increased use of these drugs has resulted in a higher incidence of local and systemic anesthetic toxicity (LAST). From the initial symptoms to the deleterious effects on cardiac and the central nervous system, LAST is an important consequence of which we should be aware. LAST is known since the introduction and use of local anesthetics; it was originally associated with seizures and respiratory failure. However, in the 1970s, side effects on the heart were also identified, as the fatal cardiac toxicity associated with bupivacaine was discovered in healthy patients. Prevention and safe administration of regional anesthesia remains primary factors in the avoidance of the toxicity of these drugs. When a patient has LAST, treatment should be started immediately to reduce seizures. If there is cardiac arrest, follow ACLS guidelines. Intravenous lipids improve cardiac conduction, contractility and coronary perfusion by removing liposoluble local anesthetic from cardiac tissue.

Keywords: local anesthetic, toxicity, mechanism of action, prevention, management, lipid emulsion

1. Introduction

Systemic toxicity due to local anesthetics (LAST) is a nightmare for each anesthesiologist. It can have catastrophic outcome in an otherwise simple procedure, such as a regional dental anesthesia, local anesthesia, nerve block either peripheral, intravenous or peridural. The clinical phenomenon of LAST has been known for more than 100 years. Historically, the introduction of cocaine as the first local anesthetic (LA) in late nineteenth century was soon accompanied by reports of its systemic toxicity. The symptoms of systemic toxicity were frequently described as seizures or respiratory failure, but some cases also included reports of adverse cardiac effects [1]. These reasons demanded medical and pharmaceutical industries to search for new less toxic LA.

At first, manipulation of existing molecular structures after analyzing natural products lead to development of few drugs. It became clear that the development of more LA of ester group did not return the desired results. The main concern was short duration of action due to instability of ester bonds. The drugs were prepared in an oily formulation to increase the duration (which proved neurotoxic locally, or by enhancing the lipophilicity of the molecule which made it more toxic to central nervous system (CNS) as well as cardiovascular system (CVS)). Lidocaine, synthesized in 1944 was the first amide LA drug to be used clinically. It gave a dependable block, but unfortunately was short acting. In search of an LA with a longer duration of action than lidocaine, a family of N-alkylpiperidines 2,6 xylidides was introduced in 1950s. It was shown that increasing N-alkyl carbon chain length (to max at C4 or C5) increased lipophilicity, which increases duration of action, but unfortunately also increased systemic toxicity. Derivatives developed for clinical use included mepivacaine, bupivacaine, ropivacaine, levobupivacaine, etc. But in subsequent year's cases of lethal LAST were documented.

Accidental intravascular injection during regional anesthesia is the most common cause of LAST. Some comorbidities may increase the risk of LAST; liver failure, heart disease, pregnancy and metabolic syndromes. In addition, patients at extreme ages have an increased risk factor of toxicity, due to the reduction in anesthetic clearance. Children under 4 months of age have low plasma concentrations of acid glycoprotein, which may result in a lower intrinsic clearance of bupivacaine [2, 3].

The incidence of LAST is extremely variable from zero events after more than 12,000 nerve blocks to 25 per 10,000 nerve blocks. One study reported seizures in 79 of 10,000 brachial plexus block procedures. This complication was due to toxicity of the CNS as a result of intravascular LA injection. Although the published data are inconsistent, the prevailing goal is to prevent LAST, and when it manifests, it must be treated quickly and effectively [4–6].

Cardiac toxicity is the most important component of LAST since, unlike the CNS toxicity, it can end in cardiac arrest and death. It is often due to an intravascu-lar injection not noticed during nerve block. LA bind and inhibit voltage dependent sodium channels. It leads to conduction disorders, contractile dysfunction and ventricular arrhythmias. The incidence of cardiac toxicity increases with bupivacaine due to its affinity for inactive sodium channels during the cardiac action potential at a concentration of 0.2 μg/mL. This is done in a fast/slow manner, which means that bupivacaine binds very rapidly to a large proportion of sodium channels during the potential for cardiac action, but is slowly released from the channels during diastole, which results in a large proportion of medication that accumulates at 60–150 beats per minute. Lidocaine at 5–10 μg/mL will also result in a substantial blockage of sodium channels during a potential for cardiac action. However, in contrast to bupivacaine, lidocaine follows the principle of rapid entry/exit, which means that it is rapidly released from sodium channels during diastole. This allows faster recovery and a lower incidence of cardiac toxicity compared to bupivacaine.

CNS toxicity is another important consequence of LAST. Although it is composed of many initial prodromal features, it is most often manifested as seizures. A mechanistic theory focuses on acid-sensitive K^+ channels. These pH-sensitive channels generate neuronal currents of leakage of potassium. LA inhibition causes membrane depolarization and increased neuronal excitability. As these channels are expressed throughout the brain, this is the suggested mechanism for seizures in this context. Consequently, it became mandatory to understand the mechanism of LAST, so that it could be prevented and managed efficiently.

This chapter reviews the mechanisms, frequency, clinical characteristics, prevention and treatment of LAST.

2. LAST mechanisms

LA agents are classic sodium channel inhibitors. LAST hypotheses are based primarily on the binding site, ion channels, signaling pathway or enzymes involved in the CNS and cardiac toxicity or its treatment. LA inhibit some components of the oxidative phosphorylation pathway, which affects the myocardium and the CNS that are poorly tolerant of anaerobic metabolism. These deleterious effects differ quantitatively between LA, doses and administration routes. It is appropriate to first review the ion channels implicated in LAST [7–9].

2.1 Sodium channel blockade

LA are sodium channel blocking acting on inactivated sodium channel state and blocking it. They affect the initial depolarization phase and slow it down, leading to slow cardiac conduction. The antiarrhythmic property of lidocaine is related to this slowed conduction as it causes fast blockade of the channels. In contrast, bupivacaine and ropivacaine cannot be used as anti-arrhythmic drugs though they have fast blockade, but slow release of sodium channel (lasting longer than 1 s in contrast to lidocaine which lasts 0.15 s) [10]. Slowed conduction leads to widening the QRS complex, prolongation of the PR interval, AV block and, eventually, ventricular fibrillation due to the unidirectional blockade and re-entry phenomenon.

2.2 Potassium channel blockade

Out of three known organized potassium channels, two groups are of interest where LA toxicity is concerned. Out of these, one group of channels are known as the inward, outward and transient rectifier potassium channels, thus plays an important role in the potassium efflux during phases 2 and 3 of the cardiac muscle action potential [11]. If these channels are blocked, it will lead to prolongation of action potential; i.e. phase 2, delay in repolarization; i.e. phase and shift the resting membrane potential more positive (phase 4) to increase automaticity [12]. The second group of potassium channels of interest are K2p. Previously known as the delayed rectifier channels, these channels are believed to be responsible for the background or leak potassium currents. In this setting, they control the resting membrane potential. A blockade of these channels shifts the resting membrane potential towards spontaneous depolarization. K2p channels are extensively spread in the body. In the CNS they are mainly located in the thalamo-cortical and striatal neurons, where blockade leads to increased neuroexitability [13]. They are also present in high concentrations in the cerebral blood vessels, where blockade leads to vasoconstriction and decreased cerebral blood flow. K2p channels are also present in neurons of the auditory system, where blockade leads to tinnitus. LA agents are also known to have K2p mediated stimulating effect on ventilation [14]. They are located in the brainstem and carotid body, where they regulate the respi-ratory response to carbon dioxide via sensing the changes of pH and expressed in the oxygen-sensing cells of the glomus body respectively. K2p channels are sensitive to changes in oxygen tension and extracellular pH and are potentiated by volatile anesthetic [13]. In the CVS K2p channel blockade predisposes the patient to re-entry dysrhythmias. It is well known that hyperkalemia exacerbates LAST, and that K^+ATP openers (which effectively lowers intracellular K^+ levels) attenuate the toxic effects of bupivacaine [15].

2.3 Ca^{2+} channel blockade

All voltage-gated Ca^{2+} channels are comprised of two subunits according to the latest research: α and β subunit. The α subunit has fairly constant chemical structure for all voltage gated Ca^{2+} channels and is the main pore- forming element of the channel. The β subunit has highly variable structure that depends on the location and function of the channel for e.g. in cardiac conduction tissue β1 subunit completes the ion channel structure. The role of the β1 subunit seems to be the modulation of channel opening and membrane ion trafficking [16]. In terms of their physiological effect, the heart has two distinct types of channels namely the T-type (transient) that are low voltage activated channels (LVA), and L-type (long lasting). On the other hand, are high voltage activated channels (HVA).

The T-type channels are mainly located in the pacemaker cells of the sinoatrial node, and the opening of these channels completes the prepotential required for the pacemaker potential. L-type channels are present on the surface of the myocytes of both atrium and ventricle, and are closely associated with the T-tubules. The plateau phase (phase 2) of cardiac muscle action potential is produced by opening of these L-type channels. LA bind to these channels and predispose them to an inactivated state. The consequence of this is prolongation of the action potential (phase 2) and depressed contractility [9].

3. LAST risk factors

Risk factors to develop LA toxicity are related to kind of LA used, the type of nerve block, and the patient.

3.1 LA related

The most important and most studied factors in the development of LAST are undoubtedly the type and dose of LA.

3.1.1 Type of LA

The kind of LA injection influence toxicity risk. Animal studies showed that [17] more levobupivacaine than bupivacaine was required to induce cardiac arrest and levobupivacaine caused fewer convulsions and arrhythmias than bupivacaine, at similar doses [18]. Ropivacaine may cause less motor block, but whether it is clini-cally significantly less toxic is unknown. Other property differentiating the toxicity of LA is their intrinsic effect on vessels, where levobupivacaine and ropivacaine have intrinsic vasoconstrictors properties (that may prolong duration of action and slow systemic absorption), whereas bupivacaine is an intrinsic vasodilator. The clinical significance of this difference remains unclear. Another important concept in the study of LAST is the ratio of the dose required to produce cardiovascular collapse to that required to induce seizures, the so called CC/CNS ratio (ratio of dose causing cardiovascular collapse to the dose causing seizures). Bupivacaine has a CC/CNS ratio of 2.0 compared with 7.1 for lidocaine. Therefore, progression from CNS signs and symptoms to cardiovascular collapse can occur more readily with bupivacaine than with lidocaine.

3.1.2 Dose of LA

Determining the optimal dose of LA to use is complex and always a topic of debate. Using the lowest effective dose is always prudent and advisable practice along with consideration of patient characteristics and site of administration. Some may argue that the recommended doses provide a rough guide for clini-cal use. The maximum weight-based doses have lost rationale in others view as such dosing does not correlate to the resulting blood level and does not take into account relevant patient factors or the site of injection. Other factors that question the maximum weight based doses are variation between different texts and countries, no recommendation whether dose calculation is based on actual body weight or ideal body weight and such hard and fast dosing rules do not take into account the complete clinical context [19]. As a result, if dosing is calculated on actual body weight, the obese, pregnant, or both patients may receive a dangerously high dose.

3.2 Block-related

Inadvertent intravenous injection of LA can occur during any regional anesthetic technique, but tends in becoming LAST only if larger volumes (5–10 mL) are injected, or small doses during face and neck procedures. Symptoms usually occur within 3–5 min and can be severe if appropriate measures are not taken. LAST resulting from the gradual systemic absorption of LA is characterized by a late presentation (20–30 min or more after a bolus injection), and usually occurs when a relatively high dose of LA has been administered in the presence of another risk factor. Local anesthetic systemic toxicity may also occur in the context of continuous LA infusion, in which case the onset may be hours to days after starting the infusion. The symptoms last until the drug metabolism reduces concentrations plasma levels below the toxic threshold. Prolonged monitoring and supportive therapy are essential.

3.2.1 Site of block

Blocking site is important since rate of absorption, chances of direct intravascular injections and thus chances of toxicity depends on the anatomical location. For example, interscalene block, stellate ganglion block, intercostal nerve block have a higher risk of direct intravascular injection and other blocks like scalp, bronchial mucosa, inter pleural cavity carry an increased risk of rapid absorption and toxicity due to the injection being in a highly vascularized area. The classic order of sites propensities to lead to toxicity, in order from lowest to highest: subcutaneous injec-tion, brachial plexus, epidural, caudal, and finally intercostal blocks and topical mucosal anesthesia.

3.2.2 Conduct of the block

Performing the block in a safer way decreases the chances of toxicity by manifolds. The practice of giving the dose of LA in incremental injections, after frequent aspiration, adding test dose and most important is using ultrasound-guided needle placement to give the LA reduces the risk of toxicity.

3.3 Patient-related factors

3.3.1 General principles

Various factors are related to toxicity of LA. Most common being the free peak plasma concentration, perfusion at the site of injection, co-morbidities (renal, liver, metabolic, and cardiac diseases). As already discussed earlier, more the perfusion at the site of injection, more will be the peak plasma concentration as systemic absorption is accelerated. A low α1-acid glycoprotein (AAG) titer results in a higher concentration of free LA.

In patients with severe renal impairment there may be slightly increased risk of toxicity as these patients typically have a reduced clearance of LA, hyper dynamic circulation but increased AAG. So, it is prudent to reduce the initial dose by 10–20% according to severity of renal impairment.

In patients with liver disease, single dose blocks are unaffected, but the doses for repeat boluses and continuous infusions should be reduced. Such patients may also have renal or cardiac disease. AAG is synthesized in patients with end-stage liver disease, offering some protection against LAST. Patients with severe cardiac failure are particularly susceptible to LA-induced myocardial depression and arrhythmias.

Further, lower liver and renal perfusion slows metabolism and elimination, so safe initial and maintenance doses of LA are correspondingly lower too. On the other hand, poor perfusion at the injection site may decrease peak plasma concentrations.

3.3.2 Age related factors

Extremes of age have different physiological changes making them different from young and adolescent age group. In elderly patients; there is a safety benefit in dose reduction without altering the clinical efficacy. In the geriatric patient's nerves appears to be more sensitive to LA due to various factors like altered nerve morphology, there is less fat tissue surrounding the nerves, and axonal function is also reduced. Moreover, this age group has multiple co-morbidities and decreased muscle mass; blood flow to organs is reduced, decreased clearance and organ function. In patients older than 65 years' involuntary overdoses being responsible for some cases of LAST. When considering the use of LA in geriatric patients, it is mandatory to pay special attention to the presence of systemic disease and muscle wasting [20].

In neonates and infants, the risk of accumulation of LA with continuous infusions is more than in adults as AAG levels are reduced (about half that of adult at birth). Children have an increased elimination half-life of LA, which in neonates is increased to 2–3 times that of an adult. Bupivacaine accumulates with continuous infusion and 2-chloroprocaine can be used as an alternative. LAST has the highest incidence in infants less than 6 months of age and is associated with bolus dosing and penile nerve blocks [21].

3.3.3 Pregnant patients

Pregnancy is one of several clinical settings in which LAST can be potentiated. Pregnant patients are at an increased risk of toxicity as they have increased perfusion as well as decreased AAG levels; thus high peak free plasma concentration of LA. Some of the earliest anecdotal reports of LAST-related fatal cardiac arrests involved pregnant women [1]. Notably, several of the original anecdotal reports of LAST-related fatal cardiac arrests involved pregnant women. It has since been proven that pregnancy increases the risk for LAST, and subsequent guidelines preclude use of 0.75% bupivacaine in late gestation because this concentration was involved in cases of fatal toxicity in parturients [22–24].

4. Clinical presentation of LAST

Most of the LAST events happen a few minutes after the LA injection and present with signs of the CNS, which may or may not be accompanied by changes in the CVS (**Figure 1**). Sometimes, the manifestations are atypical in terms of time and clinical picture. The onset of symptoms may be delayed up to 60 min after a bolus injection, and signs of CVS toxicity may appear in the absence of any CNS characteristics. This last scenario may be more common in patients who are very sedated or under general anesthesia. High plasma concentrations during LAST can occur in three circumstances: inadvertent intra-arterial injection, intravenous injection or systemic absorption, each of which has a characteristic temporal course. LAST associated with intra-arterial injection occurs classically during nerve blockages in the head and neck (stellate ganglion, interscalene or deep cervical plexus blocks) in which there is an involuntary injection of LA in an artery that supplies the brain. The symptoms of the CNS, usually seizures, occur almost immediately. When the injected dose is small, progression to CVS collapse is uncommon. Recovery

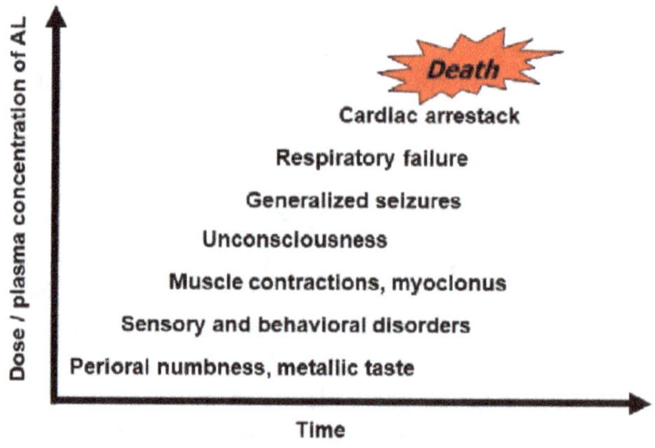

Figure 1.
Scheme showing the most important clinical manifestations of LAST.

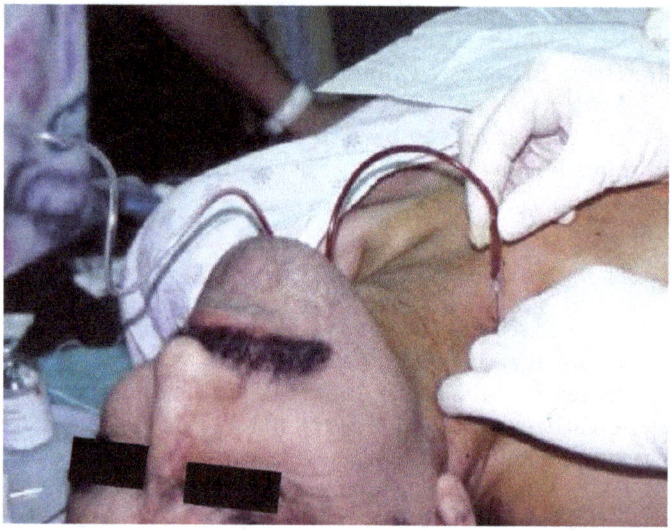

Figure 2.
Accidental arterial puncture during a stellate ganglion block in a patient with postherpetic neuropathy.

is equally rapid since LA quickly redistributes from the cerebral circulation [25]. **Figure 2** shows an intra-arterial puncture detected during the blockage of the stellate ganglion in a patient with herpes zoster neuropathy.

4.1 Central nervous system toxicity

Central nervous system toxicity could be presumed as a two-stage process in which initial blockade of Na^+ channels occurs in the inhibitory neurons thus allowing excitatory neurons to act unopposed which culminates in generalized convulsions. Higher concentrations of LA agent affect all neurons, leading to global CNS depression, which is clinically seen as coma and evident on EEG as slowing and ultimately silent EEG. In most cases, convulsions, although an impressive clinical entity, can be handled safely without permanent brain damage. Clinical manifestations of the systemic neurotoxicity of LA usually occur in stages; in the initial phase there is perioral numbness, confusion, tinnitus followed by an exciting phase that shows seizures and, finally, a depressive phase where there is loss of consciousness and respiratory depression.

4.2 Cardiovascular system toxicity

Both the direct and indirect effects of the LA drugs on myocardium are involved in the mechanism of cardiovascular toxicity [26].

Clinical presentation includes hypertension and tachycardia in initial phase (during CNS excitatory phase), followed by intermediate phase showing myocardial depression, decreased cardiac output and thus hypotension, followed by sinus bradycardia, peripheral vasodilatation, conduction defects and dysrhythmias in terminal phase.

5. Management of LAST

All medical and paramedical personnel working in operating theaters and hospi-tal locations where LA are used should be prepared to recognize, diagnose and treat patients with signs and symptoms of LAST in a timely manner. The ASRA has pub-lished and updated the guidelines recommended by experts for the management of LAST (**Table 1**) [4, 5]. The initial treatment of LAST should focus on keeping the airways permeable with adequate ventilation, circulatory support and the reduction of systemic side effects. Immediate ventilation and oxygenation to prevent hypoxia and acidosis can facilitate resuscitation and reduce the likelihood of progression to seizures or cardiovascular collapse [24, 25].

5.1 Preparation

All patients receiving LA injections in doses potentially to trigger LAST should have oxygen, standard monitoring which is to be continued at least 30 min after completion of injection to detect delayed presentation if any, and intravenous access applied [27, 28]. Immediate access to LAST Management Checklist is advisable, and all medications and resuscitation equipment required should be immediately avail-able, preferably in the form of a “LAST Rescue Kit”.

5.2 Immediate management

Immediate management involves the general safety and resuscitation measures that are essential in any emergency. First, stop LA injection and call for help. The immediate priority is to manage the airway, breathing, and circulation. Avoid factors potentiating LAST like hypoxia, hypercarbia, and acidosis (metabolic or respiratory [24, 25, 29]).

5.2.1 Intravenous lipid emulsion therapy

Use of intravenous lipid emulsion as a therapeutic modality comes with several advantages. Theories suggest that it improves cardiac conduction, contractility and coronary perfusion by removing the liposoluble LA from cardiac tissue. Better understanding of the mechanism of action of lipid emulsion with recent advances underlines its importance as therapeutic modality in the management of LAST. First advantage is that lipid emulsion may shuttle any LA agent from high blood flow organs to detoxification organs such as the liver [30]. Secondly, lipid emulsion therapy may also improve the cardiac output and blood pressure. Post conditioning myocardial protection may also occur [31–34]. There is an unavailability of large scale data collection and other prospective studies to demonstrate efficacy of lipid

Checklist for LAST treatment	
The pharmacologic treatment of LAST is different from other cardiac arrest scenarios	
Reduce individual epinephrine boluses to ≤1 mcg/kg	
Avoid vasopressin, calcium channel blockers, beta blockers, or other local anesthetics	
• Stop injecting local anesthetic • Get help ○ Consider lipid emulsion therapy at the first sign of a serious LAST event ○ Call for the LAST rescue kit ○ Alert the nearest cardiopulmonary bypass team – resuscitation may be prolonged • Airway management ○ Ventilate with 100% oxygen / avoid hyperventilation / advanced airway device if necessary • Control seizures ○ Benzodiazepines preferred ○ Avoid large doses of propofol, especially in hemodynamically unstable patients • Treat hypotension and bradycardia—if pulseless, start CPR	
Lipid emulsion 20% (precise volume and flow rate are crucial)	
Greater than 70 kg patient	**Less than 70 kg patient**
Bolus 100 mL lipid emulsion 20% rapidly over 2–3 min	Bolus 1.5 mL/kg lipid emulsion 20% rapidly over 2–3 min
• Lipid emulsion infusion 200–250 mL over 15–20 min	• Lipid emulsion infusion ~0.25 mL/kg/min (ideal body weight)
If patient remains unstable:	
• Re-bolus once or twice at the same dose and double infusion rate; be aware of dosing limit (12 mL/kg) • Total volume of lipid emulsion can approach 1 L in a prolonged resuscitation (e.g., > 30 min) • Continue monitoring ○ At least 4–6 h after a cardiovascular event ○ Or, at least 2 h after a limited CNS event • Do not exceed 12 mL/kg lipid emulsion (particularly important in the small adult or child) ○ Much smaller doses are typically needed for LAST treatment	
With permission from www.anestesia-dolor.org.	

Table 1.
Checklist for LAST treatment [4, 5].

emulsion therapy due to various difficulties [24, 35, 36]; however various animal studies provide strong support for use of lipid emulsion therapy to reduce mortality when used along with resuscitative measures [37]. Early administration of 20% intravenous lipid emulsion therapy should, therefore, be an immediate priority after airway management in any LAST event that is judged to be potentially seri-ous. A bolus of 1.5 mL/kg of 20% lipid emulsion and the subsequent infusion of 0.25 mL/kg per minute should be administered. The infusion should be continued for 10 min after reaching hemodynamic stability. An additional bolus and an infu-sion rate increase to 0.5 mL/kg per minute can be administered if stability is not achieved. The maximum recommended dose for initial administration is approxi-mately 10 mL/kg for 30 min (**Table 1**) [4, 37, 38]. Lipid emulsion remains first-line therapy (in conjunction with standard resuscitative measures) in LAST. However, more research in humans is necessary to establish its real usefulness [36].

5.2.2 Seizure management

Prompt seizure prevention and termination is crucial to avoid injury and acidosis. Benzodiazepines are first line therapy for management of seizures due to their cardio stable profile. Propofol or thiopental can be used in low doses, although these drugs may worsen the hypotension or cardiac depression associated with LAST. It should be avoided in patients with cardiovascular compromise. Neuromuscular blockade can be considered in cases of ongoing seizures; small doses of succinylcholine should be administered intermittently to stop muscle activity and increased acidosis. Early termination of seizure activity helps to avoid metabolic acidosis and hypoxia that occurs due to repeated muscular contractions [24].

5.2.3 Cardiovascular support

The treatment of LA-induced cardiac arrest focuses on restoring cardiac output, to restore tissue perfusion, prevent and treat underlying acidosis. Chest compressions should be started without delay and to be continued till return of spontaneous circulation (as per ACLS algorithms for cardiopulmonary resuscitation). If epinephrine is used, small initial doses of ≤ 1 μg/kg are preferred to avoid impaired pulmonary gas exchange and increased afterload [39]. Vasopressin is not recommended, as it can cause pulmonary hemorrhage. If myocardial LA levels is more than the threshold that corresponds to ion channel blocking concentrations, then the ionotropic effect of lipid emulsion therapy remains questionable. Chest compressions ensure the coronary perfusion that is sufficient to reduce tissue LA levels. In the absence of rapid recovery following ACLS measures and intravenous lipid emulsion therapy, early consideration should be given to cardiopulmonary bypass for circulatory support. For other deleterious CVS effects—such as arrhyth-mias, conduction block, progressive hypotension, and bradycardia – standard ACLS algorithms should be followed with the omission of LA, such as lidocaine and procainamide. Amiodarone is the first-line antiarrhythmic in the event of ventricu-lar dysrhythmia. In addition, calcium channel blockers and B-adrenergic receptor blockers are not recommended.

5.2.4 Post-event management

Report the case of LAST to the registry at www.lipidrescue.org [39]. Monitoring is mandatory for at least 2 h in isolated and recovering CNS event but for 6 h for LAST with CVS features.

6. Prevention

The primary objective of every anesthesiologist is always patient safety. Pre-anesthetic evaluation, patient preparation, complete monitoring before starting administration of LA, and continuing this monitoring during surgery and the immediate postoperative period are mandatory.

6.1 Pre-procedure

- During preoperative assessment, evaluate the patient for co-morbidities, evaluation of the risks and benefits of regional anesthesia for that individual should be discussed, patient should be explained regarding procedure and appropriate consent to be obtained.

- Preparation includes selection of type of LA, prior calculation of doses, labeling all syringes.
- All monitoring facilities to be available along with LAST rescue kit and resusci-tative measures.

6.2 Intra-procedure

- Block to be performed with continuous monitoring attached, with a capable help nearby.
- The method of administration of LA should include the administration of incremental doses with frequent aspiration, ultrasound-guided needle placement, administration of test doses. This can help in the early detection of accidental intravascular placement of the needle or catheter and thus avoid erroneous administration of the LA, avoiding toxic plasma concentrations.
- Continuous communication with the patient to detect early signs of intravascular injection like perioral numbness, tinnitus etc.

6.3 Post-procedure

Clearly label any kind of spinal/epidural catheter or peripheral nerve block catheter; it should be documented well in patient chart also. Drug and dose already administered or to be administered should be well informed in instructions to the medical staff responsible for post-operative care of the patient. Continuous monitoring of vital signs in the postoperative period in suspected case of delayed LAST to be considered.

7. Conclusion

LAST is a serious life-threatening emergency, with protean manifestations, that can happen after administering LA. Anesthesiologists must understand its risks, prevention, and safe management. Promptly recognition and timely manage-ment of LAST can dramatically change the clinical course. In addition to the usual advanced cardiac resuscitation maneuvers, the current treatment focuses on the administration of lipid emulsion. While the development of new treatment plans can help limiting the associated morbidity and mortality, prevention remains vitally important. It is mandatory for all the practitioners using LA to understand patho-physiological basis, mechanisms, risk factors, prevention and treatment modalities of LAST.

Acknowledgements

We thank www.anestesia-dolor.org for allowing us to publish **Figures 1** and **2**.

Author details

Divya Garg*, Shikha Soni and Rakesh Karnawat
Department of Anaesthesia and Critical Care, Dr. S.N. Medical College, Jodhpur, Rajasthan, India

*Address all correspondence to: drdivya.garg12@gmail.com

References

[1] Albright GA. Cardiac arrest following regional anesthesia with etidocaine or bupivacaine. Anesthesiology.1979;**51**(4): 285-287. DOI:10.1097/00000542-197910000-00001

[2] Bina B, Hersh EV, Hilario M, Alvarez K, McLaughlin B. True allergy to amide local anesthetics: A review and case presentation. Anesthesia Progress. 2018;**65**(2):119-123. DOI: 10.2344/anpr-65-03-06

[3] Aydin G. Unexpected local anesthesia toxicity during the ultrasonography-guided peripheral nerve block. Journal of Clinical Anesthesia. 2018; **50**:26.DOI:10.1016j.jclinane.2018.06.039

[4] Neal JM, Woodward CM, Harrison TK, The American Society of Regional Anesthesia and Pain Medicine. Checklist for managing local anesthetic systemic toxicity: 2017 version. Regional Anesthesia and Pain Medicine. 2018;**43**(2):150-153. DOI: 10.1097/AAP.0000000000000726

[5] Neal JM, Barrington MJ, Fettiplace MR, Gitman M, Memtsoudis SG, Mörwald EE, et al. Practice advisory on local anesthetic systemic toxicity: Executive summary 2017. Regional Anesthesia and Pain Medicine. 2018;**43**(2):113-123. DOI: 10.1097/AAP.0000000000000720

[6] Barash PG, Cullen B, Stoelting RK. Clinical Anesthesia. 5th ed. Philadelphia: Lippincott, Williams & Wilkins; 2005. pp. 449-469

[7] Haskins SC, Tanaka CY, Boublik J, Wu CL, Sloth E. Focused cardiac ultrasound for the regional anesthesiologist and pain specialist. Regional Anesthesia and Pain Medicine. 2017;**42**(5):632-644. DOI: 10.1097/AAP.0000000000000650

[8] Bentov I, Damodarasamy M, Spiekerman C, Reed MJ. Lidocaine impairs proliferative and biosynthetic functions of aged human dermal fibroblasts. Anesthesia and Analgesia. 2016;**123**(3):616-623. DOI: 10.1213/ANE.0000000000001422

[9] Graf B. The cardiotoxicity of local anesthetics: The place of ropivacaine. Current Topics in Medicinal Chemistry. 2001;**1**:207-214. DOI: 10.2174/1568026013395164

[10] Ganong WF. Review of Medical Physiology. 18th ed. Stanford, Connecticut: Appleton and Lange; 1997

[11] Sommers de K. Pharmakologie. 6th ed. Johannesburg: Heinemann; 1999. pp. 184-194

[12] Kindler C, Yost CS. Two pore potassium channels: New sites for local anesthetic action and toxicity. Regional Anesthesia and Pain Medicine. 2005;**30**(3):260-274. DOI: 10.1016/j.rapm.2004.12.001

[13] Nisenbaum ES, Wilson CJ. Potassium currents responsible for inward and outward rectification in rat spiny projection neurons. The Journal of Neuroscience. 1995;**15**:4449-4463

[14] Gross JB, Cadwell CB, Shaw LM, Laucks SO. The effects of lidocaine on the ventilatory response to carbon dioxide. Anesthesiology. 1983;**59**:521-525

[15] de La Coussaye JE, Eledjam JJ, Peray P, Bruelle P, Lefrant JY, Bassoul B, et al. Lemakalim, a potassium channel agonist, reverses electrophysiological impairments induced by a large dose of bupivacaine in anaesthetized dogs. British Journal of Anaesthesia. 1993;**71**(4):534-539. DOI: 10.1093/bja/71.4.534

[16] Yue DT. The dawn of high-resolution structure of the queen of ion channels. Neuron. 2004;**42**:357-361. DOI: 10.1016/s0896-6273(04)00259-4

[17] Mazoit J, Boico O, Samii K. Myocardial uptake of bupivacaine: II. Pharmacokinetics and pharmacodynamics of bupivacaine enantiomers in the isolated perfused rabbit heart. Anesthesia and Analgesia. 1993;**77**:7-82

[18] Huang Y, Pryor M, Mather L, Veering BT.Cardiovascular and central nervous system effects of intravenous levobupivacaine and bupivacaine in sheep. Anesthesia and Analgesia. 1998;**86**:797-804. DOI: 10.1097/00000539-199804000-00023

[19] Rosenberg PH, Veering BT, Urmey WF. Maximum recommended doses of local anesthetics: A multifactorial concept. Regional Anesthesia and Pain Medicine. 2004;**29**:564-575

[20] Waldinger R, Weinberg G, Gitman M. Local anesthetic toxicity in the geriatric population. Drugs & Aging. 2019. DOI: 10.1007/s40266-019-00718-0

[21] Boretsky KR. A review of regional anesthesia in infants. Paediatric Drugs. 2019. DOI: 10.1007s40272-019-00360-8

[22] Santos AC, Pedersen H, Harmon TW, Morishima HO, Finster M, Arthur GR, et al. Does pregnancy alter the systemic toxicity of local anesthetics? Anesthesiology.1989;**70**(6):991-995.DOI: 10.1097/00000542-198906000-00018

[23] Santos AC, DeArmas PI. Systemic toxicity of levobupivacaine, bupivacaine, and ropivacaine during continuous intravenous infusion to nonpregnant and pregnant ewes. Anesthesiology. 2001;**95**:1256-1264

[24] Bern S, Weinberg G. Local anesthetic toxicity and lipid resuscitation in pregnancy. Current Opinion in Anaesthesiology. 2011;**24**(3):262-267. DOI: 10.1097/ACO.0b013e32834654df

[25] El-Boghdadly K, Chin KJ. Local anesthetic systemic toxicity: Continuing professional development. Canadian Journal of Anaesthesia. 2016;**63**(3):330-349. DOI: 10.1007/s12630-015-0564-z

[26] Plowman AN, Bolsin S, Mather LE. Central nervous system toxicity attributable to epidural ropivacaine hydrochloride. Anaesthesia and Intensive Care. 1998;**26**(2):204-206. DOI: 10.1177/0310057X9802600214

[27] Gitman M, Barrington MJ. Local anesthetic systemic toxicity: A review of recent case reports and registries. Regional Anesthesia and Pain Medicine. 2018;**43**(2):124-130. DOI: 10.1097/AAP.0000000000000721

[28] Vasques F, Behr AU, Weinberg G, Ori C, di Gregorio G. A review of local anesthetic systemic toxicity cases since publication of the American Society of Regional Anesthesia recommendations: To whom it may concern. Regional Anesthesia and Pain Medicine. 2015;**40**(6):698-705. DOI: 10.1097/AAP.0000000000000320

[29] Mochizuki T, Sato S. Hypocapnia prolongs bradycardia induced by bupivacaine or levobupivacaine in isolated rat hearts. Canadian Journal of Anaesthesia. 2008;**55**(12):836-846. DOI: 10.1007/BF03034055

[30] Fettiplace MR, Lis K, Ripper R, Kowal K, Pichurko A, Vitello D, et al. Multi-modal contributions to detoxification of acute pharmacotoxicity by a triglyceride micro- emulsion. Journal of Controlled Release. 2015;**198**:62-70. DOI: 10.1016/j. jconrel.2014.11.018

[31] Rahman S, Li J, Bopassa JC, Umar S, Iorga A, Partownavid P, et al. Phosphorylation of GSK-3β mediates intralipid-induced cardioprotection against ischemia/reperfusion injury. Anesthesiology. 2011;**115**(2):242-253. DOI: 10.1097/ALN.0b013e318223b8b9

[32] Lou PH, Lucchinetti E, Zhang L, Affolter A, Schaub MC, Gandhi M, et al. The mechanism of Intralipid®-mediated cardioprotection complex IV inhibition by the active metabolite, palmitoyl-carnitine, generates reactive oxygen species and activates reperfusion injury salvage kinases. PLoS One. 2014;**9**(1): e87205. DOI: 10.1371/journal.pone.0087205

[33] Stehr SN, Ziegeler JC, Pexa A, Oertel R, Deussen A, Koch T, et al. The effects of lipid infusion on myocardial function and bioenergetics in l-bupivacaine toxicity in the isolated rat heart. Anesthesia and Analgesia. 2007;**104**(1):186-192. DOI: 10.1213/01.ane.0000248220.01320.58

[34] Fettiplace MR, Ripper R, Lis K, Lin B, Lang J, Zider B, et al. Rapid cardiotonic effects of lipid emulsion infusion. Critical Care Medicine. 2013;**41**(8):e156-e162. DOI: 10.1097/CCM.0b013e318287f874

[35] Weinberg G. Current evidence supports use of lipid rescue therapy in local anaesthetic systemic toxicity. Acta Anaesthesiologica Scandinavica. 2017;**61**(4):365-368. DOI: 10.1111/aas.12870

[36] Harvey M, Cave G. Lipid emulsion in local anesthetic toxicity. Current Opinion in Anaesthesiology. 2017;**30**(5):632-638. DOI: 10.1097/ACO.0000000000000498

[37] Fettiplace MR, McCabe DJ. Lipid emulsion improves survival in animal models of local anesthetic toxicity: A meta-analysis. Clinical Toxicology (Philadelphia, Pa.). 2017;**55**(7):617-623. DOI: 10.1080/15563650.2017.1288911

[38] Whizar-Lugo VM. Tratamiento de la toxicidad por anestésicos locales. Uso de lípidos intravenosos. Anest Mex. 2009;**21**:73-76

[39] Association of Anaesthetists of Great Britain and Ireland. AAGBI Safety Guideline: Management of Severe Local Anaesthetic Toxicity. Available at: https: // www. aagbi org /sites/default/files/la_toxicity_2010_0.pdf [Accessed: 08 July 2018]

8

Adjuvant Drugs to Local Anesthetics

Nandita Mehta and Sayyidah Aasima tu Nisa Qazi

Abstract

Local anesthetics have a potential to be used in a wide variety of situations including central neuraxial blocks, peripheral nerve blocks, intravenous, and local infiltration both for surgeries and acute and chronic pain management. Their use can be limited by their duration of action and the dose-dependent adverse effects on the cardiac and central nervous system. Adjuvants are drugs which, when co-administered along with local anesthetic agents, improve the latency of onset and duration of analgesia and counteract disadvantageous effects of local anesthetics. There is a wide armamentarium of adjuvant drugs to choose to be added in neuraxial and peripheral nerve blocks. They can be broadly divided into non-opioids and opioids, with non-opioids being vasoconstrictors, α2-adrenoceptor agonists, anti-inflammatory agents, acetylcholine esterase inhibitors (neostigmine), adenos-ine, ketorolac, midazolam, magnesium, and sodium bicarbonate and opioids being lipophilic (fentanyl and sufentanil) and hydrophilic (morphine).

Keywords: local anesthetics, adjuvants, neuraxial blocks, peripheral nerve blocks, opioids, neurotoxicity

1. Introduction

Local anesthetics (LA) are widely used in clinical practice for regional anesthe-sia or analgesia in various locations like central neuraxial blockade, peripheral nerve block, intravenously, and local infiltration. Infiltration with LA around the nerve produces analgesia by interrupting pain signals to the brain. The analgesic effect of a nerve block with LAs lasts only a few hours. Therefore, after surgery patients may suffer from moderate to severe acute pain. The duration of the action of LA can be prolonged by either increasing the dose or administering a continuous infusion of the drug, which can lead to dose-dependent side effects on the cardiovascular sys-tem and/or central nervous system (CNS) [1, 2]. The popularity of peripheral nerve blocks for surgical anesthesia as well as for postoperative analgesia has increased significantly due to anesthetists becoming more familiar with ultrasound-guided techniques. While the use of catheters for continuous infusions allows for sustained pain relief during the perioperative period, they can increase the challenges related to patient management, catheter displacement, and the potential for increased infection risk. In the case a long-acting LA or continuous block is used, sensory block is also associated with prolonged motor block in the postoperative period. Prolonged motor blockade in the postoperative period is undesirable as it leads to delayed mobilization of the patient and hence increased risk of complications.

The adjuvant drugs of regional LAs improve the quality and duration of anesthe-sia and analgesia and patient safety, thus increasing patient satisfaction and comfort [3, 4]. The aim of this chapter is to discuss the past, present, and future trends in the use of adjuvants, as well as their benefits and side effects.

2. Adjuvants drugs

Adjuvants are drugs which, when administered along with LA agents, may improve the latency of onset and duration of analgesia and counteract the undesirable effects associated with large doses of LAs. The use of adjuvant drugs has the potential to improve the efficacy of peripheral and central neuraxial blocks and decrease LA systemic toxicity by chiefly prolonging the duration of sensory block,

Opioids
• Morphine • Pethidine • Fentanyl • Sufentanil • Hydromorphone • Buprenorphine • Diamorphine • Tramadol
Vasoactive agents
• Epinephrine • Phenylephrine
Alpha-2 adrenergic agonists
• Clonidine • Dexmedetomidine
Steroids
• Dexamethasone
Nonsteroidal anti-inflammatory drugs
• Parecoxib • Lornoxicam
Other agents
• Ketamine • Midazolam • Neostigmine • Droperidol • Magnesium sulfate • Sodium bicarbonate • Potassium chloride • Adenosine • Dextran

Table 1.
Classification of adjuvant drugs.

enhancing motor blockade, and limiting the overall dose requirement of LAs. An ideal adjuvant should not only shorten the speed of onset of action of the LA drug but also reduce its dosage along with providing hemodynamic stability, optimal sedation, and minimum adverse effects.

A wide variety of adjuvant drugs have been used for both neuraxial and peripheral nerve blocks (**Table 1**). They can be broadly divided into non-opioids and opioids.

Current research is directed toward a search for agents and techniques which would prolong LA action while limiting its side effects and giving the patient its maximum benefit. These include techniques like the use of charged molecules to produce LA action (tonicaine and n-butyl tetracaine), newer delivery mechanisms for prolonged bioavailability (liposomal, cyclodextrin, and microsphere systems), and the use of other drugs (dextrans, adenosine, neuromuscular blockers) [3, 4].

While the use of LA adjuvants in regional anesthesia [5, 6] is in widespread clinical off-label use and has been subject to multiple clinical trials, we would like to emphasize on the fact that only a few adjuvants have been approved by the Food and Drug Administration (FDA), so absolute caution must be exercised while using these adjuvants.

3. Opioids

Opioids are the most common and the earliest used LA adjuvants. Their use in neuraxial and peripheral nerve blocks has evolved greatly over the last 30 years. It is advisable to use specific opioids, at appropriate doses and routes of administration that result in a primarily spinal site of action rather than a systemic opioid [7]. Afferent noxious stimuli from peripheral tissues converge in the dorsal horn of the spinal cord, where the primary nociceptive neuron synapses with the interneurons and the second-order nociceptive neuron in the spinothalamic tract. Blockade of these opioid receptors by agonists helps to suppress afferent nociceptive input from pain sites by modulating the release of pain-pathway associated peptides [8]. Opioids produce analgesia by mimicking the actions at specific receptors of endogenous opioid peptides. These peptides are beta-endorphin, met-enkephalin, and dynorphin. The three main types of opiate receptors, each with its own subtypes, are mu (μ), delta (δ), and kappa (κ) [9]. The most important target for opioids is the μ-receptor (endorphin), and intrathecal opioids appear to selectively modulate C- and A-fibers with minimal impact on dorsal root axons. The enkephalins are the primary endogenous ligands of the delta receptor and are involved with spinal analgesia. Dynorphin is the ligand for the kappa receptor. Activation of the kappa receptor results in segmental spinal analgesia and sedation. Most of the mixed agonist–antagonist opioids like butorphanol bind to the kappa receptor.

The exact mechanism of action of opioids at peripheral nerve is still uncertain. Evidences have begun to support the presence of peripheral opioid receptors [10]. The possible mechanism of prolonged analgesia by peripheral opioid administration could be through direct binding at opioid receptors of dorsal nerve root aided by axonal flow, diffusion through brachial plexus sheath to extradural or subarachnoid space to dorsal horn, and central action after peripheral systemic uptake [11].

3.1 Morphine

The first opioid to be used intrathecally was morphine with the initial clinical study published in 1979 [12]. Morphine being relatively less hydrophobic than other opioids remains in the CSF for a longer time and therefore occupies the rostral receptor sites for a longer duration than other opioids [13]. Consequently, morphine produces a long-lasting and adequate analgesia with intrathecal use [14]. However, this huge advantage is offset by the increased risk of adverse effects, especially post-operative respiratory depression [15], which remains a particular concern among anesthetists. Intrathecal and epidural morphine are associated with a high incidence of side effects like nausea, vomiting, pruritus, urinary retention, sedation, and delayed respiratory depression [13, 16]. The recommended dose for intrathecal administration is 50–300 μg, while as 2–5 mg of epidural loading dose is considered adequate. The risk of side effects increases exponentially with the increase in the dose [16, 17].

3.2 Pethidine

Pethidine (meperidine) is a lipophilic phenylpiperidine derivate that is 30 times more lipid soluble and 10 times less potent than morphine, leading to a faster onset and a shorter duration of action than morphine. Pethidine possesses some local anesthetic properties (motor and sensory fiber block) which lets it stand out from the rest of the opioid agents. Pethidine is a popular choice for obstetric analgesia used mainly in epidural analgesia during labor. Intrathecal use of pethidine is not recommended. The incidence of nausea, vomiting, and hypotension is more with pethidine than with morphine. Pethidine can be injected as a loading dose of 25–50 mg in the epidural space.

3.3 Fentanyl

In addition to acting on the spinal cord receptors and peripheral receptors, fentanyl is also reported to have a local anesthetic like action, but this requires a very high concentration (50 g/mL) which is not clinically feasible [18]. Fentanyl as an adjuvant to LA causes significant prolongation of duration of analgesia but delays the onset of both sensory and motor blockade compared to LAs alone [19]. The change in pH of the anesthetic solution resulting in slower penetration of nerve membrane by LA is considered to be responsible for this effect [20]. The recom-mended intrathecal dose is 10–25 μg, and the epidural loading dose is 50–100 μg. Fentanyl as adjuvant does not prolong motor block, so it allows early ambulation, thereby reducing the morbidity. The duration of action is 2–4 h, and the risk of respiratory depression is very low and of short duration [17].

3.4 Sufentanil

A potent agonistic opioid was synthesized in the mid-1970s. A piperidine derivative is 6–10 times more potent than fentanyl, depending on the route of administration; it has been registered for intravenous, epidural, and subarachnoid administration. It is considered to be more lipid soluble than its counterparts, a bet-ter μ receptor ligand. It is an extremely potent opioid with a faster onset of action than its counterparts. Its use in clinical practice is limited by its short duration of action and high side effect profile. The recommended intrathecal dose is 2.5–10 μg, and epidural loading dose is 10–50 μg [17].

3.5 Hydromorphone

This opioid has intermediate lipid solubility. Due to its hydrophilicity, epidural hydromorphone can cross the blood-brain barrier faster and provide fast onset and modest duration of action.

3.6 Buprenorphine

Buprenorphine is a highly lipophilic partial opioid receptor agonist. It is also considered to have local-anesthetic-like capacity by blocking voltage-gated sodium channels. Buprenorphine and its metabolite nor-buprenorphine have been shown to act on κ and δ opioid receptors in addition to μ receptors which account for its anti-hyperalgesic effects. The risk of side effects like postoperative nausea and vomiting (PONV) is more with the use of perineural buprenorphine [21].

3.7 Diamorphine

It is a diacetylated analogue of morphine with a potency of approximately 1.5–2 times that of morphine. This leads to a faster onset and slightly shorter duration of action than morphine. It is a lipophilic semi-synthetic opioid and is a prodrug that is converted to its active metabolites (morphine and 6-monoacetyl morphine) by deacetylation in the liver and neural tissues. The recommended intrathecal dose is 300–400 μg, and epidural loading dose is 2–5 mg [17, 22].

3.8 Tramadol

Tramadol is a weak centrally acting opioid. A potency ratio of oral morphine to oral tramadol has been reported to be between 1:4 and 1:10. It has been shown to have Na^+ and K^+ channel blocking properties and can block motor and nocicep-tive signals similar to that of LAs. The central and peripheral analgesic effects of tramadol have not been fully explained, but it is a selective agonist of μ-receptors. Tramadol also prevents reuptake of noradrenaline and enhances both serotonin and noradrenaline release. The monoaminergic activity of tramadol increases the inhibitory activity of the descending pain pathways, resulting in a suppression of nociceptive transmission at the spinal level [23].

4. Vasoactive agents

Vasoactive drugs are the oldest adjuvants that have been used, although at the beginning their action was attributed more to the fact that their vasoconstric-tor effect prolonged the anesthetic and analgesic results of LAs by decreasing the blood flow of the site where they were injected. Adrenaline was the first vasopressor used.

4.1 Epinephrine

Epinephrine has been used along with LA in neuraxial and peripheral nerve blocks since Heinrich Braun first experimented with its use as a "chemical tourniquet" in the early 1900s [24]. Epinephrine potentiates the LA action. The substantia gelatinosa of the dorsal horn of the spinal cord houses alpha-2 adrenoreceptors wherein the epinephrine by its direct action mediates its antinociceptive properties resulting in presynaptic inhibition of transmitter release from Aδ and C fibers. Also its vasoconstrictive properties limit the systemic absorption of LA leading to prolonged duration of action. There are concerns about epinephrine being a potent vasoconstrictive agent can place the blood supply of the spinal cord at risk and may lead to ischemia of the spinal cord leading to permanent damage. Epinephrine is typically administered in doses of 0.2–0.3 mg [25].

4.2 Phenylephrine

Phenylephrine has a mechanism of action similar to that of epinephrine. It has vasoconstrictive abilities, thus limiting the uptake of LA and prolonging their duration of action. Phenylephrine in the dose of 2–5 mg prolongs both lidocaine and tetracaine spinal anesthesia to a similar extent as epinephrine. The use of phenylephrine has declined in popularity because of its association with transient neurologic symptoms (TNS) [26].

5. Alpha-2 adrenergic agonists

Alpha-2 adrenergic receptor agonists have recently been the focus of interest for their sedative, analgesic, perioperative sympatholytic, anesthetic sparing, and hemodynamic stabilizing properties. The central α-2-AR agonists inhibit nociceptive impulses by activating post-junctional α-2-adrenoceptors in the dorsal horn of the spinal cord. These receptors are located on primary afferent terminals (both at peripheral and at spinal endings), on neurons in the superficial lamina of the spinal cord, and within several brainstem nuclei responsible for analgesia. They block the conduction of C- and A-delta fibers and increase potassium conductance, thus intensifying conduction block. They also cause local vasoconstriction, thereby reducing vascular uptake of the LA from around the neural structures and in turn prolonging the duration of action [27–29].

5.1 Clonidine

Clonidine is an imidazole derivative with selective partial agonist properties which inhibit the nociceptive impulses by acting on the post-junctional alpha-2 adrenoreceptors in the dorsal horn of the spinal cord. In neuraxial blocks, it has a local effect leading to decreased sympathetic outflow, while in peripheral nerve blocks it prolongs the duration of analgesia by hyperpolarization of cyclic nucleotide-gated cation channels. Clonidine enhances and prolongs sensory and enhances motor blockade when used along with LA for epidural or peripheral nerve blocks [30]. The alpha-2 adrenergic agonists also enhance analgesia from intraspinal opioids by interactions with both pre- and post-synaptic receptors within the spinal cord.

Although there is no agreement on the doses of intrathecal clonidine [31], the most commonly used doses vary widely. The most recommended dose for intrathecal use is 15–150 μg, with the incidence of adverse effects (bradycardia, sedation, hypotension) increasing with doses above 150 μg. Clonidine can be used via epidural route with a bolus dose of 75–150 μg. In pediatric anesthesia, the use of clonidine (1 μg/kg) as an adjuvant along with LA for caudal blocks doubles the duration of analgesia when compared to LA alone but causes marked sedation [17].

Clonidine has been found to prolong the action of local anesthetics in peripheral blocks in the postoperative period. This effect of clonidine is dose-related. After brachial plexus block with mepivacaine, the minimum doses which significantly prolong analgesia and anesthesia are 0.1 and 0.5 μg/kg, respectively [32].

5.2 Dexmedetomidine

Dexmedetomidine is seven times more selective agonist to alpha-2 receptor than clonidine (seven times more specific for alpha-2 than alpha-1) but has a similar mechanism of blocking hyperpolarization-activated cation channels. When used as an adjuvant to LA for neuraxial block, dexmedetomidine leads to reduced onset time of sensory and motor block, increased duration of sensory block, and delayed recovery from motor blockade. It leads to prolongation of postoperative analgesia, decreased requirement of additional analgesics, delayed first rescue analgesic, and decreased postoperative shivering. Dose in spinal anesthesia varies from 3 to 15 μg as an adjuvant to LA [33]. For caudal epidural block, 1–2 μg/kg of dexmedetomidine along with bupivacaine can lead to prolonged analgesia without significant side effects [34].

The most common reported adverse effects are bradycardia and hypotension. Bradycardia due to dexmedetomidine is resistant to atropine, and higher doses are needed; although rare, even cardiac arrest can occur.

It has been shown that clonidine and dexmedetomidine administered orally, intramuscularly, and intravenously also prolong the anesthetic effect of intrathecal LA [35–40].

6. Steroids: dexamethasone

Acute inflammation from tissue injury has an important role in surgical pain, and glucocorticoids may be useful for its anti-inflammatory effect. Johansson et al. [41] investigated the corticosteroid effect on the plantar nerve of rats finding that methylprednisolone suppresses transmission in thin unmyelinated C fibers but not in myelinated A-beta fibers. The effect was reversed when the corticosteroid was removed, suggesting a direct action in the membrane.

Dexamethasone-induced prolongation of peripheral nerve blockade follow-ing LA injection is commonly attributed to its anti-inflammatory action. It also improves the quality and duration of analgesia over LAs alone. This is thought to be mediated by its capacity to alter the release of inflammatory mediators, reduce ectopic neuronal discharge, and inhibit potassium channel-mediated discharge of nociceptive C fibers [41]. Its action on glucocorticoid receptor is considered to alter the functioning of ion channels and produce acidosis around the nerve cell, thereby reducing the concentration of LA required to produce blockade of signal transmission or trapping the highly ionized bupivacaine molecule into the neuronal cell. Studies using dexamethasone for postoperative pain relief have produced positive results mainly in surgery involving large amounts of tissue trauma. A systematic review and meta-analysis included 1695 patients distributed in 29 controlled clinical trials where dexamethasone 4 and 8 mg perineural was used as adjuvant to LA. These authors found that dexamethasone increased the mean (95% CI) duration of analgesia by 233 (172–295) min when injected with short- or medium-term action LA and by 488 (419–557) min when injected with long-term action LA, $p < 0.00001$ for both. However, these results should be taken with caution due to the great heterogeneity of results, with I2 exceeding 90% for both analysis. Meta-regression did not show an interaction between dose of perineural dexa-methasone (4–10 mg) and duration of analgesia ($r2 = 0.02$, $p = 0.54$). There were no differences between 4 and 8 mg dexamethasone on subgroup analysis [42]. After reviewing the current literature, Wiesmann et al. [43] prefer a systemic application mode (intravenously) over a perineural route of dexamethasone administration as a complement to peripheral nerve blocks. A single dose of dexamethasone could be a useful complement to prolong peripheral nerve blocks. In a randomized controlled triple-blind crossover study in 24 male volunteers, the authors used ultrasound-guided ulnar nerve blocks (ropivacaine 0.75% wt/vol, 3 ml, with saline 1 ml with or without dexamethasone 4 mg) which were performed on three occasions in each volunteer along with an IV injection of saline 1 ml with or without dexamethasone 4 mg. The median [inter-quartile range (IQR)] duration of sensory block was 6.87

(5.85–7.62) h in the control group, 7.37 (5.78–7.93) h in the perineural group, and 7.37 (6.10–7.97) h in the IV group ($P = 0.61$). There was also no significant difference in block onset time between the three groups. Dexamethasone 4 mg had no clinically significant effect on the duration of sensory block provided by ropivacaine applied to the ulnar nerve [44]. The role of dexamethasone as an adjunct in peripheral nerve blockades is still unclear.

7. Nonsteroidal anti-inflammatory drugs (NSAIDs)

Several studies have demonstrated that the presence of COX-2 receptors in the dorsal horn of the spinal cord could regulate spinal nociceptive transmission [45]. Some studies suggest that administering a COX-2 antagonist directly on the central or peripheral nerve might have a better analgesic profile than intravenous administration of the same drug [46]. Basically COX-2 inhibitors reduce inflammation and pain sensation by inhibiting prostaglandin production. However, the role of COX-2 in the central nervous system is of more importance. Inflammation can induce COX-2 production and will lead to the release of prostanoids that sensitize the peripheral nociceptor terminals and produce localized hyperalgesia. It is hence thought that the administration of COX-2 antagonist on spinal or peripheral nerves may be a more effective mode of pain relief than the intravenous or intramuscular route. There are very less studies on this subject. Further research and studies need to be conducted to verify the use of NSAIDs as adjuvants.

8. Miscellaneous agents

8.1 Ketamine

Ketamine is a noncompetitive antagonist of NMDA receptor that has been shown to have local anesthetic properties. Ketamine acts on more than one region. It has actions at monoaminergic receptors, opioid receptors, voltage-sensitive calcium channels, and muscarinic receptors, in addition to local anesthetic actions through sodium channel blockade. Systemic ketamine causes central summation in the second-order pain neuron and decreases severe pain [3, 47, 48]. Epidural administration of ketamine at 0.5–1 mg/kg has been shown to reduce intraoperative and postoperative analgesic requirements without increased side effects [25]. Preservative-free S(+)-ketamine administered during caudal block for children at a dose of 0.5 mg/kg has been shown to extend analgesia time by several hours [17]. Intrathecal administration of ketamine is not recommended.

The risk of psychomimetic adverse effects such as hallucinations is a worrying factor for most anesthetists, limiting its use, but it can be easily overcome by using intravenous benzodiazepines as premedication prior to the block.

8.2 Midazolam

Midazolam, a water-soluble benzodiazepine, an indirect agonist of the gamma-aminobutyric acid (GABA) receptor, has been studied primarily as an adjuvant for neuraxial anesthesia. Addition of preservative-free midazolam to 0.5% hyperbaric bupivacaine for subarachnoid block in infraumbilical surgery has been found to prolong the duration of effective analgesia as compared to the same concentra-tion of bupivacaine alone and delays the need for postoperative rescue analgesics without having any reported significant side effects or hemodynamic instability. The use of intrathecal midazolam also decreases the incidence of postoperative nau-sea and vomiting. A small diluted intrathecal dose (1–2.5 mg) of preservative-free midazolam is reported to have few systemic side effects and is free of short-term neurotoxicity [49]. An infusion of epidural midazolam at 10–20 μg/kg/h for up to 12 h is considered safe.

8.3 Neostigmine

Neostigmine is an acetylcholinesterase inhibitor that can enhance analgesia by acting on muscarinic receptors and increasing endogenous acetylcholine at the nerve terminal. It produces spinal analgesia in the preclinical models. Intrathecal neostigmine produces analgesia by the inhibition of (endogenous spinal neurotransmitter) acetylcholine destruction via muscarinic and cholinergic receptors located at dorsal horn of spinal cord, substantia gelatinosa, and in lesser amounts at laminae III and V [50]. There is a high incidence of nausea and vomiting and prolongation of recovery from spinal anesthesia following intrathecal administration of neostigmine, implying that it may not be a useful additive for ambulatory spinal anesthesia. The dose of intrathecal neostigmine ranges from 10 to 50 μg with the side effects increasing as the dose rises.

8.4 Magnesium sulfate

Magnesium is an N-methyl-D-aspartate (NMDA) antagonist that plays a role in moderating calcium influx into neurons. Research has demonstrated that magnesium decreases peripheral nerve excitability and enhances the ability of lidocaine to raise the excitation threshold of A-beta fibers.

Intrathecal and epidural use of magnesium has shown variable results. It may prolong LA/opioid block in women in labor at a dose of 50 mg, but a very high dose of magnesium has been reported to produce transient neurological toxicity [17]. Farzanegan et al. compared the combination of bupivacaine 12.5 mg and morphine 2 mg versus bupivacaine 12.5 mg and morphine 2 mg and magnesium 50 mg versus placebo epidurally for postoperative analgesia after thoracotomy. These authors achieved better analgesia and lower consumption of postoperative morphine significantly in the magnesium group [51]. In preeclamptic parturients doses of 50 mg of intrathecal magnesium with epidural ropivacaine significantly prolonged postoperative analgesia compared with 1 mg intrathecal midazolam without any complications [52]. In a recent meta-analysis, 11 studies showed that the use of epidural magnesium as an adjuvant to bupivacaine is still controversial. Although epidural magnesium prolonged the time of the first rescue analgesic and reduced the number of patients who required rescue analgesics, as well as the requirement of these analgesics, further studies are needed to assess their usefulness [53].

8.5 Sodium bicarbonate

Local anesthetic agents are usually packed at low pH to enhance their shelf life. In anesthetic practice, there has been considerable interest in studying the effect of pH on the onset, duration, and potency of blockade of LAs. It is proven that alkalinization of the LA improves the quality of block by influencing the portioning coefficient of anesthetic between aqueous solution and biological membranes [20]. Adding sodium bicarbonate to lidocaine decreases the latency of onset and enhances the depth of epidural blockade by increasing the concentration of non-ionized drug. The alkaline pH increases the extraneural amount of non-ionized LA, which is the form that diffuses through the lipid phase of the neural membrane leading to more rapid diffusion across perineural tissue barriers [54]. CO_2 produced by the addition of bicarbonate and bicarbonate per se reduces the margin of conduction safety of the neural membrane. Moreover, CO_2 penetrates into the nerve, where it may determine trapping of the active cationic form of LA by acidifying the axoplasm [55].

8.6 Potassium chloride

Movements of ions through the nerve membrane are considered one of the main steps in the process of excitation and propagation of nerve stimuli. A nerve impulse can be effectively blocked by accumulation of potassium ions outside the neuron [56]. Thus, administration of exogenous potassium chloride will reinforce and prolong the blockade produced by LA. The addition of potassium chloride to LA increases the extracellular concentration and depolarizes the nerve membrane and thus blocks the conduction of nerve impulses. Potassium chloride up to 4 mmol/l to isotonic solutions of lidocaine enhances the clinical effectiveness of the combina-tion [57]. The addition of physiological amounts of potassium chloride shortens the latency period and prolongs the duration of the blockade.

8.7 Adenosine

Adenosine receptors are expressed on the surface of most cells. Five classes of adenosine receptors have been identified. The A1 and A2 receptors are present centrally and peripherally, with agonism of the A1 receptor leading to antinociceptive response and that of the A2 receptor being algogenic (i.e., activation results in pain). The diagnostic and therapeutic role for intrathecal adenosine in acute and chronic pain states is under investigation by several research groups. Intrathecal adenosine decreases the spontaneous and evoked pain intensity in patients with neuropathic pain involving hyperalgesia/dysesthesia/allodynia [58]. Its interaction along with spinal LA is just beginning to be studied.

8.8 Dextran

Low molecular weight dextran (LMWD) was used as an adjuvant with LA as early as in the 1970s, but the efficacy of dextrans including LMWD remained controversial, as several studies reported an absence of any substantial difference in analgesic duration with their addition. That might have been due to poor techniques of regional anesthesia. The use of USG regional blocks has rekindled the use of LMWD as adjuvant. The addition of LMWD to a LA and epinephrine mixture when used as an infiltration anesthesia [59], or to a LA alone when performing a regional block [33], safely prolongs the effective action by reducing systemic absorption. More studies need to be conducted to elicit the exact mechanism and dosing ranges.

A word of caution regarding the use of additives in LAs is that only preparations without preservatives should be used, since these can be neurotoxic. Also, only adjuvants in clinically safe doses should be used in order to avoid getting the side effects due to excessive dosages.

Hence further research is required to find the exact mechanism of action and the safe dose of various adjuvants in order to avoid cardiovascular and neurological complications. The practice of making off-label use of drugs without getting FDA approval should be discouraged.

9. Conclusion

Locoregional anesthesia is increasingly used as it has demonstrated efficacy, safety, and low costs. Patients and surgeons have realized its enormous advantages. Although the use of LA in the management of locoregional anesthesia, postopera-tive pain, and chronic pain is limited by its duration of action and dose-dependent adverse effects that mainly affect the cardiovascular and CNS systems, this has been improved with the use of various LA adjuvant drugs. Adjuvants are medications that work synergistically with LAs to improve the onset, duration, and quality of anesthesia-analgesia in regional techniques, as well as greatly reducing the use of opioid analgesics.

The arsenal of adjuvants has developed from adrenaline, opioids, to a large group of non-opioid medications with various mechanisms of action. Opioids are the most commonly used adjuvants and range from morphine, fentanyl, and sufent-anil to hydromorphone, buprenorphine, and tramadol with very different results. Its use has been limited by its adverse effects such as respiratory depression, nausea, vomiting, and pruritus, especially with its neuraxial use. Other adjuvants include alpha-2 agonists such as clonidine and dexmedetomidine, midazolam, NMDA antagonists including ketamine and magnesium, neostigmine, sodium bicarbonate, and nonsteroidal anti-inflammatory drugs. Concern regarding the safety profile of these adjuvants is due to their potential neurotoxicity and neurological complications that may limit their use and require further investigation.

Conflict of interests

The authors declare no conflict of interest.

Author details

Nandita Mehta* and Sayyidah Aasima tu Nisa Qazi
Department of Anaesthesia and Critical Care, ASCOMS Jammu, J&K, India

*Address all correspondence to: drnanditamehta@gmail.com

References

[1] Becker DE, Reed KL. Local anesthetics: Review of pharmacological considerations. Anesthesia Progress. 2012;**59**(2):90-101. DOI: 10.2344/0003-3006-59.2.90

[2] Shah J, Votta-Velis EG, Borgeat A. New local anesthetics. Best Practice & Research. Clinical Anaesthesiology. 2018;**32**(2):179-185. DOI: 10.1016/j.bpa.2018.06.010

[3] Swain A, Nag DS, Sahu S, Samaddar DP. Adjuvants to local anesthetics: Current understanding and future trends. World Journal of Clinical Cases. 2017;**5**(8):307-323. DOI: 10.12998/wjcc.v5.i8.307.x

[4] Schäfer M, Mousa SA, Shaqura M, Tafelski S. Background and current use of adjuvants for regional anesthesia: From research to evidence-based patient treatment. Der Anaesthesist. 2019;**68**(1):3-14. DOI: 10.1007/s00101-018-0522-6

[5] Krishna Prasad GV, Khanna S, Jaishree SV. Review of adjuvants to local anesthetics in peripheral nerve blocks: Current and future trends. Saudi Journal of Anaesthesia. 2020; **14**:77-84. DOI: 10.4103/sja.SJA_423_19

[6] Prabhakar A, Lambert T, Kaye RJ, Gaignard SM, Ragusa J, Wheat S, et al. Adjuvants in clinical regional anesthesia practice: A comprehensive review. Best Practice & Research. Clinical Anaesthesiology. 2019;**33**(4):415-423. DOI: 10.1016/j.bpa.2019.06.001

[7] Bujedo BM. Current evidence for spinal opioid selection in postoperative pain. The Korean Journal of Pain. 2014;**27**(3):200-209. DOI: 10.3344/kjp.2014.27.3.200

[8] Buvanendran A, Kroin JS. Useful adjuvants for postoperative pain management. Best Practice & Research. Clinical Anaesthesiology. 2007;**1**:31-49. DOI: 10.1016/j.bpa.2006.12.003

[9] Guany Y, Borzan J, Meyer RA, Raja SN. Windup in dorsal horn neurons is modulated by endogenous spinal mu-opioid mechanisms. The Journal of Neuroscience. 2006;**26**:4298-4307.DOI: 10.1523/JNEUROSCI.0960-06.2006

[10] Stein C, Lang LJ. Peripheral mechanisms of opioid analgesia. Current Opinion in Pharmacology. 2009;**9**:3-8. DOI: 10.1016/j. coph.2008.12.009

[11] Wajima Z, Shitara T, Nakajima Y, Kim C, Kobayashi N, Kadotani H, et al. Comparison of continuous brachial plexus infusion of butorphanol, mepivacaine and mepivacaine-butorphanol mixtures for post-operative analgesia. British Journal of Anaesthesia. 1995; **75**:548-551. DOI: 10.1093/bja/75.5.548

[12] Wang JK, Naus LA, Thomas JE. Pain relief by intrathecal applied morphine in man. Anaesthesiology. 1979;**50**:149-151

[13] Ummenhofer WC, Arends RH, Shen DD, Bernards CM. Comparative spinal distribution and clearance kinetics of intrathecally-administered morphine, fentanyl, alfentanil and sufentanil. Anaesthesiology. 2000;**92**:739-753. DOI:10.1097/00000542-200003000-00018

[14] Liu SS, Block BM, Wu CL. Effects of post-operative central neuraxial analgesia on outcome after coronary artery bypass surgery: A meta-analysis. Anesthesiology. 2004;**101**:153-161. DOI: 10.1097/00000542-200407000-00024

[15] Bromage PR, Camporesi EM, Durant PA, Nielsen CH. Rostral spread of epidural morphine. Anesthe-siology. 1982;**56**:431-436. DOI: 10.1097/00000542-198206000-00004

[16] Yurashevich M, Habib AS. Monitoring, prevention and treatment of side effects of long-acting neuraxial opioids for post-cesarean analgesia. International Journal of Obstetric Anesthesia. 2019;**39**:117-128. DOI: 10.1016/j.ijoa.2019.03.010

[17] Musokota MJ, Kasandji KF, Tshebeletso NC. Pharmacology of local anaesthetics and commonly used recipes in clinical practice. In: Hakan ER, editor. Current Topics in Anesthesiology. Croatia: IntechOpen; 2017. pp. 5-27. DOI: 10.5772/67048

[18] Gissen AJ, Gugino LD, Datta S, Miller J, Covino BG. Effects of fentanyl and sufentanil on peripheral mammalian nerves. Anesthesia and Analgesia. 1987;**66**(12):1272-1276

[19] Kaniyil S, Radhakrishnan P. Does fentanyl prolong the analgesia of local anaesthetics in brachial plexus block? A randomized controlled study. International Journal of Research in Medical Sciences. 2017;**5**:583-587

[20] Capogna G, Celleno D, Costantino P, Muratori F, Sebastiani M, Baldassini M. Alkalinization improves the quality of lidocaine-fentanyl epidural anaesthesia for caesarean section. Canadian Journal of Anaesthesia. 1993;**40**: 425-430

[21] Kosel J, Bobik P, Tomczyk M. Buprenorphine—The unique opioid adjuvant in regional anesthesia. Expert Review of Clinical Pharmacology. 2016;**9**(3):375-383. DOI: 10.1586/17 512433.2016.1141047

[22] Elrazek EA. The analgesic effects of epidural diamorphine and levobupivacaine on established lower limb post-amputation stump pain—A comparative study. Middle East Journal of Anaesthesiology. 2005;**18** (1):149-160

[23] Bravo L, Mico JA, Berrocoso E. Discovery and development of tramadol for the treatment of pain. Expert Opinion on Drug Discovery. 2017;**12** (12):1281-1291. DOI: 10.1080/174 60441.2017.1377697

[24] Braun H. Ueber die bedeutung des adrenalins fur die chirurgie. Munchener Medizinische Wochenschrift.1903;**50**: 352-353

[25] Abdalla IA. Additives for spinal anaesthesia. Sudan Medical Journal. 2016;**52**(3):109-113

[26] Miller RD, editor. Miller's Anesthesia. New York: Elsevier, Churchill Livingstone; 2005

[27] Christiansson L. Update on adjuvants in regional anaesthesia. Periodicum Biologorum. 2009;**111**:161-170

[28] Llorca-Torralba M, Borges G, Neto F, Mico JA, Berrocoso E. Noradrenergic locus Coeruleus pathways in pain modulation. Neuroscience. 2016;**338**:93-113. DOI: 10.1016/j. neuroscience.2016.05.057

[29] Valenzuela-Harrington M, Negrete-Díaz V, Rodríguez-Moreno A. Núcleo Coeruleus. Neurotransmisores, funciones y patología. Anest Mex. 2007;**19**:155-166

[30] Dobrydnjovi A, Guptaa L, Holmstrom B, Granath B. Improved analgesia with clonidine when added to local anesthetic during combined spinal-epidural anesthesia for hip arthroplasty: A double-blind, randomized and placebo-controlled study. Acta Anaesthesiologica Scandinavica. 2005;**49**:538-545

[31] Whizar LV, Flores CJC, Preciado RS. Intrathecal clonidine as spinal anaesthesia adjuvant. Is there a magical dose? In: Topics in Spinal Anaesthesia. Croatia: IntechOpen; 2014. DOI: 10.5772/58712

[32] Singelyn FJ, Gouverneur JM, Robert A. A minimum dose of clonidine added to mepivacaine prolongs the duration of anesthesia and analgesia after axillary brachial plexus block. Anesthesia and Analgesia. 1996;**83**:1046-1050

[33] Gupta M, Shailaja S, Hegde KS. Comparison of intrathecal dexmedetomidine with buprenorphine as adjuvant to bupivacaine in spinal anaesthesia. Journal of Clinical and Diagnostic Research. 2014;**8**(2):114-117. DOI: 10.7860/JCDR/2014/7883.4023

[34] El-Hennawy AM, Abd-Elwahab AM, Abd-Elmaksoud AM, El-Ozairy HS, Boulis SR. Addition of clonidine or dexmedetomidine to bupivacaine prolongs caudal analgesia in children. British Journal of Anaesthesia. 2009;**103**(2):268-274. DOI: 10.1093/bja/aep159

[35] Dziubdziela W, Jałowiecki P, Kawecki P. Prolongation of bupivacaine spinal anaesthesia by oral and intramuscular clonidine. Wiadomości Lekarskie. 2003;**56**:520-526

[36] Rhee K, Kang K, Kim J, Jeon Y. Intravenous clonidine prolongs bupivacaine spinal anesthesia. Acta Anaesthesiologica Scandinavica. 2003;**47**:1001-1005. DOI: 10.1034/j.1399-6576.2003.00158.x

[37] Whizar-Lugo V, Gómez-Ramírez IA, Cisneros-Corral R, Martínez-Gallegos N. Intravenous dexmedetomidine vs. intravenous clonidine to prolong bupivacaine spinal anesthesia. A double blind study. Anest Mex. 2007;**19**:143-146

[38] Reddy VS, Shaik NA, Donthu B, Reddy Sannala VK, Jangam V. Intravenous dexmedetomidine versus clonidine for prolongation of bupivacaine spinal anesthesia and analgesia: A randomized double-blind study. Journal of Anaesthesiology Clinical Pharmacology. 2013;**29**(3):342-347. DOI: 10.4103/0970-9185.117101

[39] Kaya FN, Yavascaoglu B, Turker G, Yildirim A, Gurbet A, Mogol EB, et al. Intravenous dexmedetomidine, but not midazolam, prolongs bupivacaine spinal anesthesia. Canadian Journal of Anaesthesia. 2010;**57**(1):39-45. DOI: 10.1007/s12630-009-9231-6

[40] Srinivas DB, Lakshminarasimhaiah G. Comparison of subcutaneous dexmedetomidine versus clonidine as an adjuvant to spinal anesthesia: A randomized double blind control trial. Local and Regional Anesthesia. 2019;**12**:29-36. DOI: 10.2147/LRA.S197386

[41] Johansson A, Hao J, Sjölund B. Local corticosteroid application blocks transmission in normal nociceptive C-fibres. Acta Anaesthesiologica Scandinavica. 1990;**34**(5):335-338. DOI: 10.1111/j.1399-6576.1990.tb03097.x

[42] Albrecht E, Kern C, Kirkham KR. A systematic review and meta-analysis of perineural dexamethasone for peripheral nerve blocks. Anaesthesia. 2015;**70**(1): 71-83. DOI: 10.1111/anae.12823

[43] Wiesmann T, Volk T, Steinfeldt T. Glucocorticoids as an adjunct in peripheral regional anesthesia. Move to the "holy grail of perineural analgesia". Der Anaesthesist. 2016;**65**(4):295-298. DOI: 10.1007/s00101-016-0143-x

[44] Marhofer P, Columb M, Hopkins PM, Greher M, Marhofer D, Levi Bienzle MR, et al. Dexamethasone as an adjuvant for peripheral nerve blockade: A randomised, triple-blinded crossover study in volunteers. British Journal of Anaesthesia. 2019;**122**(4):525-531. DOI: 10.1016/j. bja.2019.01.004

[45] Resnick DK, Graham SH, Dixon CE, Marion DW. Role of cyclooxygenase-2 in

acute spinal cord injury. Journal of Neurotrauma. 1998;**15**(12):1005-1013

[46] Liu X, Zhao X, Lou J, Wang Y, Shen X. Parecoxib added to ropivacaine prolongs duration of axillary brachial plexus blockade and relieves postoperative pain. Clinical Orthopaedics and Related Research. 2013;**471**(2):562-568

[47] Reboso Morales JA, González MF. Ketamina. Revista Española de Anestesiología y Reanimación. 1999;**46**(3):111-122

[48] Tawfic QA. A review of the use of ketamine in pain management. Journal of Opioid Management. 2013;**9**(5): 379-388. DOI: 10.5055/jom.2013.0180

[49] Shadangi BK, Garg R, Pandey R, Das T. Effects of intrathecal midazolam in spinal anaesthesia: A prospective randomised case control study. Singapore Medical Journal. 2011;**52**(6):432

[50] Lauretti GR, Lima IC. The effects of intrathecal neostigmine on somatic and visceral pain: İmprovement by association with a peripheral anticholinergic. Anesthesia and Analgesia. 1996;**82**(3):617-620

[51] Farzanegan B, Zangi M, Saeedi K, Khalili A, Rajabi M, et al. Effect of adding magnesium sulphate to epidural bupivacaine and morphine on post-thoracotomy pain management: A randomized, double-blind, clinical trial. Basic & Clinical Pharmacology & Toxicology. 2018;**123**(5):602-606. DOI: 10.1111/bcpt.13047

[52] Paleti S, Prasad PK, Lakshmi BS. A randomized clinical trial of intrathecal magnesium sulfate versus midazolam with epidural administration of 0.75% ropivacaine for patients with preeclampsia scheduled for elective cesarean section. Journal of Anaesthesiology Clinical Pharmacology. 2018;**34**(1): 23-28. DOI: 10.4103/joacp.JOACP_74_17

[53] Li LQ , Fang MD, Wang C, Lu HL, Wang LX, Xu HY, et al. Comparative evaluation of epidural bupivacaine alone and bupivacaine combined with magnesium sulfate in providing postoperative analgesia: A meta-analysis of randomized controlled trials. BMC Anesthesiology. 2020;**20**(1):39. DOI: 10.1186/s12871-020-0947-8

[54] Strobel GE, Bianchi CB. The effects of pH gradients on the action of procaine and lidocaine in intact and desheathed sciatic nerves. The Journal of Pharmacology and Experimental Therapeutics. 1970;**172**:1-17

[55] Wong K, Strichartz GR, Raymond SA. On the mechanisms of potentiation of local anesthetics by bicarbonate buffer: Drug structure-activity studies on isolated peripheral nerve. Anesthesia and Analgesia. 1993;**76**:131-143

[56] Aldrete JA, Barnes DR, Sidon MA, et al. Studies on effects of potassium chloride to lidocaine. Anesthesia & Analgesia. 1969;**48**(2):269-276

[57] Kircha S, Barsa J, Fink BR. Potentiation of nerve block in vivo by physiological adjuvants in the solution. British Journal of Anaesthesia. 1983;**55**(6):549-553

[58] Belfrage M, Segerdahl M, Arner S, Sollevi A. The safety and efficacy of intrathecal adenosine in patients with chronic neuropathic pain. Anesthesia and Analgesia. 1999;**89**:136-142

[59] Ueda W, Hirakawa M, Mori K. Inhibition of epinephrine absorption by dextran. Anesthesiology. 1985;**62**:72-75

9

Introduction to Local Anesthetics

Víctor M. Whizar-Lugo, Karen L. Íñiguez-López, Ana C. Cárdenas-Maytorena and Cristian D. Ramírez-Puerta

Abstract

The fascinating history of local anesthetics (LAs) began in South America with the herbal and traditional use of cocaine leaves by the indigenous peoples of Peru and Bolivia, the sacred plant of the Incas *Erythroxylum coca*. The use for anesthetic purposes dates back to 1884. Since then, the evolution of LAs has been closely related to research motivated by its efficacy and safety versus toxicity. According to their chemical structure, these drugs are classified into two main groups: esters and amino amides; however, there are three LAs with different characteristics: articaine, sameridine, and centbucridine. The pharmacological and toxic mode of action is primarily in the voltage-dependent sodium channels located in the cell membrane, which clinically produces analgesia, anesthesia, seizures, arrhythmias, and cardiac arrest. The quality of anesthesia and analgesia depends on the type of LA, dose, and application technique, while the deleterious effects are secondary to its plasma concentration. Nonanesthetic properties of LAs such as their antimicrobial, antineoplastic, antiarrhythmics, antitussive, and antiasthmatics effects have been described and are briefly reviewed.

Keywords: local anesthetics, pharmacology, toxicity

1. Introduction

Local anesthetics (LAs) are drugs commonly used in medicine and especially in anesthesiology, which when administered in the vicinity of peripheral neural tissue produce changes in the conformation of voltage-dependent sodium channels that depolarize the neural tissue and produce analgesia, anesthesia, and sympathetic and motor block in the dermatomes of the affected nerves without altering consciousness. This inhibitory phenomenon is reversible and transitory and is known as regional anesthesia and is classified into local, peripheral nerves, nervous plexuses, peridural, subarachnoid, and intravenous anesthesia.

LAs are safe and effective drugs, although when wrongly managed, they can reach high plasma concentrations and produce systemic toxicity (LAST) that manifests primarily in the central nervous system (CNS) and cardiovascular system (CVS), causing side effects that can occasionally lead to death. Local neuro toxicity has also been described when injected in the vicinity of the peripheral nervous system or at subarachnoid or epidural space. Myotoxic effects have also been described.

The main clinical use of LAs is to achieve pain insensitivity, although they have other pharmacological uses such as antiarrhythmic, anti-asthmatic, anti-inflammatory, antithrombotic, bacteriostatic, and bactericidal effects that have been demonstrated, as well as antitumoral agent enhancer activity [1–3]. LAs are grouped into two categories: those of the ester type and those of the amino-amide group. They are the only drugs used in regional anesthesia, although it has been described that other drugs with different molecular structure such as amitriptyline, meperidine, eugenols, beta-adrenergic antagonists, $alpha_2$ agonists, spasmolytics, anticonvulsants, and antihistamines have local anesthetic effects [4–6]. There are three LAs that due to their chemical structure differ from the classic LAs: articaine, sameridine, and centbucridine. Articaine is classified into the amide group, it is fat soluble and short acting and has intermediate potency, with rapid metabolism due to an ester group in its structure. Sameridine, on the other hand, has mixed effects as an opioid agonist and LA properties under investigation for intrathecal use [7, 8]. Centbucridine is a nonester, nonamide drug still under clinical investigation [9].

In this introductory chapter, the most important properties of LAs are detailed, emphasizing their pharmacological classification, pharmacokinetic profile, action mechanisms, side effects, and some relevant clinical aspects, as well as their nonanesthetic uses.

2. Brief history of the discovery and evolution of LAs

In the Andean Mountains, centuries ago, the Incas began using cocaine leaves which they chewed or ingested in the form of potions that provided them with plenty of energy to carry out their religious rituals. In addition, as a powerful stimulant, the coca leaf was chewed to mitigate the effects derived from altitude, hunger or fatigue and as a medicine for gastrointestinal discomfort, colds, or bruises. This sacred plant of the Incas, *Erythroxylum coca*, caught the attention of Europeans who took it to the old continent at the end of the 16th century. It was until 1859 when Paulo Mantegazza, an Italian physiologist, wrote *Sulle virtu igieniche e Medicinale della Coca* (On the hygienic and medicinal properties of coca and on nervine nourishment in general) where he pointed out its healing properties. The German chemist Albert Niemann isolated the active substance from these leaves and called it cocaine, noting its power to anesthetize the tongue. In 1884, Sigmund Freud wrote his famous monograph entitled *Ueber coca*. Like some of his contempo-raries, Freud acknowledged that cocaine had local anesthetic effects when applied to the mucous membranes, but it was Karl Köller who used it for the first time for anesthetic purposes when applied in various mucous membranes and in the con-junctiva for surgical purposes. It is Köller to whom it is attributed the beginning of local anesthesia [10–12].

The knowledge of the toxic and additive effects of cocaine became public quickly; it went from being the LA in vogue to a potent CNS stimulant that until today is a social stigma. This fired the investigation toward new LAs, and safer drugs were found. Benzocaine was synthesized in 1890, and in 1904, Alfred Einhorn introduced procaine by degrading cocaine, which was later marketed as novocaine® and was the most widely used LA in the world. Tetracaine was synthesized in 1928 and introduced into clinical anesthesia in 1932. In 1943 Löfgren discovered lidocaine that was introduced for clinical use in 1947 and is currently the most used LA. Mepivacaine appeared in 1956, and in 1963, the clinical use of bupivacaine was introduced, while etidocaine began to be used in 1972. Other LAs appeared during the following years but were withdrawn from the market due to their toxic effects. In 1970, Albrigth [13] mentioned some deaths attributed to bupivacaine and etidocaine. His editorial was enough to start basic and clinical research in search of new drugs with a better safety profile. The result was the introduction of ropivacaine in 1997 and levobupivacaine in 1999, both levoisomeric drugs. It is noteworthy that these two LAs had been discovered in 1957 and 1972, respectively (**Table 1**).

Local anesthetics	Year of synthesis	Introduction in clinic
Cocaine	1860	1884
Procaine	1904	1905
Dibucaine	1925	1930
Tetracaine	1928	1932
Lidocaine	1943	1947
Chloroprocaine	1950	1952
Mepivacaine	1956	1957
Prilocaine	1959	1960
Bupivacaine	1957	1963
Etidocaine	1971	1972
Ropivacaine	1957	1997
Levobupivacaine	1972	1999

Table 1.
Chronological appearance of local anesthetics.

The levoisomeric LAs did not replace other LAs but are complementary to the therapeutic armamentarium in regional anesthesia. Both ropivacaine and levobupivacaine have been conquering a special place in regional anesthesia techniques, but their toxicity is still superior to procaine, chloroprocaine, and lidocaine. While these LAs are not comparable in potency and duration, they still have a place in anesthesiology, with the exception of intrathecal lidocaine. The history of these drugs will continue to be written as new results on therapeutic effectiveness and toxicity are obtained.

3. Basics data

It is necessary to know some elementary aspects of the structure and function of the cell membrane, as well as to understand the role of voltage-dependent sodium channels, which are protein structures that are located in the cell membrane and play a paramount role in cellular electrical activity and impulse transmission.

3.1 Cellular membrane

The cell membrane is a barrier of lipids and proteins, which forms the outer surface of eukaryotic cells. The lipid part of the membrane is formed by a bilayer with a thickness of 60–100 Å, which gives it structure and constitutes a barrier that prevents the passage of water-soluble substances. It has three important types of lipids: phospholipids, glycolipids and cholesterol. The membrane proteins are suspended individually or in groups within the lipid structure and shape the various channels. The selectivity of transmembrane protein channels allows the cell to control the entry and exit of substances, as well as transport between cell compartments. Membrane proteins not only facilitate selective transport, but in addition, they are able to carry out active transport against the concentration gradient with special pumps, such as the sodium-potassium pump. Other functions of the membrane, such as the recognition and binding of certain substances on the cell surface, are also determined by the protein part of the membrane. These proteins are called cell receptors.

Cellular receptors are connected to internal systems that only act when certain substances bind to the membrane surface. Many of the cell controls act through this mechanism. Some metabolic pathways do not take action unless the "signal" molecule—for example—a hormone, has reached the cell surface. Glycoproteins are located in the membrane that identify other cells as members of an individual or as strangers. The interactions between the cells that make up a tissue are based on membrane proteins. In this manner, the structure of the membranes depends on the lipids, while the functions depend on the proteins.

3.2 Physiology of nerve transmission

The resting cell membrane maintains a voltage difference of 40–90 mV between the inner and outer layers, the inside being negative and the outside positive. This is the so-called resting potential, which is maintained by an active mechanism of the Na/K pump. The polarized membrane does not allow the passage of sodium ions (Na $^{+)}$ through the voltage-dependent sodium channels that are in resting state. When an electrical stimulus arrives, the membrane depolarization begins by activating the sodium channels that open to give way to the Na^+, which enter the intracellular medium, transforming the negativity of the transmembrane potential. This initiates a cycle of changes of sodium channels in four functional stages: resting, activated, inactivated, and deactivated. In the resting state, the outer gate of the sodium channel is closed, and the internal gate or closing gate is open. When a stimulus reaches the membrane, the sodium channel is activated by opening the external gate and letting Na^+ pass. When the membrane potential rises to +20 mV, the closure of the internal gate is triggered, and it enters an inactive state. The channel is deactivated when the membrane potential reaches -60 mV. When the passage of Na $^{+}$ ceases through the pore of the sodium channel, the potassium channel increases its permeability, allowing this ion to pass inside the cell due to differences in concentration (concentration gradient). Then the initial phase is restored; the Na-K pump mobilizes Na^+ outside and K^+ inside the cell. Sodium channels pass from the inactive-deactivated state to the initial resting state. All these movements of Na^+ and K^+ are manifested in changes in the transmembrane electrical potential, generating the action potential that is propagated along the nerve fiber (**Figure 1**) [14]. Because there is a potential difference across the cell membrane, the membrane is said to be polarized. If the membrane potential becomes more positive than it is at the resting potential, the membrane is said to be depolarized. This whole process lasts 1 millisecond; 30% is consumed by the depolarization phase. According to the electrical instant, the sodium channels dependent on voltage exist in four stages; resting (-90 mV), activated (-60 mV), inactivated (+20 mV) and deactivated (-60 mV).

3.3 Voltage-dependent sodium channels

Hodgkin and Huxley proposed that cell membranes contained channels that facilitated ionic passage through them, which was confirmed when ionic currents that selectively flow through these transmembrane pores were directly measured. In 1972, Singer and Nicolson [15–17] proposed the "Fluid Mosaic Model" in the structure of the cell membranes were they described the cell membrane as a two-dimensional liquid that restricts the lateral diffusion of membrane components and includes the integral proteins inserted in the lipid bilayer, some of which completely cross it and others cross it partially. Of these membrane proteins, three primary groups stand out: the channels, pumps, and receptors that constitute the transport system through cell membranes and regulate the movements of small molecules and ions that cannot pass through the lipid bilayer.

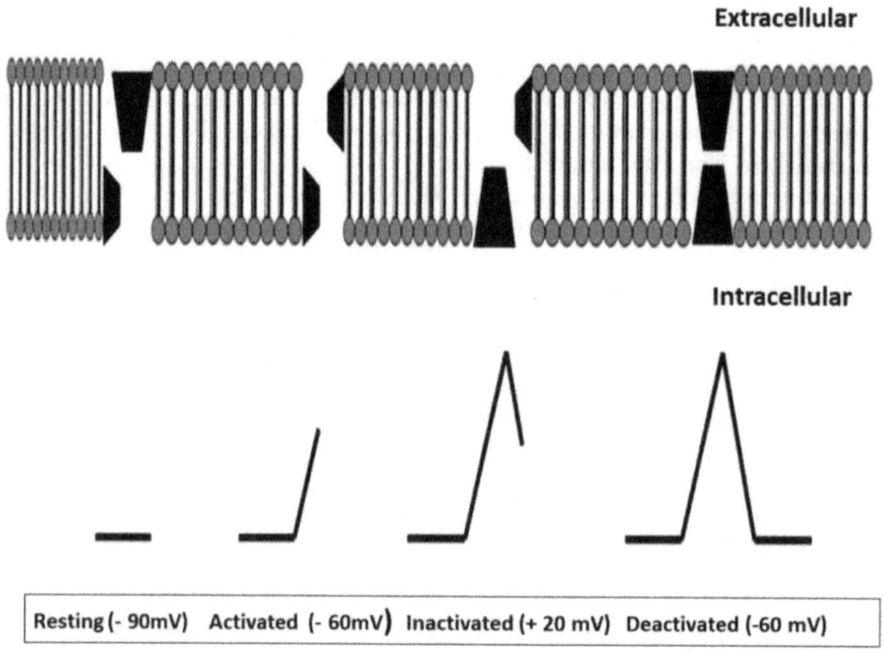

Figure 1.
Representation of the four structural phases of sodium channels and their relationship with the action potential. Modified from Columb MO, MacLennan K. Local anesthetics agents. Anaesth Intensive Care Med 2007; 8: 159–162 [14].

Sodium channels are protein structures that are integrated into the lipid bilayer of the cell membrane and are responsible for orchestrating the electrical signals that are transmitted by certain tissues, such as nerves and the heart's electrical conduction system. They are tubular-shaped components that resemble pores filled with water and are distributed through the whole cell membrane, primarily at the beginning of axons and in Ranvier nodes. This ion channels are divided into three types; those regulated by voltage, those regulated by extracellular ligand and those regulated by intracellular ligands, although other authors classify them into only two groups; those regulated by voltage and those operated by receptors [18–20]. The family of voltage-regulated sodium channels is composed of nine members that have been described in mammals and a tenth component related to a protein. All of them are members of a super family of ion channels that also includes potassium and calcium channels. Its nomenclature is complex and the chemical symbol of sodium Na^+ is used first, followed by V indicating voltage regulated (Na^+ V). The next number indicates the subfamily gene (Na^+ V1), and the next number identifies the specific isoform of the channel, for example Na^+ V1.1. This last number was assigned in the chronological order in which the genes were discovered. There are variants that come together or splice in each family member, which are told apart from each other by a lowercase letter, for example Na^+ V1.1. a. [18, 19].

The sodium channels are formed by an alpha subunit, a simple polypeptide with a relative molecular mass of ~260,000 and are responsible for the selectivity and gate voltage. Some sodium channels have beta 1 and 2 subunits. These sodium ionophores are made up of four homologous domains; each of these four domains contains six transmembrane segments known as alpha-helices. This causes each sodium channel to cross the cell membrane 24 times. The center of this structure is the channel pore through which the Na^+ passes into the interior of the cell and also the LAs in their hydrophilic form on their way to be fixed in the internal pore of the sodium channel, where the voltage sensor is located. This voltage sensor is located in the fourth segment of each domain, where the LAs are fixed in the sixth segment of Domains 3 and 4. The voltage sensor has a very high positive charge, and these four domains are connected to each other by segments or hydrophilic bridges formed by amino acids that are located on the extracellular side of the membrane. The bridge that joins segments 5 and 6 of each domain is known as a pore handle and covers the pore of the channel to allow only the passage of Na^+. This channel structure is responsible for selectivity and is vulnerable to certain toxins that can inactivate the sodium channel, although another description mentions that the selectivity filter is given by a narrowing of the ionic pore located below its gate [19].

The gate of the ionic pore is the initial portion of the sodium channel on the outer side of the cell membrane, is made up of protein "walls" and has an aqueous cavity similar to an irregular cylinder, where the external vestibule is located, which contains the selectivity filter and the voltage sensor. The closure gate is located in the most distal portion of the sodium channel, on the intracellular side of the cell membrane. The sodium channel inlet measures about 1.2 nm and narrows to about 0.3 to 0.5 nm at the site where the selectivity filter is located, which consists of aspartic acid, glycine, lysine, and alanine. The exact mechanism of how these channels discriminate between different cations is not known [19].

Figure 2 shows a representation of a voltage-dependent sodium channel, which is in the lipid bilayer of the cell membrane. Its four domains (D1, D2, D3, and D4) are each made up of six segments (alpha helices) that cross the entire cell membrane, emphasizing segment 4, colored in black and corresponding to the voltage sensor, which has a positive charge. On the extracellular face of the cell membrane there are two types of structures that connect the six segments, the one marked with T between segments 5 and 6 of each domain represent the site where some toxins act. The FS selectivity filter in the initial portion of the ionic pore is shown. The site where LAs act is marked with an X. This site has been highly

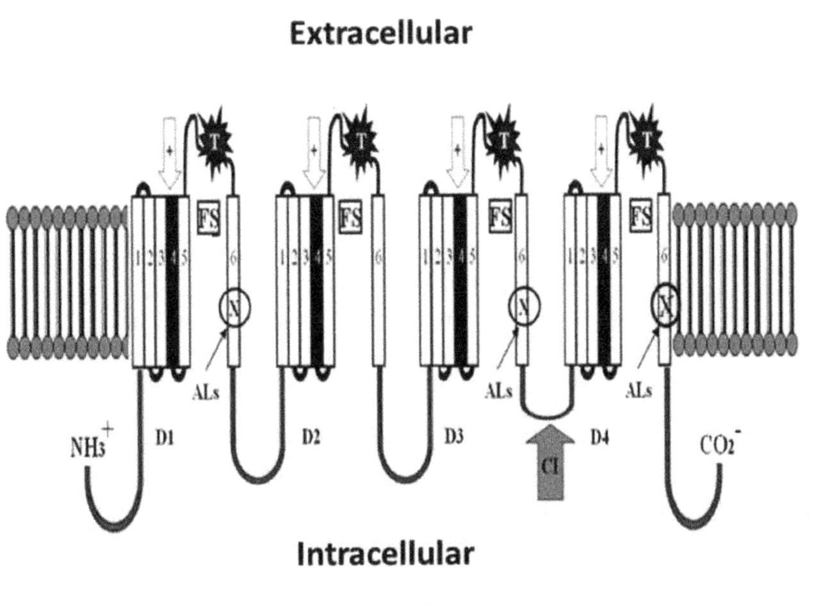

Figure 2.
Diagram of the voltage-dependent sodium channel with its 4 domains. Each domain has 6 helices that cross the cell membrane. The black stars located at the junctions of the helices 5 and 6 of each domain (pore handle) are the sites where cellular toxins (TTX) act. The sodium channel inactivation gate (IC) is located on the intracellular face between domain 3 and 4. The effector site of local anesthetics is located on helix 6 (or segment 6) of domains 3 and 4, although some schemes also draw it in domain 1.

controversial and is located in the final portion of the ionic pore near the intracellular surface of the membrane. The available information suggests that domains 3 and 4 appear to contain this point in segment 6, although some references also place it in segment 6 of Domain 1.

Among other tissues, sodium channels are located in excitable membranes such as the CNS membranes, peripheral nervous system, and the conduction system of the heart. During a nervous impulse, the cell goes through three different phases; it first depolarizes as the sodium channels open, then a refractory period follows until the cell finally repolarizes when the sodium channels become impermeable to Na^+. The intracytoplasmic junction between Domain III and Domain IV (CI in **Figure 2**) is responsible for this inactivation according to the "ball and chain" model.

4. Mechanism of action of LAs

As mentioned before, LAs inhibit the electrical impulse by selectively interfering with the function of voltage-dependent sodium channels by preventing the transport of Na^+ through the ionic pore of sodium ionophores, from outside to inside of the cells. When an electrical impulse reaches the excitable cell, the sodium channel opens for a millisecond and about 7000 Na^+ pass. A refractory period continues until the ionophores become impermeable to Na^+, and the membrane repolar-izes again and enters a phase of inactivation, which is due to the activation of the intracytoplasmic junction between Domain III and IV. Unlike the tetrodotoxin and saxitoxin that act outside the cell membrane, LAs are temporarily fixed to the alpha helices 6 of Domains 3 and 4, which alters the voltage sensor and closes the inactivation gate, which obstructs the sodium channel and results in blockage of the initial phase of the action potential [14, 21–23].

There are two ways by which LAs reach the internal gate of the sodium channel and reach their site of action;

a. It has been postulated that LAs in their neutral, lipophilic (hydrophobic, B) form easily enter the lipid cell membrane in free form and from there contribute to the closure of sodium channels by the expansion of the cell membrane. From this location, LAs also pass into the cellular interior where they ionize and transform into their charged form (hydrophilic, BH^+), which reaches the site where they interact (segment 6 of Domains 3 and 4) in the internal gate of the sodium channel.

b. LAs in their cationic or hydrophilic form (BH^+) enter the cell cytoplasm through the sodium channels when they are open and reach their site of action by closing the sodium channel [14, 20, 23, 24]. LAs have no effect on the resting phase or on the potential threshold, although they can prolong the refractory period and repolarization.

Figure 3 illustrates these two routes of arrival of LAs to their receptor site in segments 6 of Domains 3 and 4.

Another factor that determines the action of LAs is the impulse frequency, the basis of the modulated receptor hypothesis, which suggests that these drugs bind more closely to the receptor within the ionic gate of voltage-dependent sodium channels when these are in an open or inactive state, that is in the depolarization phase, that when they are in a resting state, at which time they are separated from them. LAs that bind and dissociate rapidly such as lidocaine are little affected by this phenomenon, which is not the case with molecules such as bupivacaine,

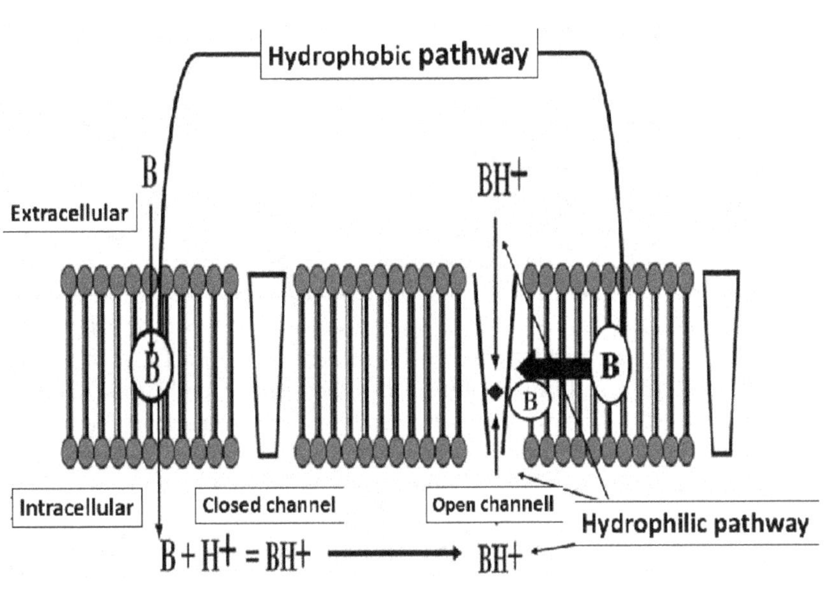

Figure 3.
Arrival pathways of LAs to the sodium channel. The hydrophobic pathway refers to the passage of LAs in their neutral (lipophilic) form that easily penetrate the cell membrane. Once in the cell membrane, the LA (B) expands it and by mechanical effect closes the sodium channel. This same neutral form of LA penetrates the cell, where it is protonized by incorporating an H+, (BH+ cationic form) that easily reaches the internal gate of the sodium channel and attaches to segment 6 of domains 3 and 4, activating the closure of the sodium channel. The hydrophilic pathway exemplified in the right portion of the scheme illustrates how a cationic LA (BH+) penetrates through and is fixed in the sodium channel.

ropivacaine, or etidocaine that are benefitted when the stimulation frequency is high, since it does not give time to recover to their resting state. This phenomenon explains the greater toxicity of some LAs [24, 25].

The affinity of LAs for the sodium channel is what determines their pharmacological action and also their toxic effects. The most important clinical outcome of these events at the level of voltage-dependent sodium channels and their interaction with LAs molecules are two results: regional anesthesia-analgesia and/or deleterious toxic effects.

5. Chemical structure of LAs

LAs are divided into two groups according to their chemical structure: the amino esters (cocaine, procaine, chloroprocaine, and tetracaine) and the amino amides (lidocaine, bupivacaine, mepivacaine, ropivacaine, and prilocaine). The typical molecule of a LA consists of three components: a) an aromatic lipophilic ring, usually benzene, b) an amphipathic intermediate chain of about 6 to 9 Å, and c) a terminal tertiary amine, hydrophilic, which is a base proton acceptor (H^+). The intermediate chain binds the basic amine with the aromatic ring and has an ester (CO)- or amide (CNH)-type bond. Each of these three parts of the LA formula contributes to different properties. The aromatic ring of the molecule improves the liposolubility of the compound that can be increased by aliphatic substitutions at certain sites (R). When the liposolubility of LAs is increased, its diffusion is increased through nerve structures (nerve sheaths and axonal membranes), which improves their anesthetic and toxic potency since a greater proportion of the drug enters the neural tissue and is fixed there with higher affinity. An example of this phenomenon is bupivacaine which has greater potency than lidocaine; the first is prepared at 0.5% (5 mg/mL) and the second at 2% (20 mg/mL). The terminal amine may exist in tertiary form (3 junctions) that is liposoluble and facilitates cell membrane penetration, or as a quaternary form (4 junctions) that is positively charged and makes the molecule water soluble, which makes it difficult to pass through the lipid membranes [11, 25].

As stated before, the aromatic ring determines the degree of lipoafinity of the LA, and the terminal amine acts as an *on-off switch,* allowing the LA to exist as either lipoafin or water soluble. Both the tertiary and quaternary forms play a very important role in the sequence of events that lead to nerve conduction blockage. The tertiary hydrophilic amine, which is kept charged to the physiological pH and gives it its condition of weak bases with a positive charge, is the part that will be fixed to the receptor in the sodium channel of the cell membrane to exert the pharmacological effect. The presence of an ester or amide group in the intermediate chain provides the basis for their classification and also determines the metabolism of these substances. LAs with ester binding are readily hydrolyzed in the plasma by cholinesterase; instead, those with an amide junction are biotransformed by liver microsomes via the microsomal system. **Figure 4** shows the elementary chemical structure of LAs.

If the size of the molecule of a LA is increased, its potency and duration of action increase but also its toxicity. There is a direct correlation between potency, duration of effect, lipophilic character, molecular size and toxicity. Chloroprocaine is the least toxic, followed by procaine, prilocaine, lidocaine, mepivacaine, etidocaine, ropivacaine, bupivacaine, tetracaine and dibucaine, with cocaine being the most toxic LA.

Another aspect of capital importance is the stereoisomerism that some LAs have. It refers to the existence of molecules with the same structural and molecular formula, but with different spatial orientation around a particular atom, the chiral center. It is like a reflection in a mirror, like placing one hand next to the other; they are the same but cannot be superimposed, they are mirror images. LAs of the pipeco-loxylidide family (mepivacaine, bupivacaine and ropivacaine), as well as etidocaine and prilocaine are chiral compounds, with an asymmetric carbon atom, which can exist in their enantiomeric form, such as mirror images. When the compound deflects the polarized light to the left it is an S-isomer (Sinus) or levo-isomer, if the light is rotated to the right it is an R-isomer (Rectus) or dextro-isomer. Although the S and R isomers have a similar pharmacological activity, the clinical importance of the isomerism is that the same drug can have different biological activity. For example, the S-enantiomers of amino-amide LAs produce greater vasoconstriction and have less systemic toxicity than D-isomer. The typical example of stereoisomerism is

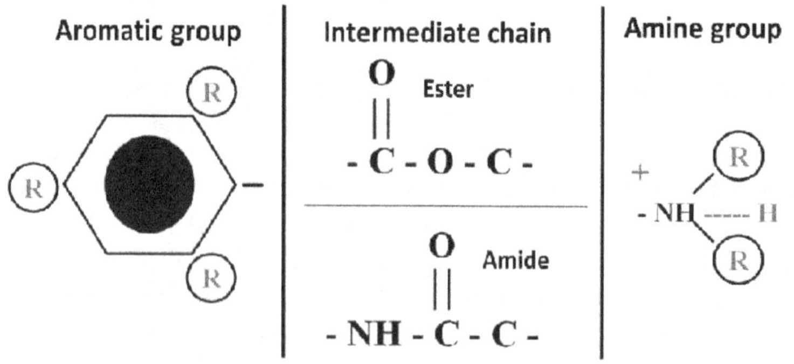

Figure 4.
Typical structural formula of a local anesthetic.

Amino ester	Amino amide
Cocaine	Dibucaine
Benzocaine	Lidocaine
Procaine	Mepivacaine
Tetracaine	Prilocaine
2-cloroprocaine	Bupivacaine
	Etidocaine
	Ropivacaine
	Levobupivacaine

Table 2.
Chemical classification of local anesthetics.

bupivacaine, which contains the dextro-isomer and levo-isomer. The mixture of both is known as racemic combination. Ropivacaine only has a L-isomer. Lidocaine and ametocaine are aquirales since they do not have stereoisomers. D-isomers have more affinity for sodium channels than L-isomers, this makes the former more toxic [26, 27]. **Table 2** shows the chemical classification of LAs.

6. Physical properties, activity, and potency

LAs are small molecules 220–350 Daltons weight, weak bases, poorly soluble and unstable in water, and therefore, they must be combined with a strong acid to obtain a stable salt that is soluble in water at pH 4.7. The solubility in water is directly related to the degree of ionization and inversely related to the fat solubility. In solution, LAs exist in two forms: basic, nonionized (B) and acidic, cationic, ionized (BH^+). The ratio between these two forms depends on the dissociation constant (Ka) of the conjugated acid and on the local concentration of H^+ ions. At a specific pH for each LA, the concentration of B is equal to that of BH^+. This pH is called pKa. The relationship can be expressed like this: pKa = pH-log (B) / (BH^+). At a pH of 7.40, the percentage of BH^+ form will be higher the higher the pKa. Diffusion of a LA is passive. In order to act they must contact the axon and for this they must pass through the epineurium, perineurium and endoneurium of the peripheral nerve, as well as the myelin layer in the myelinated fibers (lipid-rich structures), and finally cross the cell membrane to be in contact with the receptor site on sodium channels. The fat-soluble basic form B diffuses easily through the perineural structures and the axonal membrane; once inside the cell it is protonized and it is this ionized form that occupies the aforementioned receptor site [23, 25].

The minimum inhibitory concentration (MIC) is necessary to block the conduction of a nerve impulse along a nerve fiber within a certain period. The MIC is different for each LA and allows to differentiate them according to their potency. Several factors can determine the Cm: the size of the fibers (higher MIC for the thicker ones), the pH (lower MIC at higher pH), calcium concentration (higher MIC at higher calcium concentration), and frequency of nerve stimulation (smaller MIC at higher frequency).

Due to the characteristics of the nerve fibers, LAs first block the unmyelinated fibers (C fibers, which correspond to the postganglionic neurons of the autonomic nervous system), those of nociceptive conduction (analgesia), proprioceptive, tactile sensitivity, and pressure (anesthesia), and finally, the motor fibers (motor block).

The latency period of a nerve block is not linked to the potency of the LA, but seems to depend on its lipid solubility and pKa, that is, on the pH in which 50% of the molecules are in ionized form and 50% in nonionized form. The higher the pKa, the greater the latency time of a LA. On the other hand, the decrease in tissue pH can lengthen the latency time by limiting the formation of free base; instead, carbonation of a LA solution shortens its latency time. Alkalinization has also been shown to produce a better sensory and motor quality nerve block and may increase diffusion of block height. By alkalinizing LAs, their ionization increases and the percentage of fat solubility of the LA increases, facilitating its diffu-sion through the lipid structures of the nerves, including the axonal membrane. The addition of 1 mL of sodium bicarbonate to 10 mL of lidocaine improves the onset of extradural or peripheral block for 3–5 min, also increasing its duration of action.

With the exception of cocaine and ropivacaine, LAs produce vasodilation. Adding a vasoconstrictor to LAs is an acceptable routine since two basic actions were demonstrated: increased duration of action and decreased absorption. It also increases the intensity of sensory and motor block in neuroaxial anesthesia. Epinephrine was one of the first drugs to be injected into the subarachnoid space: however, its use was not widespread as the initial results were disappointing. The local vasoconstriction produced by adrenaline favors the decrease in the absorp-tion of LAs, which favor a longer interaction, in addition to decreasing blood concentrations levels and thus their potential for systemic toxicity. On the other hand, epinephrine has an effect on $alpha_2$ receptors in the CNS, especially in the spinal cord, which could be another factor for the improvement it has in neuroaxial blocks. Higher concentrations of adrenaline 2: 000,000 (5 μg/mL) do not offer major advantages in terms of prolonging anesthesia or reducing plasma concentra-tions. Never use solutions with adrenaline to infiltrate areas with terminal arterial circulation such as the fingers, the penis, the nasal tip, or other areas with critical arterial circulation, since it may promote ischemia and local necrosis.

	Physico-chemical characteristics				Relative potency in different blocks		
Anesthetic	**pKa**	**Ionized % at pH 7.4**	**Partition coefficient**	**% protein binding**	**Epidural**	**Spinal**	**Peripheral nerve**
• Bupivacaine	8.1	83	3420	95	4	9.6	3.6
• Levobupivacaine	8.1	83	3420	97	4	9.6	3.6
• Etidocaine	7.7	66	7317	94	2	6.7	0.7
• Lidocaine	7.9	76	366	64	1	1	1
• Mepivacaine	7.6	61	130	77	1	1	2.6
• Prilocaine	7.9	76	129	55	1	¿	0.8
• Ropivacaine	8.1	83	775	94	4	4.8	3.6
• Chloroprocaine	8.7	95	810	—	0.5	—	—
• Procaine	8.9	97	100	6	—	—	—
• Tetracaine	8.5	93	5822	94	—	—	—

**Modified from Salinas FV, Liu SL, Schlz AM. Analgesics. Ion channel ligands/sodium channels blockers/local anesthetics. Chapter 30. In: Evers AS, Maze M. Editors. Anesthetic pharmacology. Physiologic principles and clinical practice. Editorial Churchill-Livingstone. Philadelphia, USA. 2004 pag 507–537.*

Table 3.
*Physical and chemical characteristics and relative potency of some local anesthetics **

The phenomenon of tachyphylaxis or acute tolerance to LAs is characterized by a decreased effectiveness of a LA with repeated administration of the same dose. Its prevalence and mechanisms have not been well defined. This phenomenon occurs with different anesthetics, with different application techniques, and has been seen to develop more frequently when redosing is administered after the analgesic effect of the previous dose has ended [28, 29]. It has been mentioned that it could be due to a progressive acidification of the injection site that is established more rapidly with weak pKa LAs. A central mechanism through spinal cord sensitization that could be avoided by pretreatment with NMDA or nitric oxide antagonists has also been described [29–31].

The potency of LAs refers to the sensitivity of the neural tissue to the different LAs. This potency increases with increasing affinity for lipids. The binding capacity of LAs to the phospholipid membrane as a result of the physicochemical characteristics and the interaction in vivo is directly related to their potency. Other factors affecting the potency of a LA include: hydrogen ion balance, fiber size, type, and myelination, vasodilator/vasoconstrictive properties (affects vascular absorption rate), frequency of nerve stimulation, tissue pH, and electrolyte concentrations (hypokalemia and hypercalcemia antagonize the block).

Table 3 shows some physical and chemical characteristics as well as the relative potency of some frequently used LAs.

7. Pharmacokinetics

The anesthetic and analgesic results of the injection of a LA in the vicinity of the neural tissue depend on the factors that have already been described. Plasma levels are affected by the injection site, the degree of absorption, its tissue distribution, its metabolism, and elimination, among other factors that have already been discussed.

7.1 Absorption

The quantity of LA that is absorbed from its application site and reaches the bloodstream is an important toxicity and elimination factor. LAs with poor absorption are safer. The absorption depends, on one hand, on the characteristics of the tissue; it increases in very vascularized territories and diminishes in fatty tissue. The plasma concentration depends on the total dose administered rather than the concentration, for most LAs there is a linear relationship between total dose and blood concentration [32]. On the other hand, the physicochemical characteristics also modulate the absorption of the drug, for example, the most lipophilic LAs and with greater affinity for proteins will be absorbed more slowly than those with less affinity for fatty tissue. Remember that the most lipophilic are also the most potent LAs. The decrease in absorption when adrenaline is added is more effective for LAs of short action and lower potency [33, 34]. With this, gradual absorption is achieved, the duration of action is prolonged and plasma levels are decreased as well as hemorrhage in the operative field.

7.2 Distribution

It depends on the physicochemical characteristics of each LA, its coefficient of solubility and plasma protein binding. A higher coefficient of solubility together with a lower degree of protein binding favors an easier distribution in peripheral tissues and a lower plasma concentration. LAs cross the blood-brain and placental barriers by simple diffusion; this diffusion is greater when the ability to bind to plasma proteins is lower. Variable levels bind to plasma proteins in the bloodstream, particularly alpha-1- glycoprotein acid. This protein-binding property correlates with its affinity for sodium channels and predicts the duration of neural blockage. Bupivacaine has the highest percentage of protein binding and is therefore the LA with the longest duration of action.

7.3 Metabolism and elimination

LAs differ in their metabolism according to their chemical structure; those with ester-type binding (except cocaine) are rapidly hydrolyzed by plasma esterases, so the duration of their action increases with the deficit of this enzyme or the presence of atypical cholinesterase. Cocaine is hydrolyzed in the liver. The metabolites of the esters are eliminated by the kidney.

Amide LAs are metabolized in the liver. This is a slow process, which favors a longer half-life than esters and can accumulate when repeated doses or infusions are administered. Liver function interferes with the elimination of these drugs; extrac-tion, perfusion and hepatic metabolism are definitive factors, as it is the degree of protein binding. The metabolites and the nonmetabolized drug are eliminated by urine and a small amount by feces. Elimination is favored by an acid urinary pH. Prilocaine is metabolized outside the liver.

The fact that amino ester-type LAs are rapidly metabolized favors that they remain in the blood for a short period of time, including placental blood and the fetus. Those of the amino-amide type pass more easily to the fetus, especially those with lower affinity to plasma proteins such as lidocaine, which can result in fetal toxicity. When the fetus has been compromised by any pathology and is acidotic, more ionization of the LA that has passed into its fetal circulation is favored. In this way the LA will remain longer in the fetus with the possibility of severe toxicity. In the newborn, this toxicity can be accentuated since there is no hepatocellular maturity.

8. Clinical aspects

LAs are one of the most commonly used drugs in clinical anesthesia; either by the neuroaxial route, in the vicinity of nerves and nerve plexuses, subcutaneous, transcutaneous, trans mucosal, intraarticular, and intravenously. The introduction of levoisomeric LAs, the evolution of regional anesthesia techniques with the recommendations of epidural test dose with a vasoactive marker, fractional peridural doses, low and intrathecal minidose, multiple injections with low volumes for nerve plexuses blocks, the use of nerve stimulator, guides with ultrasound and other imaging techniques, as well as the addition of adjuvant drugs such as opioids, $alpha_2$ agonists, NMDA receptor antagonists, among others have done regional anesthesia safer. **Tables 4** and **5** categorize the most important formulas and characteristics of LAs most commonly used in anesthesiology.

8.1 Amino ester LAs

The precursor of this group is cocaine. They are characterized by being metabolized by plasmatic esterases, short half-life and being related to allergic reactions. The most commonly used are procaine, chloroprocaine, and tetracaine. Benzocaine has no use in regional anesthesia.

Formulae	Important features
Cocaine 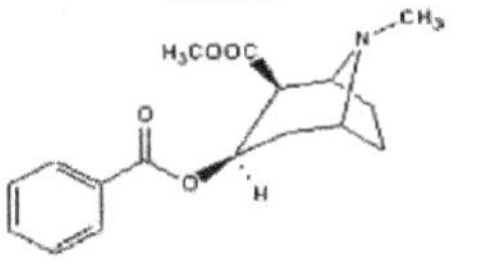	In addition to blocking the impulse of axonal conduction, it has the ability to inhibit neurotransmitter recapture in adrenergic neuronal endings, which means accumulation of norepinephrine in sympathetic synapses inducing vasoconstriction and cardiac stimulation. In the CNS, the accumulation of norepinephrine causes stimulation; however, some adrenergic neurotransmitters in the CNS are inhibited, in particular the dopamine recapture resulting in euphoria and abuse potential. Its clinical utility is limited to topical anesthesia, in solutions 4 and 10%. Due to its vasoconstrictor action, it has been used in anesthesia of the nasal mucosa to facilitate nasotracheal intubation.
Procaine 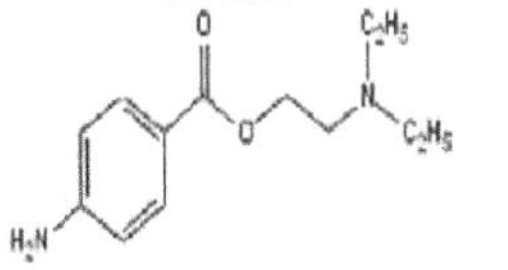	It has been used at 0.5, 1, 2, 5, and 10% for infiltration, peripheral, and spinal blocks. Procaine is of special interest in dentistry in 2% solution with 1:50,000 adrenaline. The allergic capacity of para-aminobenzoic acid (PABA) limits its clinical utility. The maximum doses are 750 mg with adrenaline and 500 mg without vasoconstrictor. It has been used by the subarachnoid route in increasing concentrations to establish the differential diagnosis in some painful syndromes.
Chloroprocaine 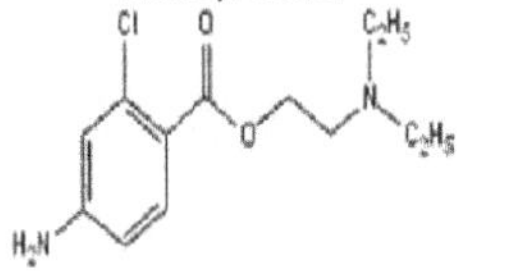	It is used in solutions 1, 2, and 3% for infiltration, peripheral blockages, and epidural anesthesia. Due to its brief time of action, it is very useful in peridural block in cesarean section. The neurotoxicity observed after intrathecal injection, attributed to the sodium bisulfite in the solution, has limited the wide use caused by its low systemic toxicity. The maximum recommended doses are 800 mg with adrenaline and 600 mg without it. There are studies that favor intrathecal injection of chloroprocaine without methylparaben.
Benzocaine 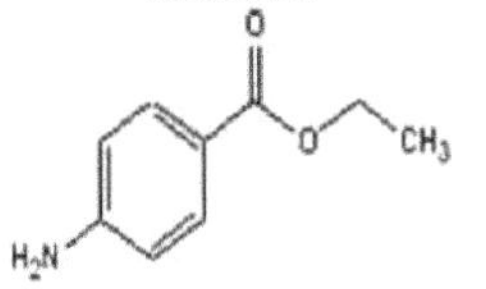	Useful in topical anesthesia in the form of ointment, chewable tablets, and gel. It is poorly soluble and remains in the place of its application. It is not used in regional anesthesia.
Tetracaine 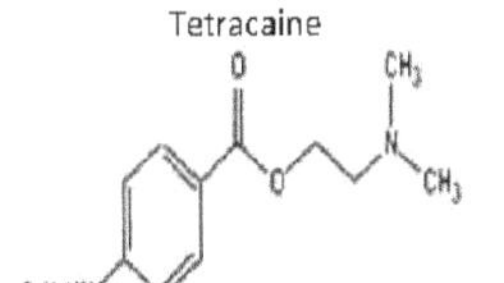	It has pKa of 8.46, plasma protein binding of 75.6% and N-heptane / water partition coefficient of 4.1. Despite its high systemic toxicity, it has been used in subarachnoid anesthesia in hyperbaric solutions 1 and 2% due to its high efficacy. Its latency is not very long, and the duration of the anesthetic effect is 2 to 3 hours, because its plasma hydrolysis is quite slow. Its use has been replaced by levoisomeric anesthetics.

Table 4.
Formulae and characteristics of amino ester local anesthetics.

8.2 Amino amide LAs

They are the most used in regional anesthesia. Lidocaine is the typical anesthetic with which almost all new drugs in this group have been compared. Even when they have differences such as latency time, duration, and toxicity they have a mechanism of action common to all LAs. They can be divided into two large groups: those of short duration and those of long duration.

Slow long-release of LAs are recent advances that have improved the management of postoperative pain. Nanostructured carriers, such as liposomes and polymers, facilitate the prolonged release of LAs. Exparel® was the first approved liposomal LA to combine racemic bupivacaine with liposomes. Polymersomes have advances over liposomes with complementary profiles, inspiring the emergence of hybrid carriers [35, 36]. Also, multilamellar vesicles with ropivacaine are being investigated to prolong its analgesic effect [37].

Formulae	Most important features
Lidocaine 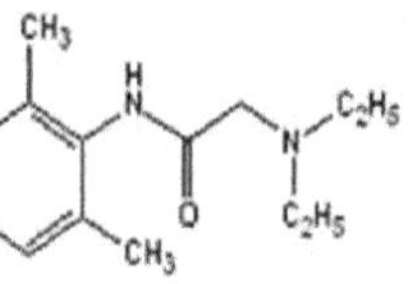	It is the prototype in this group. After intravenous administration, the apparent volume of distribution is 92 L. Its alpha half-life is 8.3 min, its beta half-life is 108 min, and its plasma clearance 0.77 L/min. Its metabolism is hepatic, with an extraction coefficient of 0.7. The addition of adrenaline decreases its passage to the blood by 30%. It has a duration of action that varies from 2 to 3 hours depending on the site of administration and the addition of adrenaline. The toxic neurological manifestations of lidocaine are directly proportional to plasma levels. If these are low (0.5 to 4 mg / mL); lidocaine is anticonvulsant, at higher levels (8 mg/mL) it can cause seizures. In the heart, lidocaine blocks sodium channels, decreasing contraction (V max), the amplitude and duration of the action potential, and increases the duration of the refractory period. These effects are only observed with elevated plasma levels. The action on the heart can be summarized in: dose automatism: below 5 mg/mL, onset of sinus bradycardia; conduction: no modification (atrioventricular or intraventricular) at usual doses; contractility: decrease, but only at doses that cause frank toxicity. At low plasma levels, lidocaine increases vascular tone; at higher levels vasodilation occurs. Direct intravascular injection does not produce obvious hemodynamic alterations as long as the dose is not greater than 3 mg/kg. From 4 to 8 mg/kg, cardiovascular depression occurs, which is dangerous if the dose is greater than 8 mg/kg. If there is heart failure, the toxicity threshold decreases.
Prilocaine 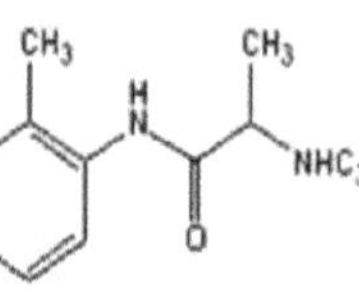	Its pharmacokinetic properties are similar to those of lidocaine, although it is less vasodilator. It is used in infiltration for peripheral nerve and in epidural anesthesia. The usual concentrations range between 0.5 and 2%. It is 40 times less toxic than lidocaine. An ideal use is intravenous regional anesthesia. A potential risk is the appearance of methemoglobinemia (total doses greater than 500 to 600 mg), so its use in obstetrics is restricted or contraindicated.
Articaine 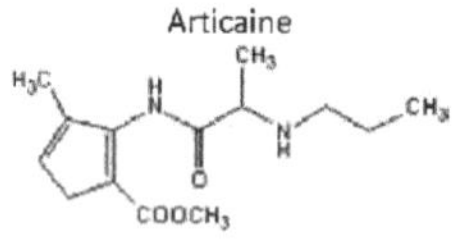	First approved in Germany in 1976, in Canada in 1982 and in 2000 by the FDA. It has a thiophene group, an ester group and also an amide group. It has been classified in the amide group by its intermediate chain and because it is metabolized in the liver. However, its ester portion allows it to be degraded by plasma pseudocholinesterase. The mean maximum plasma drug concentration is about 400 μg/L for articaine with epinephrine 1:200,000 and 580 μg/L without epinephrine. The elimination half-time is approximately 20 min. The rapid breakdown to the inactive metabolite articainic acid is related to a very low systemic toxicity and consequently to the possibility of repeated injections. It has been associated with paresis and long-lasting paraesthesia, which are more frequent than those produced by lidocaine. It is commonly used in dentistry.
Mepivacaine 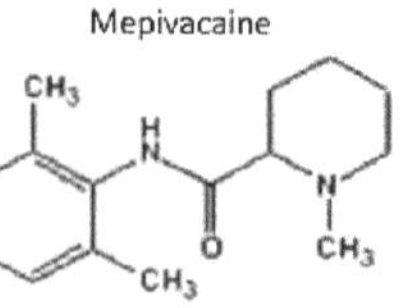	Its molecular formula is C15H22N2O-HCL, soluble in water and very resistant to acid and alkaline hydrolysis. It is available in concentrations of 1%, 1.5% and 2%. The latency and duration of action are similar to those of prilocaine and its potency resembles lidocaine. Useful concentrations range between 0.5 and 2%. It diffuses well through tissues, which allows favorable blocking despite a less optimal needle placement. It produces an intense motor block. It is used to perform infiltration, peridural and spinal anesthesia (with a lower incidence of neurological alterations than lidocaine). Its use is not advised in obstetrics based on its prolonged metabolism in the fetus and in the newborn. It is recommended for peripheral nerve blocks in certain conditions: patients with cardiac risk or with drugs that potentiate toxicity. Adrenaline decreases the absorption of mepivacaine but does not prolong its duration of action.

Formulae	Most important features
Etidocaine 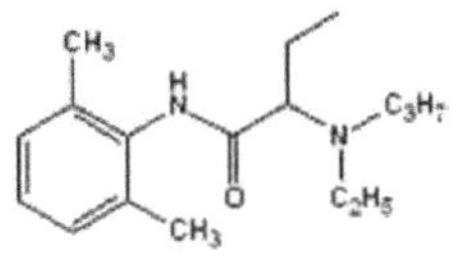	It is more fat-soluble and has a higher degree of affinity to plasma proteins than lidocaine, has a short latency and longer duration. Epidural route is used at 0.5 to 1%. It produces greater motor blockage than sensitive which makes it useful in abdominal surgery, its use in obstetric analgesia anesthesia is not advised. Its beta half-life is 2.5 hours, and care should be taken in liver disorders because of the prolonged action.
Bupivacaine 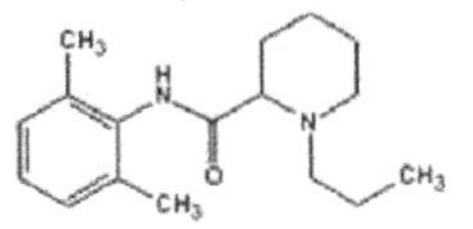	It is a racemic mixture, long-acting drug that produces a differential sensory-motor block at low concentrations. It has a limited placental transfer, so it is widely used in obstetrics in concentrations of up to 0.5%. Higher concentrations are not recommended in obstetrics. It is the LA with greater cardio and neuro toxicity and greater difficulty in resuscitation since it has a great affinity for voltage-dependent sodium channels. However, after lidocaine, it is the most used. It is widely used in pain clinic.
Levobupivacaine 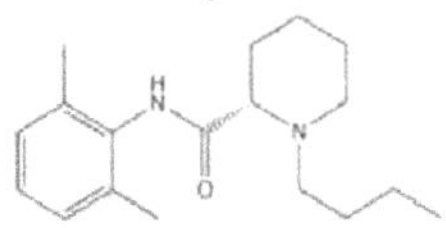	It is bupivacaine levoisomer. It has pharmacological properties similar to bupivacaine but less toxicity. Its toxicity depends on the route of administration and the dose, its pharmacokinetic is similar to bupivacaine and its plasma peak is 30 min after epidural administration, with an alpha-glycoprotein and albumin binding greater than 97% at concentrations of 0.1 at 1 ug/mL. It is metabolized in the liver and the kidney does not seem to intervene in its elimination. Produces differential blockade similar to bupivacaine, which depends on the dose and concentration, which will be less than 0.25% such as 0.0625 and 0.125% for epidural analgesia, and 0.5% to 0.75% for neuroaxial anesthesia and peripheral nerve blocks.
Ropivacaine 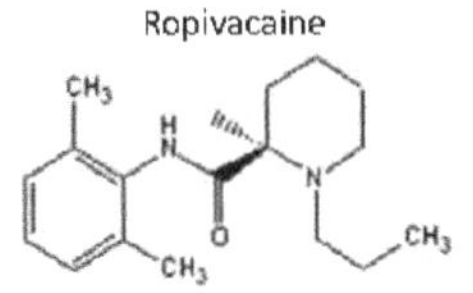	The first levoisomeric LA for clinical use. The plasma alpha glycoprotein binding is 95%, with a pKa of 8.1 and a partition coefficient of 141. Due to its low absorption, it has a longer elimination half-life and its pharmacokinetic has a linear proportional to the dose, with a volume of distribution of 47 liters. Like bupivacaine, it has a greater effect on C fibers than A, which produces a sensory rather than motor block. The clinical experience is excellent in neuroaxial anesthesia and peripheral nerve blocks. It is of great value by epidural route (obstetrics), and in postoperative analgesia. It is characterized by a block of greater latency and long duration. Less analgesic potency than bupivacaine and levobupivacaine. It is less cardiotoxic and neurotoxic than bupivacaine with a better response to resuscitation. Usefull in pain clinic.

Table 5.
Formulae and characteristics of local amino-amide type anesthetics.

8.3 There are 3 LAs: articaine, sameridine, and centbucridine, which due to their special physico-chemical characteristics deserve a brief description

8.3.1 Articaine

It is a short-acting LA with intermediate potency. It has been included in the amide group, but it contains an additional ester group that is quickly hydrolyzed by esterases, a chemical characteristic that accelerates its metabolism. The plasma protein binding rate of articaine and articainic acid is 70%. I.V. articaine 80 mg does not produce toxic effects in healthy individuals. It has been used neuraxially, ocularly, intravenously, and in regional blocks. It is suitable and safe for procedures requiring a short duration of action in which a fast onset of anesthesia is desired, e.g., dental procedures and ambulatory spinal anesthesia. Its most frequent use is in dentistry, where it has demonstrated efficacy and safety. Complete anesthesia is achieved in 90% of cases, using articaine 4% 60–80 mg with epinephrine 1: 200,000. It diffuses well through soft tissue and bone; concentration in the alveolus of a tooth in the upper jaw after extraction was about 100 times higher than that in systemic circulation. In comparative clinical trials, its effects were not gener-ally significantly different from those of other short-acting LAs like lidocaine, prilocaine, and chloroprocaine. There is no conclusive evidence demonstrating above average neurotoxicity, although cases of frequent persistent paresthesia after articaine use have been described [38–41]. Saralaya et al. compared 4% articaine with 1:100,000 epinephrine versus 2% lidocaine with 1: 100,000 epinephrine in 50 patients operated on the third molar. These authors found that the mean onset time for articaine and lidocaine was 3.16 ± 0.55 and 3.2 ± 0.48 min, respectively. Postoperative analgesia was longer in the articaine group and its duration of action was 289.04 ± 40 and 361.88 ± 40 min, respectively, compared to lidocaine, which is 144.2 ± 12 and 197.44 ± 25 min, respectively. These authors recommend articaine since it was more potent and with a longer duration of action with better postopera-tive analgesia and could be considered as an alternative to lidocaine [42]. Even in the presence of pulpitis, articaine proved to be more effective than lidocaine in patients undergoing root canal treatment [43]. There is no information available on the use of articaine during lactation, so its use is not entirely recommended yet.

8.3.2 Sameridine

This drug has mixed characteristics: LA and μ-opioid partial agonist. It is structurally similar to meperidine. It is a compound that is still under investigation (N-ethyl-1-hexyl-N-methyl-4-phenyl-4-piperidine carboxyamide hydrochloride) mainly for spinal anesthesia. Liver hydroxylation is the primary metabolic pathway, and no local neurotoxicity has been found in animal studies. Its effect on respiration is directly related to plasma levels. In healthy volunteers [44] 25 mg vs. intrathe-cal bupivacaine 15 mg has similar effects on resting ventilation. The ventilatory response to hypoxia and hypercarbia were found to be discreetly diminished in the group treated with sameridine. Intravenous doses of 0.73 mg/kg depress the ventilatory response to hypercarbia [45]. The clinical doses of 150 μg/kg have no significant effects on ventilation [46]. Intrathecal doses of 15–25 mg of sameridine are sufficient for inguinal and orthopedic surgery, respectively. Doses of 5–20 mg are comparable with 100 mg of intrathecal lidocaine. The advantage is that sameri-dine produces residual analgesia and reduces the need for opioids in the first hours of the postoperative period [7, 8], so it could have a role in the management of postoperative pain.

8.3.3 Centbucridine

It is a nonester, nonamide LA, chemically known as 4-N-butylamino-1,2,3,4-tetrahydroacridine hydrochloride. It is a quinolone derivative drug with LA effects synthesized in 1982 by Patnaik et al. [47–49]. It is 5 to 8 times more potent than lidocaine, while its LD50 is one fourth that of lidocaine. It has vasoconstrictor and antihistamine effects, rapid onset of action (1–3 min), duration of action is prolonged (2.5 hours), and no events of cardiotoxicity or neurotoxicity have been reported. Centbucridine has been investigated for infiltration, conjunctival sur-face, in peripheral nerves, neuroaxial anesthesia, intravenous regional anesthesia; however, the majority of studies are in dental anesthesia [9, 50–52]. Most studies compare 0.5% centbucridine vs. 2% lidocaine, with similar anesthetic results, although some have found longer anesthetic duration in patients who were treated with centbucridine [51, 53]. Centbucridine can be used with confidence in dental patients who cannot tolerate other LAs or when epinephrine is contraindicated.

8.4 Maximum dose of LAs

Another clinical aspect of capital interest is the maximum doses of each LA. The maximum recommended doses have been established arbitrarily by the pharmaceutical industry [54] and vary according to the route of administration, the type of anesthetic, with or without vasoconstrictors, as well as the type of patient and surgery. **Table 6** shows the maximum recommended doses for the most com-monly used LAs, without these doses having been established by studies conducted specifically to determine the safest and most effective amounts of each. Note the variants, sometimes with important ranges; 200 mg of lidocaine is recommended in Europe, while in the United States this dose reaches 300 mg when epinephrine is not used. Notwithstanding these differences, it is advisable to stay below the maximum recommended dosage range to avoid undesirable toxic effects.

8.5 Adequate anesthetic technique

Regional anesthesia techniques are important not only in the expected results, but to reduce undesirable side effects of LAs. It is known that spinal anesthesia produces lower plasma concentrations of LAs, unlike interpleural injection that in theory results in higher concentrations, and therefore, could be the procedure that produces more toxic events. However, this situation is hypothetical, since toxic events occur more frequently in peripheral blockages and peridural injections. For different types of nerve blocks, the same total injected dose produces different blood concentrations for mepivacaine, lidocaine, prilocaine and etidocaine, with the intercostal block being the one that produces the highest blood absorption, followed by injections in the peridural space. Plexus nerve blocks and subcutaneous injection are those that have a lower degree of absorption of LAs.

8.6 Undesirable side effects

The anesthetic and analgesic effects of LAs and their toxicity originate in the same mechanism of action; its interaction in the sodium channels. The therapeutic efficacy and safety of LAs has been proven from the moment of their discovery and it was precisely the deleterious effects that prompted the search for safer agents.

Maximum dose of lidocaine: Without epinephrine 200 mg (in Europe), 300 mg (in USA) With epinephrine (5 μg/mL) 500 mg in both regions
Maximum dose of PPX anesthetics: Bupivacaine 150–175 mg Levobupivacaine 150 mg Ropivacaine 200–300 mg
Epinephrine 1: 200,000 reduces absorption of subcutaneous lidocaine by 50%, intercostal, epidural and brachial by 20–30%

Table 6.
Maximum dose of LAs [54].

In 1905 Braun mentioned the characteristics that a new LA should have: *In addition to producing local anesthesia, any new drug in this abundant group should have the following properties: be less toxic than the standard available, it should not irritate or damage tissues, it must be soluble in water, and stable in solution, it must be able to mix with adrenaline, and must be rapidly absorbed into the cell membrane* [55]. More than a century of these recommendations have passed, and we still use LAs that do not meet these characteristics. LAs are used with an acceptable safety margin, without being the ideal drug. The following paragraphs briefly describe the most interesting side effects due to their magnitude and frequency. For more information on toxicity read chapter 10 of this book.

8.6.1 Toxicity

The history of LAs toxicity began at the end of the 19th century, when clinicians of that time realized the deleterious effects of cocaine and began the search for better drugs. Albright's editorial in 1979 [13] commented on six deaths due to cardiovascular collapse after the administration of bupivacaine or etidocaine whipped up this investigation in such a rapid way that currently there are safer drugs. The most important systemic toxic reactions are on CNS and the cardiovascular system. The CNS is affected with lower plasma concentrations than those that cause cardiovascular toxicity and is manifested by alterations in cognition, seizures, and coma. Arrhythmias with or without cardiovascular collapse of difficult management and death occur in the cardiovascular system. The incidence of systemic toxicity has been reduced to 0.01%, with regional blockages being the most associated with these events (7.5/10,000). The current use of ultrasound-guided nerve blocks is likely to reduce these statistics. Toxic effects can be grouped into two large groups:

1. Toxic reactions to:
   a. Systemic and local
   b. Not related to the LAs
2. Allergic reactions
   a. To the LA
   b. To conservatives or antioxidants

Events due to toxicity still occur in expert hands and are more related to the type of block and the dose injected. Various factors have been described:

- Potency of the LA. The greater the fat solubility, the greater potency and more possibility of cardio and neuro toxicity.
- Isomerism. LAs that contain a dextroisomer are more toxic than levoisomers. The former have been shown to have a higher affinity for the effector site of sodium channels.
- Total administered dose (plasma concentration). Toxicity is related to plasmatic concentration of AL, and this depends directly on the total administered dose. Epidural blocks and tumescent subcutaneous infiltrations use the highest doses of LAs and have been linked to toxic events.

- Injection site. In general terms, the blood absorption of LAs varies according to the injection site, although it is modified by factors such as the type of anesthetic injected, the addition of vasoconstrictors, and the speed and frequency of injec-tion. The interpleural route favors high absorptions due to the large injection surface and its vascularity. However, this route has not been more frequently related to systemic toxicity, perhaps due to the lung capacity to fix and eliminate the concentration of LA up to ~40%. Spinal administration does not produce systemic toxicity from small doses and decreased vascularity. Injections close to the brain (facial, nasal, oral, neck) have larger possibility of neurological systemic toxicity, either by direct intra-arterial injection or by retrograde flow that transports small doses of the LA directly to the brain tissue than induces seizures and coma [56].

- Patient's health/ASA. Factors such as age, liver and kidney dysfunction, hypoxemia, acidosis, pregnancy, and pharmacological interactions (cytochrome P450 inhibitors) modify the possibility of systemic toxicity.

In the ester group, cocaine remains the most toxic LA, and procaine and chloroprocaine are the least potent and least toxic potency, not only in the ester group, but among all known LAs. In the amino-amide group racemic bupivacaine, etidocaine, and mepivacaine are more toxic than levobupivacaine and ropivacaine. Lidocaine and prilocaine are the least toxic in this group.

Cardiotoxicity. The toxic effects of LAs on the cardiovascular system are divided into two groups; the physiological changes that are generated with some regional anesthesia techniques and the effects that derive from the actions of these drugs on sodium, potassium, calcium channels, and beta myocardial receptors. These side effects on the cardiovascular system can be explained by the following four mechanisms:

1. Regional effect due to the blockage of sympathetic preganglionic fibers secondary to the neuroaxial injection of the LA.

2. A direct cardio depressant/arrhythmogenic effect due to sudden and elevated plasma concentrations of local anesthetic by intravascular injection or exaggerated absorption from the injection site.

3. Cardio depressant effect mediated through the CNS.

4. Systemic absorption of toxic dose can cause spinal depression and secondary circulatory collapse.

8.6.2 Neurotoxicity

The toxicity of LAs on the nervous system manifests itself in two areas; those that are triggered by high blood concentrations and are due to their action on sodium channels in the CNS, and those that are caused by the direct application of the anesthetic on or in the vicinity of neural structures, especially the injection of lidocaine in the subarachnoid space.

8.6.3 Myotoxicity

It is well known that continuous perineural injection and direct intramuscular injection of LAs have toxic effects on the striated muscle causing inflammatory changes. These drugs act on external cell membranes and on the membranes of intracytoplasmic organelles, especially on the double mitochondrial membrane. Bupivacaine produces alterations in active intracellular oxidative metabolism by depolarizing the mitochondrial membrane and oxidation of the pyridine nucleo-tide. This results in the opening of permeability transition pore (PTP), a type of channel located in intracellular membranes that plays an important role in various forms of cell death. Injury mechanisms involved early and late abnormalities to cytoplasmic calcium (Ca^{2+}) homeostasis by the sarcoplasmic reticulum Ca^{2+} ATPase and cytochrome C release. All of these alterations were dependent on bupivacaine concentration and were only found in voluntary striated muscle mitochondria, while mitochondria from esophageal muscle were resistant to bupivacaine [57]. In rabbits, continuous axillary block with placebo vs. 0.25% bupivacaine, at 24 hours neutrophilic infiltration was found in the placebo group, while the group receiv-ing bupivacaine had a large amount of eosinophils. One week later, lymphocytes, plasma cells, macrophages and fibroblasts were found with data of muscle regenera-tion [58]. Zink et al. [59] compared bupivacaine vs. ropivacaine and demonstrated that the former induced necrosis and apoptosis of muscle fibers, while the latter produced less severe changes in porcine skeletal muscle. These same researchers [60] confirmed their initial results that bupivacaine 0.5% is more myotoxic than ropivacaine 0.75%, by inducing irreversible myonecrosis with calcium deposits, scar formation, and muscle regeneration. The incidence of myotoxicity in ophthal-mic studies was 0.77%. Inflammatory changes within a few days after exposure marked the onset of myotoxicity, and muscle degeneration continued within the first week after exposure. Recovery time in human muscles ranged from 4 days to 1 year. None partial and complete recovery was observed in 61% and 38% of patients, respectively [61]. All LAs that have been studied have a similar myotoxic potential in terms of the tissue alterations produced, but they differ in the intensity of these lesions. Bupivacaine and chloroprocaine are the most toxic and procaine and tetracaine are the ones that produce minor alterations.

8.6.4 Allergies

True allergies to LAs are rare and generally occur more with ester-type, although allergies have been reported with amino-amide LAs, including new levoisomeric anesthetics [62]. These allergies have a highly variable frequency that ranges from 1: 350 to 1:20,000 and fortunately most are trivial, although occasionally they are factors of significant morbidity and mortality. The incidence of true IgE-mediated LA allergy remains unclear and is presumed to be as low as 0.7–1%. On some occasions these reactions have been attributed to preservatives (methylparaben) or antioxidants (bisulfites) that are contained in some commercial presentations [63, 64]. When someone is reactive to a LA, they will be allergic to it for the rest of their life due to the response of mast cells that release chemical mediators that are responsible for the clinical responses in each patient. These mediators include histamine, leukotrienes, chemotactic substances, lysosomal enzymes, prostaglan-dins, kinins, and platelet activating factors that facilitate capillary permeation with plasma leakage in the surrounding area. The manifestations of true allergy range from mild to severe and sometimes are deadly. The faster the clinical manifesta-tions occur, the more severe the reaction. The most frequent expression is contact dermatitis, but they can also manifest as urticaria, rash, rhinitis, bronchial spasm, angioneurotic edema, tachycardia, and hypotension and lead to anaphylactic shock. Immunoglobulin E-mediated anaphylaxis can induce respiratory failure and cardiopulmonary collapse. The treatment of true allergies to LAs depends on their severity; mild or moderate reactions disappear spontaneously. In severe reactions it is recommended to use steroids, H1 blockers, antihistamines, or epinephrine. When there is a probable or proven history of allergy to LAs, caution should be exercised: if allergy to an ester compound is found, it should be switched to an amino-amide anesthetic, preferably one without methyl paraben or metabisulfite. When the allergy is to an amino-amide anesthetic, it is advisable to change to another anes-thetic from the same group.

8.6.5 Methemoglobinemia

Prilocaine is metabolized to O-toluidine which can cause methemoglobinemia in susceptible individuals, especially when more than 500 mg is used. In pregnant women, this problem is even more critical since fetal blood poorly reduces methemoglobin. Management is with 1–5 mg of methylene blue.

8.6.6 Rebound pain

When the analgesic effect of a peripheral nerve block performed with LAs, a state of hyperalgesia known as rebound pain may occur 12–24 hours postoperatively, with intensity disproportionate for the type of the performed surgery. It has been classified as a complication of peripheral nerve blocks, the etiology of which is unknown. Several factors have been considered, including neurotoxicity of LAs, its effects on nociceptors, direct neurotrauma, the possibility of hyperalgesia induced by systemic opioids before or during the block. Its frequency is unknown, although it seems to be increasing, especially in outpatient surgery where it has been reported in up to 40%. It is a relevant complication since it hinders the postoperative evolu-tion, disturbing sleep, increasing the opioid requirement and delaying hospital discharge. Preventive analgesia before the blockage subsides, intra-articular or intravenous anti-inflammatory drugs, and the use of adjuvants added to nerve-block or systemic solutions can reduce rebound pain [65–67].

9. Nonanesthetic uses of LAs

Some nonanesthetic (off-label) uses of LAs have been described. Although these investigations have not been precisely determined, this topic deserves a brief description.

9.1 Cough, laryngospasm, and asthma

Lidocaine has been used successfully to prevent or treat cough and laryngospasm induced during tracheal extubation, as well as in patients with asthma and chronic cough difficult to treat [68–70]. The meta-analysis of Yang et al. found that iv lidocaine decreases postoperative airway complications [71]. Nebulized lidocaine has been used with encouraging results in patients with asthma, chronic cough, and laryngospasm; doses ranging from 10 to 400 mg are a therapeutic alternative in asthma and cough that is difficult to manage [72]. Its mechanism of action has been related to the decrease in airway inflammation via downregulation of TLR2 [73].

9.2 Effects of LAs on cancer

Regional anesthesia is preferably used in oncological surgery since it does not interfere with the immune system, and the postoperative outcome of these patients is better. On the other hand, there is evidence that LAs could have direct antineoplastic effects [74, 75]. Some malignancies have increased voltage-dependent sodium channel activity. Blocking these channels with LAs may help inhibit tumor progression [76]. Zheng et al. found an anti-melanoma activity of ropivacaine and lidocaine but not bupivacaine, via targeting small GTPases [77].

9.3 Antibiotics

Besides pain insensitivity, it has been shown that the in vitro and in vivo use of LAs have bacteriostatic, bactericidal, fungistatic, and fungicidal properties against a wide spectrum of microorganisms, this action being attributed to the interruption of the membrane permeability of microbial cells, leading to leakage of cellular components and subsequent cell lysis. Different LAs showed varying degrees of antimicrobial capacity; bupivacaine and lidocaine, for example, inhibit growth to a significantly greater extent than ropivacaine. Higher concentrations, prolonged exposure, and higher temperature correlate with a proportional increase in inhibition of microbial growth. Reducing the incidence of endophthalmitis after intravitreal injection, prophylaxis for surgical wound infections, preventing the incidence of catheter-associated infections, reducing oral biofilms in the oral mucosa, and preventing infection-causing bacteria nosocomial are some examples of antimicrobial application of lidocaine [2, 78–80].

10. Conclusions

The first LA anesthetic was derived from the plant *Erythroxylum coca*, and regional anesthesia began in 1884 when Karl Köller anesthetized the cornea of his patients for surgical purposes. Since then, a host of events, drugs, discoveries, and various anesthesia techniques have culminated in safer and more effective regional anesthesia. LAs have an impressive history of efficacy and safety in medical and dental practice, but still have deleterious effects that can—on rare occasions—cause the death of our patients. Knowing the basics of the substrates where LAs work makes it easier to understand the action mechanisms that these drugs have on voltage-dependent sodium channels. The sequence of events that occur from the choice of the patient, the preparation and injection of LAs to the production of regional anesthesia-analgesia and/or its toxic effects are complex. These physiological and pathophysiological events depend on features as varied as the structural and physico-chemical characteristics, total injected dose, injection site, adjuvant drugs, physical condition of the patient, among others. The safe practice of regional anesthesia definitely reduces catastrophes, but these disasters can appear at any time. LAs have an impressive history of efficacy and safety in medical and dental practice.

Author details

Víctor M. Whizar-Lugo[1*], Karen L. Íñiguez-López[2], Ana C. Cárdenas-Maytorena[3] and Cristian D. Ramírez-Puerta[4]

1 Institutos Nacionales de Salud, Lotus Medical Group, Tijuana BC, México

2 Centro Médico Nacional Siglo XXI, Instituto Mexicano del Seguro Social, México City, México

3 Lotus Med Group, Tijuana BC, México

4 School of Medicine, Campus Tijuana, Universidad Autónoma de Baja California, Tijuana BC, México

*Address all correspondence to: vwhizar@anestesia-dolor.org

References

[1] Hollmann MW, Durieux ME, Graf BM. Novel local anaesthetics and novel indications for local anaesthetics. Current Opinion in Anaesthesiology. 2001;**14**:741-749. DOI:10.1097/00001503-200112000-00023

[2] Razavi BM, Fazly Bazzaz BS. A review and new insights to antimicrobial action of local anesthetics. European Journal of Clinical Microbiology & Infectious Diseases. 2019;**38**: 991-1002. DOI: 10.1007/s10096-018-03460-4

[3] Lagadinou M, Onisor MO, Rigas A, Musetescu DV, Gkentzi D et al. Antimicrobial properties on non-antibiotic drugs in the era of increased bacterial resistance. Antibiotics (Basel). 2020;**9** (3). pii: E107. DOIi: 10.3390/antibiotics9030107

[4] Norris MC, Honet JE, Leighton BL, Arkoosh VA. A comparison of meperidine and lidocaine for -spinal anesthesia for postpartum tubal ligation. Regional Anesthesia. 1996;**21**:84-88

[5] Patel D, Janardhan Y, Merai B, et al. Comparison of intrathecal meperidine and lidocaine in endoscopic urological procedures. Canadian Journal of Anaesthesia. 1990;**37**:567-570

[6] Sangarlangkarn S, Klaewtanong V, Jonglerttrakool P, Khankaew V. Meperidine as a spinal anesthetic agent: A comparison with lidocaine-glucose. Anesthesia and Analgesia. 1987;**66**: 235-240

[7] Westman L, Valentin A, Eriksson E, Ekblom A. Intrathecal administration of sameridine to patients subjected to arthroscopic joint surgery. Acta Anaesthesiologica Scandinavica. 1998;**42**: 691-697

[8] Mulroy MF, Greengrass R, Ganapathy S, et al. Sameridine is safe and effective for spinal anesthesia: A comparative dose-ranging study with lidocaine for inguinal hernia repair. Anesthesia and Analgesia. 1999;**88**:815-821

[9] Samsi AB, Bhalerao RA, Shah SC, Mody BB, Paul T, Satoskar RS. Evaluation of centbucridine as a local anesthetic. Anesthesia and Analgesia. 1983;**62**(1):109-111

[10] Hugin W. La planta divina de los incas; estimulante, curativa, encantadora. La anestesia local. En Hugin W. Anestesia. Descubrimientos, avances, hitos históricos. Bazilea, Suiza. Ediciones Roche. 1989. Pag 75-96

[11] Fink RB. Leaves and needles: The introduction of surgical local anesthesia. Anesthesiology. 1985;**63**:77-83

[12] Whizar LV, Carrada PS. Anestesia subaracnoidea. Cien años después. Revista Mexicana de Anestesiología. 1999;**22**:1-4

[13] Albrigth GA. Cardiac arrest following regional anesthesia with etidocaine or bupivacaine. Anesthesiology. 1979;**51**:285-287

[14] Columb MO, MacLennan K. Local anaesthetics agents. Anaesthesia and Intensive Care Medicine.2007;**8**:159-162

[15] Singer SJ, Nicolson GL. The fluid mosaic model of the structure of cell membranes. Science. 1972;**175**:720-731. DOI: 10.1126/science.175.4023.720

[16] Nicolson GL. The fluid-mosaic model of membrane structure: Still relevant to understanding the structure, function and dynamics of biological membranes after more than 40 years. Biochimica et Biophysica Acta. 2014;**1838**(6):1451-1466. DOI: 10.1016/j.bbamem.2013.10.019

[17] Lombard J. Once upon a time the cell membranes: 175 years of cell boundary research. Biology Direct. 2014;**9**:32. DOI: 10.1186/s13062-014-0032-7

[18] Denac H, Mevissen M, Scholtysik G. Structure, function and pharmacology of volatage-gated sodium channels. Naunyn-Schmiedeberg's Archives of Pharmacology. 2000;**362**:453-479

[19] Catterall WA, Goldin AL, Waxman SG. International union of pharmacology. XLVII. Nomenclature and structure-function relationships of voltaged-gated sodium channels. Pharmacological Reviews. 2005;**57**: 397-409. DOI: 10.1124/pr.57.4.4

[20] Catterall WA, Swanson TM. Structural basis for pharmacology of voltage-gated sodium and calcium channels. Molecular Pharmacology. 2015;**88**(1):141-150. DOI: 10.1124/mol.114.097659

[21] Wang SY, Nau C, Wang GK. Residues in Na^+ channel D3-S6 segment modulate both batrachotoxin and local anesthetic affinities. Biophysical Journal. 2000;**79**:1379-1387

[22] Yarov-Yarovoy V, Brown J, Sharp EM, et al. Molecular determinants of voltaged-dependent gating and binding of pore-blocking drugs in transmembrane segment IIIS6 of the Na^+ channel alpha subunit. The Journal of Biological Chemistry. 2001;**276**: 20-27

[23] Scholz A. Mechanisms of local anaesthetics on voltaged-gated sodium and others ion channels. British Journal of Anaesthesia. 2002;**89**:52-61

[24] Butterworth JF, Strichartz GR. Molecular mechanisms of local anesthesia: A review. Anesthesiology. 1990;**72**:711-734

[25] Strichartz GR. Neural physiology and local anesthetic action. In: Cousins MJ, Bridenbaugh PO (Editors). Neural Blockade in Clinical Anesthesia and Management of Pain. Philadelphia, Lippincott-Raven; 1998. p. 42

[26] Burke D, Henderson DJ. Chirality: A blueprint for the future. British Journal of Anaesthesia. 2002;**88**:563-576

[27] Harrison NL. Optical isomers open a new window on anesthetic mechanism. Anesthesiology. 1998;**88**:566-568

[28] Kongsgaard UE, Werner MU. Tachyphylaxis to local anaesthetics. What is the clinical evidence? A systematic review. Acta Anaesthesiologica Scandinavica. 2016;**60**(1):6-14. DOI: 10.1111/aas.12631

[29] Lee KC, Wilder RT, Smith RL, Berde CB. Thermal hyperalgesia accelerates and MK-801 prevents the development of tachyphylaxis to rat sciatic nerve blockade. Anesthesiology. 1994;**81**(5):1284-1293. DOI: 10.1097/00000542-199411000-00024

[30] Wilder RT, Sholas MG, Berde CB. NG-nitro-L-arginine methyl ester (L-NAME) prevents tachyphylaxis to local anesthetics in a dose-dependent manner. Anesthesia and Analgesia. 1996;**83**(6):1251-1255

[31] Morrison LM, Emanuelsson BM, McClure JH, Pollok AJ, McKeown DW, Brockway M, et al. Efficacy and kinetics of extradural ropivacaine: Comparison with bupivacaine. British Journal of Anaesthesia. 1994;**72**(2):164-169. DOI: 10.1093/bja/72.2.164

[32] Miller RJ, Cameron AJ, Dimech J, Orec RJ, Lightfoot NJ. Plasma ropivacaine concentrations following local infiltration analgesia in total knee arthroplasty: A pharmacokinetic study to determine safety following fixed-dose administration. Regional Anesthesia and Pain Medicine. 2018;**43**(4): 347-351. DOI: 10.1097/AAP.0000000000000727

[33] Lagan G, McClure HA. Review of local anaesthetics agents. Anaesthesia & Critical Care. 2004;**15**:247-254

[34] Salinas FV, Liu SL, Schlz AM. Analgesics. Ion channel ligands/sodium channels blockers/local anesthetics. Chapter 30. En: Evers AS, Maze M. Editores. Anesthetic Pharmacology. Physiologic Principles and Clinical Practice. Editorial Churchill-Livingstone. Philadelphia, USA. 2004 pag 507-537

[35] He Y, Qin L, Huang Y, Ma C. Advances of nano-structured extended-release local anesthetics. Nanoscale Research Letters. 2020;**15**(1):13. DOI: 10.1186/s11671-019-3241-2

[36] Malik O, Kaye AD, Kaye A, Belani K, Urman RD. Emerging roles of liposomal bupivacaine in anesthesia practice. Journal of Anaesthesiology Clinical Pharmacology. 2017;**33**(2):151-156. DOI: 10.4103/joacp.JOACP_375_15

[37] Kao HW, Lin YY, Gwathney WJ, Hong K. Formulation and evaluation of multilamellar vesicles ropivacaine in pain management. International Journal of Nanomedicine. 2019;**14**:7891-7901. DOI: 10.2147/IJN.S215952

[38] Snoeck M. Articaine: A review of its use for local and regional anesthesia. Local and Regional Anesthesia. 2012;**5**:23-33. DOI:10.2147/LRA.S16682

[39] Kakroudi SH, Mehta S, Millar BJ. Articaine hydrochloride: Is it the solution? Dental Update. 2015;**42**(1) 88-90, 92-3. DOI: 10.12968/denu.2015.42.1.88

[40] Oertel R, Rahn R, Kirch W. Clinical pharmacokinetics of articaine. Clinical Pharmacokinetics. 1997;**33**(6): 417-425.DOI: 10.2165/00003088- 1997 33060-00002

[41] Hopman AJG, Baart JA, Brand HS. Articaine and neurotoxicity - a review. British Dental Journal. 2017 Nov;**223**(7):501-506. DOI: 10.1038/sj.bdj.2017.782

[42] Saralaya S, Adirajaiah SB, Anehosur V. 4% articaine and 2% lignocaine for surgical removal of third molar by mandibular nerve block: A randomized clinical trial for efficacy and safety. Journal of Oral and Maxillofacial Surgery. 2019;**18**(3):405- 411. DOI: 10.1007/s12663-018-1109-0

[43] Nagendrababu V, Duncan HF, Whitworth J, Nekoofar MH, Pulikkotil SJ, et al. Is articaine more effective than lidocaine in patients with irreversible pulpitis? An umbrella review. International Endodontic Journal. 2020;**53**(2): 200-213. DOI: 10.1111/iej.13215

[44] Modalen AO, Westman L, Arlander E, Eriksson LI, Lindahl SG. Hypercarbic and hypoxic ventilatory responses after intrathecal administration of bupivacaine and sameridine. Anesthesia and Analgesia. 2003;**96**:570-575

[45] Osterlund Modalen A, Arlander E, Eriksson LI, Lindahl SG. The effects on hypercarbic ventilatory response of sameridine compared to morphine and placebo. Anesthesia and Analgesia. 2001;**92**:529-534

[46] Osterlund A, Arlander E, Eriksson LI, Lindhal SG. The effects on resting ventilation of intravenous infusions of morphine or sameridine, a novel molecule with both local anesthetic and opioid properties. Anesthesia and Analgesia. 1999;**88**:160-165

[47] Patnaik GK, Rastogi SN, Anand N, Dhawan BN. Evaluation of local anaesthetic activity of 4-N-butylamino-1,2,3,4-tetrahydroacridine hydrochloride (Centbucridine)--a 4-substituted polymethylenequinoline. Indian

Journal of Experimental Biology. 1982;**20**(4):327-329

[48] Gupta PP, Nityanand S, Shipstone AC, Dhawan BN. Experimental evaluation of potential neurotoxicity of 4-N-butylamino 1,2,3,4-tetrahydroacridine hydrochloride (Centbucridine)--a new local anaesthetic agent. Indian Journal of Experimental Biology. 19 82;**20**(4):339-443

[49] Gupta PP, Tangri AN, Saxena RC, Dhawan BN. Clinical pharmacology studies on 4-N-butylamino- 1,2,3,4-tetrahydroacridine hydrochloride (Centbucridine)--a new local anaesthetic agent. Indian Journal of Experimental Biology. 1982;**20**(4):344-346

[50] Goyal A, Jain G, Jain A, Ansari T, Bumb S. A new era of local anaesththetic agent: Centbucridine. Archives of CraniOroFacial Sciences. 2013;**1**(3):40-43

[51] Gune NS, Katre AN. Comparison of 0.5% centbucridine and 2% lignocaine as local anesthetic agents for dental procedures in children: A randomised controlled trial. Indian Journal of Pediatrics. 2020;**87**(4):268-274. DOI: 10.1007/s12098-019-0316 1-6

[52] Suri YV, Patnaik GK, Nayak BC, Gupta PP, Singh D, Dhawan BN. Evaluation of centbucridine for intravenous regional anaesthesia. Indian Journal of Medical Research. 1983;**7 7**:722-727

[53] Mansuri S, Bhayat A, Omar E, Jarab F, Ahmed MS. A randomized controlled trail comparing the efficacy of 0.5% centbucridine to 2% lignocaine as local anesthetics in dental extractions. International Journal of Dentistry. 2011;**2011**:795047. DOI: 10.1155/2011/795047

[54] Per H, Rosenberg PH, Veering BT, Urmey WF. Maximum recommended doses of local anesthetics: A multifactorial concept. Regional Anesthesia and Pain Medicine. 2004;**29**:564-575

[55] Braun H. Ubre einiger neue ortliche anaesthetica (Stovain, Alypin, Novocain). Dtsch KimWochenschr. 1905;**31**: 1667-1671

[56] Aldrete JA, Romo-Salas F, Arora S, et al. Reverse arterial blood flow as a pathway for central nervous systemic toxic response following injection of local anesthtetics. Anesthesia and Analgesia. 1978;**57**:428-443

[57] Irwin W, Fontaine E, Agnolucci L, et al. Bupivacaine myotoxicity is mediated by mitochondria. The Journal of Biological Chemistry. 2002;**277**:12221-12227

[58] Pere P, Watanabe H, Pitkanen M, Wahlstrom T, Rosenberg PH. Local myotoxicity of bupivacaine in rabbits after continuous supraclavicular brachial plexus block. Regional Anesthesia. 1993;**18**:304-307

[59] Zink W, Seif C, Bohl JR, et al. The acute myotoxic effects of bupivacaine and ropivacaine after continuous peripheral nerve blockades. Anesthesia and Analgesia. 2003;**97**:1173-1179

[60] Zink W, Bohl J, Hacke N, Sinner B, Martin E, Graf BM. Long term myotoxic effects of bupivacaine and ropivacaine after continuous peripheral nerve blocks. Anesthesia and Analgesia. 2005;**101**:548-554

[61] Hussain N, McCartney CJL, Neal JM, Chippor J, Banfield L, Abdallah FW. Local anaesthetic-induced myotoxicity in regional anaesthesia: A systematic review and empirical analysis. British Journal of Anaesthesia. 2018;**121**(4):822-841. DOI: 10.1016/j. bja.2018.05.076

[62] Whizar-Lugo VM, Ontiveros-Morales P, Garfias-Flores M. Alergia

a ropivacaína peridural. Anestesia en Mexico. 2004;**16**:180-183

[63] Bhole MV, Manson AL, Seneviratne SL, Misbah SA. IgE-mediated allergy to local anaesthetics: Separating fact from perception: A UK perspective. British Journal of Anaesthesia. 2012;**108**(6):903-911. DOI: 10.1093/bja/aes162

[64] Grzanka A, Wasilewska I, Śliwczyńska M, Misiołek H. Hypersensitivity lo local anesthetics. Anaesthesiology Intensive Therapy. 2016; **48**(2):128-134. DOI: 10.5603/AIT. a20 16.0017

[65] Nobre LV, Cunha GP, Sousa PCCB, Takeda A, Cunha Ferraro LH. Peripheral nerve block and rebound pain: Literature review. Revista Brasileira de Anestesiologia. 2019;**69**(6): 587-593. DOI: 10.1016/j.bjan.2019.05. 001

[66] Dada O, Gonzalez Zacarias A, Ongaigui C, Echeverria-Villalobos M, Kushelev M, et al. Does rebound pain after peripheral nerve block for orthopedic surgery impact postoperative analgesia and opioid consumption? A narrative review. International Journal of Environmental Research and Public Health. 2019;16(18). pii: E3257. DOI: 10.3390/ijerph16183257.

[67] An K, Elkassabany NM, Liu J. Dexamethasone as adjuvant to bupivacaine prolongs the duration of thermal antinociception and prevents bupivacaine-induced rebound hyperalgesia via regional mechanism in a mouse sciatic nerve block model. PLoS One. 2015;**10**(4):e0123459. DOI: 10.1371/ journal.pone.0123459

[68] Lim KG, Rank MA, Hahn PY, Keogh KA, Morgenthaler TI, Olson EJ. Long-term safety of nebulized lidocaine for adults with difficult-to-control chronic cough: A case series. Chest. 2013;**143**(4):1060-1065. DOI: 10.1378/ chest.12-1533

[69] Truesdale K, Jurdi A. Nebulized lidocaine in the treatment of intractable cough. The American Journal of Hospice & Palliative Care. 2013;**30**(6): 587-589. DOI: 10.1177/1049909112458 577

[70] Oon Z, Ha CB, Sicinski M. Nebulized lidocaine in the treatment of refractory postoperative laryngospasm: A case report. A&A Practice. 2019;**13**(1):20-22. DOI: 10.1213/ XAA.0000000000000974

[71] Yang SS, Wang NN, Postonogova T, Yang GJ, McGillion M, Beique F, et al. Intravenous lidocaine to prevent postoperative airway complications in adults: A systematic review and meta-analysis. British Journal of Anaesthesia. 2020;**124**(3):314-323. DOI: 10.1016/j. bja.2019.11.033

[72] Slaton RM, Thomas RH, Mbathi JW. Evidence for therapeutic uses of nebulized lidocaine in the treatment of intractable cough and asthma. The Annals of Pharmacotherapy. 2013;**47**(4):578-585. DOI: 10.134 5/aph.1R573

[73] Wang L, Wang M, Li S, Wu H, Shen Q , Zhang S, et al. Nebulized lidocaine ameliorates allergic airway inflammation via downregulation of TLR2. Molecular Immunology. 2018;**9 7**:94-100. DOI: 10.1016/j. molimm.20 18.03.010

[74] Liu H, Dilger JP, Lin J. Effects of local anesthetics on cancer cells. Pharmacology & Therapeutics. 2020;**107558**. DOI: 10.1016/j. pharmthera.2020.10 7558

[75] Chamaraux-Tran TN, Piegeler T. The amide local anesthetic lidocaine in cancer surgery-potential antimetastatic effects and preservation of immune cell function? A narrative review. Frontiers in Medicine (Lausanne). 2017;**4**:235. DOI: 10.3389/fmed.2017.00235

[76] Mao L, Lin S, Lin J. The effects of anesthetics on tumor progression.

International Journal of Physiology, Pathophysiology and Pharmacology. 2013;**5**(1):1-10

[77] Zheng Q , Peng X, Zhang Y. Cytotoxicity of amide-linked local anesthetics on melanoma cells via inhibition of Ras and RhoA signaling independent of sodium channel blockade. BMC Anesthesiology. 2020;**20**(1):43. DOI: 10.1186/s12871-020-00957-4

[78] Kaewjiaranai T, Srisatjaluk RL, Sakdajeyont W, Pairuchvej V, Wongsirichat N. The efficiency of topical anesthetics as antimicrobial agents: A review of use in dentistry. Journal of Dental Anesthesia and Pain Medicine. 2018;**18**(4):223-233. DOI: 10.17245/jdapm.2018.18.4.223

[79] Johnson SM, Saint John BE, Dine AP. Local anesthetics as antimicrobial agents: A review. Surgical Infections. 2008;**9**(2):205-213. DOI: 10.1089/sur.2007.036

[80] Pelz K, Wiedmann-Al-Ahmad M, Bogdan C, Otten JE. Analysis of the antimicrobial activity of local anaesthetics used for dental analgesia. Journal of Medical Microbiology. 2008;**57**:88-94

10

Local Anesthetics for Spinal Anesthesia in Day-Case Surgery

Margaretha Barbara Breebaart

Abstract

Day-case procedures require a high turnover, high quality and low costs. Lidocaine has long been the gold standard for ambulatory spinal anaesthesia. However, the risk of transient neurological symptoms (TNS) limits its use. The perfect local anaesthetic for spinal anaesthesia in day-case surgery should have fast recovery, fast voiding time and a low risk on TNS and urinary retention. Urinary retention is a result of prolonged sensory blockade of the pelvic nerves and is local anaesthetic dose and potency dependent. As a substitute for lidocaine, several local anaesthetics have been suggested in various doses or combinations with or without additives. However, not all are registered for spinal use or have a short-acting profile. The use of additives has been subject of debate because of possible delay in the recovery of bladder. Recently, the old local anaesthetics chloroprocaine and prilocaine were reintroduced in the market. They provide rapid recovery after spinal anaesthesia in day-case surgery. This chapter gives an overview of the local anaesthetics suitable for spinal anaesthesia in day-case surgery, the advantages and disadvantages and the influence on discharge time and recovery of bladder function.

Keywords: spinal anaesthesia, ambulatory surgery, local anaesthetics, urinary retention, transient neurological symptoms, lidocaine, bupivacaine, mepivacaine, prilocaine, chloroprocaine

1. Introduction

Day-case surgical procedures require an anaesthetic technique with the possibil-ity of a high turnover, a high quality of care and low costs [1]. Spinal anaesthesia is an easy and cheap technique, has a fast onset and causes minimal side effects. Urinary retention and transient neurological symptom (TNS) are side effects of spinal anaesthesia and reason for some anaesthetists only to provide general anaesthesia in day-case surgery. Despite the fact that these side effects are mostly temporary, they affect the quality of care to a great extent.

Lidocaine is a short-acting local anaesthetic and was frequently used for spinal anaesthesia in day-case surgery until it became clear that the incidence of TNS is significantly higher than with other local anaesthetics [2].

The ideal spinal anaesthesia for day-case surgery provides a rapid onset and a short duration of action, allowing a fast turnover of patients for a double-bed planning. Spontaneous voiding is still a discharge criterion in our and many other hospitals: faster spontaneous voiding results in faster discharge.

Urinary retention after spinal anaesthesia is most often a result of a prolonged sensory blockade of the pelvic nerves. The duration of a spinal block is local anaesthetic dose and potency dependent [3]. The dose of a local anaesthetic to provide adequate surgical anaesthesia can be lowered by using spinal additive drugs [4]. Opioids and clonidine prolong the duration and increase the quality of the sensory nerve block in spinal anaesthesia. By adding spinal clonidine, the local anaesthetic dose can be reduced without increasing the risk of block failure [5]. The question rises if the benefit of lowering local anaesthetic dose outweighs the side effects of the additive administered.

The incidence of urinary retention after spinal anaesthesia has been reported with a high variability. There is neither uniformity nor consensus when to catheterise [6]. Fluid policy has also been a subject of debate. A restrictive fluid policy is a way of preventing bladder filling, but a more liberal schedule could speed up the time to void and fasten discharge time. Furthermore, there is an enormous inter-patient variability in bladder capacity and in the definition of urinary retention.

Different techniques exist to perform spinal anaesthesia, producing selective spinal anaesthesia by changing baricity, dose and position, like a saddle block or unilateral anaesthesia. Little is known about the effects of these techniques on the restoration of bladder function.

2. Spinal anaesthesia in day-case surgery

2.1 History of local anaesthetics for day-case surgery

In 1954, lidocaine was introduced and became very popular for spinal anaesthesia because of its favourable profile for day-case surgery [7]. In 1993, TNS were described after its use [8]. Subsequently, additional case reports and prospective trials were published about the appearance of TNS with lidocaine [9–11]. In 2005, a meta-analysis from Zaric et al. clearly demonstrated an increased risk when lidocaine was used for spinal anaesthesia. However, many physicians were not really concerned by these symptoms because they were transient and lidocaine remained very popular. Even up to now, some clinicians still prefer lidocaine.

The appearance of TNS did initiate a quest for the replacement of lidocaine to provide cost-effective, short-acting spinal anaesthesia with a low incidence of side effects. It should also be noted that with the progression of modern medicine, patient satisfaction became more important as an indicator of the quality of care. Temporary side effects that were not considered very important previously now became clinically relevant.

2.2 Spinal anaesthesia: advantages and disadvantages

Spinal anaesthesia is an easy technique that has proven its benefit for many years [12]. After injection of the local anaesthetic solution in the CSF, it provides good surgical anaesthesia for procedures below the umbilicus. The incidence of PONV is low and allows eating and drinking immediately after the procedure.

Although the incidence is low, spinal anaesthesia can fail by producing an insufficient block height or a patchy block [13]. The duration of spinal anaesthesia cannot be extended when the duration of surgery outlasts surgical anaesthesia. When this happens a conversion to general anaesthesia must be made.

Several side effects can occur after injection of the local anaesthetic. Sympathetic block, hypotension and cardiovascular depression can occur, especially when block height exceeds the fifth thoracic dermatome or when patients are of older age [12].

Late side effects from spinal anaesthesia are urinary retention, TNS, backache and PDPH. Bleeding or abscess formation are rare but can occur.

To prevent PDPH, smaller and non-cutting needles were developed with a pencil-point-shaped tip. This atraumatic needle tip separates the dural fibres rather than cutting them, with a lower risk of CSF leakage after puncture. After introduction of these needles, the incidence of PDPH dropped to 0.6–3% [14, 15].

TNS are described as a dull bouncing pain or dysesthesia at the gluteal region or lower limbs after spinal anaesthesia. The symptoms mostly occur within 24 h after block regression, and there is an interval of 2–5 h between mobilisation and onset of the symptoms [16]. The pain mostly disappears within 5 days, but a duration of 3 weeks has been described [17]. The aetiology of these symptoms is not well under-stood. A neurotoxic mechanism is suspected although no neurologic disorders are observed. Lidocaine and mepivacaine show the highest incidence of TNS, but they are described for other local anaesthetics as well [18]. Lidocaine concentration and osmolarity, early ambulation, age, needle size and level of puncture all have been suggested as contributing factors, but the evidence in literature is weak and contro-versial. Ambulatory anaesthesia, the lithotomy position and knee arthroscopy are known to be risk factors [10, 11, 19–22].

2.3 Comparison with other anaesthetic techniques

Spinal and general anaesthesia have frequently been compared in literature. In 2005, a meta-analysis compared different locoregional techniques with general anaesthesia for ambulatory surgery [23]. After including 23 trials with more than 1000 patients, it was concluded that general anaesthesia had a faster onset and a 40 min faster discharge time than spinal anaesthesia. However postoperative pain scores and the incidence of PONV were higher for general anaesthesia. Patients were equally satisfied with all techniques. Comparison of costs was not part of the analysis. After this meta-analysis, more recent studies confirmed the delay in discharge but also showed an increase in urinary retention for spinal anaesthesia. Less PONV and lower pain scores after spinal anaesthesia were consistent findings [24–28].

Spinal anaesthesia displays a clear advantage concerning PONV and postoperative pain scores. It is clear that we should improve recovery time and lower the incidence of urinary retention and TNS when spinal anaesthesia has to compete with general anaesthesia. It is important to realise that the choice of drugs and equipment only has a minor contribution in anaesthesia expenses compared to personnel costs. Reducing turnover times and fasten recovery and discharge have an economical benefit because of saving manpower. Unanticipated admissions and the occurrence of side effects are cost-increasing factors [29, 30].

A limitation in many studies has been the use of long-acting local anaesthetics, while short-acting local anaesthetics might provide a faster recovery [31].

When it comes to difference on the longer-term outcome, there is not much evidence of superiority of spinal or general anaesthesia. One prospective randomised trial with 200 patients suggests that success rate with in vitro fertilisation might be improved from 15 to 27% when spinal anaesthesia is used instead of general anaesthesia [32].

Postoperative cognitive dysfunction (POCD) is a decline in mental status after surgery. The mechanism is not understood. In 2007, a review by Newman showed that there is no difference in the incidence of POCD after general or spinal anaesthesia [33]. However, the author points out that many studies were underpowered and differences in surgery and testing provided difficulties in methodology. For elderly patients undergoing hip replacement, neuraxial anaesthesia lowers the risk of POCD than general anaesthesia [34].

2.4 Spinal anaesthesia and bladder function

Neuraxial anaesthesia increases the risk of urinary retention since the neurophysiology of the bladder is temporarily disturbed. The duration is dependent on the local anaesthetic used [3, 35, 36]. The temporary malfunction of the detrusor muscle and the lack of urge sensation during spinal anaesthesia increase the risk of bladder distension.

The time for the bladder function to restore relates to the duration of the block, which is determined by local anaesthetic potency and dose. When long-acting local anaesthetics are used, more time is required before bladder function is restored than short-acting substances. When local anaesthetic dose is increased, the time to void is prolonged as well. This causes variable times to void after spinal anaesthesia, ranging from 103 (chloroprocaine) to 462 min (bupivacaine) [3, 37]. To prevent bladder retention in an outpatient setting, the use of short-acting local anaesthetics and voiding before surgery is recommended [38].

In a day-case setting, the incidence of urinary retention after spinal anaesthesia varies between 0 and 30%, although there is consensus that the mean incidence is around 2% [3]. This variability can be explained by the difference in definition, catheterisation protocol and surgical procedure between the reported trials. There are a lot of studies concerning spinal anaesthesia in day-case surgery where urinary retention is not even mentioned. It is remarkable though that when trials were designed to study bladder function, high incidences like 23–30% are found [39, 40]. This may be explained by the closer monitoring of bladder volume.

2.5 Modifying spinal anaesthesia

Different aspects of spinal anaesthesia can be modified (**Figure 1**). Changing the solution for spinal injection, the anaesthetic technique or fluid policy can influence the duration of the sensory and motor block, the risk of certain side effects or discharge time. Modifying certain discharge criteria, like the necessity to void, can influence discharge time as well.

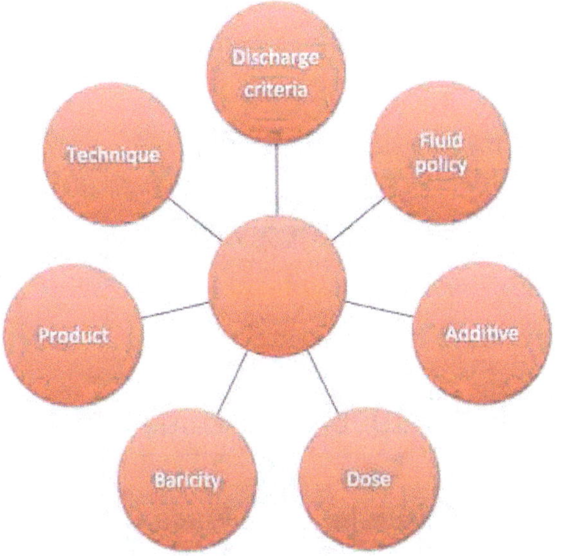

Figure 1.
Variables in spinal anaesthesia for day-case surgery.

2.5.1 Local anaesthetics

When a local anaesthetic substance is injected into the CSF, it diffuses through the lipophilic nerve membrane and reaches the sodium channel [41]. As a consequence, the sodium channel is blocked and impulses cannot be conducted along the different nerve fibres. This results in a sensory, motor and sympathetic block. After a certain period, the local anaesthetic molecules dissociate from the sodium channel and are absorbed in the blood stream to be degraded. Local anaesthetics are divided in two groups: amides and esters. Amides are degraded by the liver, and esters are rapidly hydrolysed by pseudocholinesterases in the blood stream. Every local anaesthetic has its own pharmacologic properties (pKa, liposolubility, protein binding), which not only determine the potency but also the onset and duration of the spinal block [42]. Since the first spinal anaesthesia was performed with cocaine, more local anaesthetics have been produced (**Figure 2**).

The duration of the sensory and motor block is dose dependent in neuraxial anaesthesia. Increasing local anaesthetic dose prolongs motor and sensory block. Winnie stated that locoregional anaesthesia always works provided you put the right dose of the right drug in the right place. This is also true for spinal anaesthesia. Unfortunately for spinal anaesthesia in day-case surgery, a working spinal

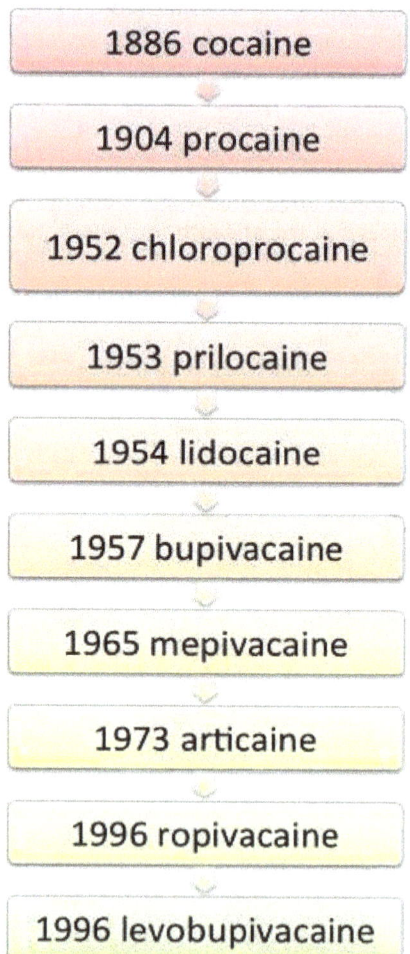

Figure 2.
Different local anaesthetics and year of production.

anaesthesia is not enough. The duration of the spinal block should be short but long enough to do provide surgical anaesthesia with a minimal risk of insufficient block height and with minimal side effects.

Lidocaine has always been a popular drug for spinal anaesthesia. It can provide 60 min of anaesthesia below the umbilicus with minimal time to achieve discharge criteria [43, 44]. The question arises if lidocaine should still be used in the twenty-first century because of its side effects, and many studies have compared it to its alternatives [45, 46].

Bupivacaine is a long-acting local anaesthetic from the amide group and has a low incidence of TNS. It has been the most common alternative for lidocaine for years. Because of its pharmacological profile, the recovery of motor and sensory block is delayed compared to short-acting local anaesthetics. The incidence of postoperative urinary retention with long-acting local anaesthetics like bupivacaine and tetracaine is higher than with short-acting local anaesthetics [3, 47]. Successful spinal anaesthesia with low doses of bupivacaine between 5 and 10 mg without additives has been described for outpatients. The incidence of urinary retention was still 3.7–16% [48, 49]. Furthermore, with these low doses, block height becomes unpredictable and the risk of block failure is high [48, 50, 51]. A meta-analysis of 17 trials looked at the use of bupivacaine for ambulatory knee arthroscopy. This paper warned for an increased risk of a failed block with doses below 7.5 mg, unless a unilateral spinal technique was used or additives were administered to the solution [52].

Other local anaesthetics like procaine and mepivacaine also have a considerable risk of TNS or have an unfavourable profile regarding block resolution and discharge times [53, 54].

Levobupivacaine and ropivacaine are both amide local anaesthetics that have similar properties to bupivacaine. Ropivacaine also is a pure enantiomer, is less potent and produces less motor block than bupivacaine. Both products are not officially registered for spinal use but used "off-label" frequently. The recovery and discharge for ambulatory surgery is not as fast as lidocaine, and micturition prob-lems are comparable [55]. There is controversy about the suggested faster recovery of ropivacaine compared to bupivacaine [56].

Although there is enough literature to support the use of these two products for spinal anaesthesia for ambulatory surgery, reintroduction of chloroprocaine and prilocaine, which are in many countries registered for spinal use, seems to have more advantages [57–59].

Chloroprocaine is a local anaesthetic from the ester group. It has a fast- and short-acting profile. It became unpopular in the 1950s after the publication of toxic neurologic symptoms, which were probably caused by the additives in the solution. The additive-free form is now approved an available for spinal use in Europe and is considered safe [60–62]. It has been shown to be suitable for spinal anaesthesia in day-case surgery and has a faster regression than long-acting local anaesthetics and available short-acting local anaesthetics [60]. The recommended dose varies between 40 and 60 mg for ambulatory surgery. Discharge times between 178 and 277 min are found. Up to date only one patient has been reported with TNS after spinal anaesthesia with chloroprocaine, demonstrating the low incidence of TNS and suitability for day-case surgery [63]. Furthermore the frequency of bladder retention is very low, even when a fluid preload is administered [64].

A meta-analyses of the advantage of the pharmacokinetic profile proofed to translate in a clinical advantage such as faster block regression, ambulation and discharge as well [65].

Prilocaine is an amide local anaesthetic with an intermediate duration of action after spinal administration. It never gained much attention because of the popularity of lidocaine. It is available in the hyperbaric form and provides anaesthesia for

75–90 min after spinal administration. The duration of the spinal block is prolonged compared to an equal dose of lidocaine, but combined with fentanyl it is a better alternative than bupivacaine for ambulatory knee arthroscopy [66]. Doses between 20 and 70 mg are described in literature, but 50 mg hyperbaric prilocaine seems sufficient for day-case arthroscopies, although rescue analgesia was necessary in 11 and 7.5% of the patients [67, 68]. The ED90 was 38 mg for bilateral spinal anaesthe-sia for knee arthroscopies [69].

The incidence of urinary retention after 60 mg prilocaine in a day-case setting was described as high as 23% [40]. Articaine is an amide local anaesthetic with intermediate potency and a short duration of action. It is an amide but differs slightly because it also contains an ester group and can be hydrolysed. Further metabolism and excretion is primarily in the kidneys [70]. Articaine provides faster motor and sensory block regression and earlier spontaneous voiding than prilo-caine; low-dose bupivacaine and lidocaine A comparison of equal doses of spinal articaine and chloroprocaine showed faster block regression for chloroprocaine [71]. Unfortunately, articaine is not available everywhere and its use is off-label.

2.5.2 *Baricity*

The baricity of a local anaesthetic is defined as its density compared to the density of the CSF. Baricity partly determines the spread of the molecules in the CSF after injection. The molecules sink or float in the CSF depending on their relative gravity. Most local anaesthetics are isobaric or slightly hypobaric. It must be remembered that an increase in temperature of the solution can change baricity, making isobaric substances slightly hypobaric once injected [72]. Hyperbaric substances are also available. These solutions contain glucose.

When hyperbaric or hypobaric substances are used for spinal anaesthesia, the spread of the local anaesthetic can be influenced by changing the position of the patient. Hyperbaric substances might have a more favourable profile because of faster block regression. Hyperbaric lidocaine, ropivacaine and bupivacaine showed faster recovery than the plain solutions and with higher or comparable cephalad spread [73–76]. No differences were found between hyperbaric and plain chloroprocaine [77]. It is believed that hyperbaric substances produce a more cephalad block spread because the molecules are dragged down over the lumbar curve to the lowest level of the thoracic kyphosis when the patient is allowed to resume the supine position. This more cephalad spread of local anaesthetic might result in a dilution of molecules in the CSF and thus a lower "mg per segment" concentration. The time necessary to absorb the local anaesthetic molecules is shorter because of a lower concentration which might explain faster block regression of a hyperbaric substance than a plain local anaesthetic [78].

2.5.3 *Additives*

Local anaesthetics can be combined with other drugs to prolong the duration of sensory or motor block or increase the level or intensity of sensory analgesia. It also allows local anaesthetic dose reduction without shortening the duration of the block but with a more favourable recovery profile. For day-case surgery, several additives were studied to reduce local anaesthetic dose in a day-case setting.

Intrathecal opioids have a direct analgesic effect after binding on the opioids receptors that are present at the spinal cord level. This is mainly through their effect on the C and A-delta fibres. The mechanism by which opioids and local anaesthetics interact is not fully understood but results in an increased somatic analgesia without influencing motor or sympathetic blockade. Intrathecal lipophilic opioids, like fentanyl and sufentanil, increase the quality and prolong the duration of sensory analgesia after spinal anaesthesia [4, 79].

For day-case surgery, the combination of a local anaesthetic with an opioid could provide fast-onset and sufficient analgesia without prolonged motor block. Side effects like respiratory depression, which can occur after spinal hydrophilic opioids, are not clinically relevant with low doses of lipophilic opioids [80].

However the incidence of pruritus after intrathecal opioids varies but can be severe [81]. A meta-analysis in 2011 evaluated the effect of intrathecal opioids. The analysis concluded that morphine provided longer postoperative analgesia up to 12 h but also increased the risk of respiratory depression and PONV. The addition of fentanyl increased the risk of pruritus but had no effect on respiration [82]. Extremely small doses such as 3 mg of bupivacaine or 20 mg of lidocaine in combination with an opioid have been described [83–85]. However as described above, opioids will also decrease the sensation of bladder fullness and weaken the detrusor contraction. This might delay voiding [86, 87]. This possible delay in voiding time could not be confirmed by all studies, but it is clear that it is dose dependent [6, 88, 89].

Clonidine binds alpha-2 receptors on the presynaptic C fibres and the A-delta fibres. It intensifies sensory and motor block, but the exact working mechanism is not known [90]. Clonidine allows local anaesthetic dose reduction. The advantage of clonidine compared to opioids is the lack of respiratory depression and pruritus as a side effect. However, marked haemodynamic changes and sedation can occur [5].

Vasoconstrictors decrease local anaesthetic uptake by reducing spinal cord blood flow. Epinephrine prolongs the duration and improves the quality of a spinal block in a dose-dependent fashion. It allows local anaesthetic dose reduction in a day-case setting but has a variable prolongation. Addition of epinephrine to lidocaine, procaine or bupivacaine caused a delay in discharge in a day-case setting [91, 92]. In combination with chloroprocaine in volunteers, it provided unexplained flu-like symptoms [93].

Several other additives, like neostigmine and magnesium, have been studied, but were not suitable because of side effects or prolonged time to ambulation [94–96].

2.5.4 Spinal anaesthetic technique

Several techniques are available to perform spinal anaesthesia. When isobaric solutions are injected, drug spread is affected by many factors, which mostly are patient dependent and can therefore not be influenced [78]. Urmey et al. showed that pointing the aperture of the spinal needle cephalad resulted in a more cephalad spread and faster block regression after 60 mg lidocaine in a day-case setting [97].

The availability of hyperbaric substances allows us to control intrathecal drug spread, by which a restriction of the sensory block to the surgical site can be obtained, like a saddle block or a unilateral block. Low doses of hyperbaric prilocaine or bupivacaine produce adequate analgesia limited to the sacral region for perianal surgery [98–101]. However a sitting position has to be obtained for at least 10 min or even more to prevent secondary spread of the local anaesthetic after repositioning the patient, what may result in an insufficient block [78].

Unilateral spinal blocks with a reduced local anaesthetic dose were compared to bilateral spinal anaesthesia in a day-case setting. Unilateral blocks resulted in faster recovery of sensory and motor block and more haemodynamic stability [102–105]. In a meta-analysis, Nair et al. concluded that a unilateral technique with small doses of bupivacaine (4–6 mg) is suitable for unilateral anaesthesia [52].

The duration of lateral decubitus, the amount of hip flexion and the position during injection were studied to improve the unilaterality and the success rate of the block [106, 107]. However, the idea that a spinal block is fixed after 15–30 min is not correct, since redistribution can be seen up to 1.5 h after injection [78]. Unilateral spinal anaesthesia has been thought to reduce bladder disturbances, as only one side of bladder innervation would be impaired. Because the physiologic function of the detrusor reflex is complex, there is still controversy whether this is really true [39, 108, 109].

2.5.5 Fluid policy

Should patients receive a 'normal' or 'restricted' amount of intravenous and oral fluids? Restricting fluid can delay bladder filling and prevent urinary retention, but it can also delay voiding and discharge, when required [110–112]. Restriction of fluids might cause minor discomfort in outpatients. A fluid load can even reduce PONV after general anaesthesia [113–115]. However, if IV fluid is not restricted, the bladder may fill too early during anaesthesia, risking overdistension [35, 116, 117].

Different amounts of fluid between 750 and 1200 ml have been suggested as a maximum in order to prevent bladder retention. However in these papers, different local anaesthetics were used, fluid loads up to 4000 ml were administered, bladder volumes were not always measured, and most procedures were considered as high risk for urinary retention, such as inguinal hernia repair and urological procedures [118, 123].

There even is controversy weather fluid load always correlates with bladder filling in such a short period. When 800–1200 ml IV fluid was administered, neither correlation with bladder filling was found nor could a difference in voiding interval or urinary retention be detected compared to a restrictive regimen [37, 113, 119, 120]. One study found a correlation between bladder volume and IV fluid when more than 900 ml was administered [121]. It may be concluded that excessive volumes should be avoided, but a restrictive policy may not be necessary to prevent urinary retention.

Moreover, with the common policy to freely allow patients to drink clear fluids up to 2 h before surgery, the bladder may fill intraoperatively regardless of restricted intravenous fluid administration.

2.5.6 Discharge criteria

Discharge time is an indicator of efficiency of an ambulatory surgery unit. For safe and good clinical practice, guidelines and criteria are useful. Depending on the healthcare system, discharge criteria can vary in different countries or regions. There are several scores that can be used to test home readiness for ambulatory surgery. The modified Aldrete score [122] and the PADSS score [123] are two of them. Voiding and oral intake are parts of the PADSS and the modified Aldrete score as discharge criteria. In both scores, readiness for discharge can be achieved without voiding or oral intake, when all other variables are optimal.

Waiting for oral intake and voiding can delay discharge for both general and spinal anaesthesia. A large trial of 1184 patients showed that spinal anaesthesia was responsible for a 44 min delay in discharge for women [49, 124, 125]. There is agree-ment in literature that after general anaesthesia and absence of patient or surgery-related risk factors, patients can be discharged without voiding [126].

However, guidelines available are not clear weather voiding should be required after spinal anaesthesia. In the day-case and short-stay surgery guidelines from the British association of day surgery, the following guideline can be found: "Voiding is also not always required, although it is important to identify and retain patients who are at particular risk of developing later problems, such as those who have experienced prolonged instrumentation or manipulation of the bladder" [127].

The American Society of Anesthesiologists (ASA) guidelines recommend void-ing before discharge only when risk factors are present as well [128]. Since spinal anaesthesia is regarded as a risk factor on its own, the guidelines are subject to different interpretation [121]. Patients operated for urogenital surgery, hernia repair, those who had experienced bladder problems in the past, patients with prostate disease and aged persons should void before discharge [35, 37, 129, 130], regardless of anaesthetic technique.

An often-quoted abstract concludes that even high-risk patients can be discharged without voiding. Although 1719 patients were included in the study, only 30 patients were identified as high risk. Those patients could not void and were discharged and followed by a home nurse. Three patients had to be catheterised at home. No bladder volumes were measured [131]. Mulroy et al. compared an accelerated protocol where low-risk patients could be discharged after neuraxial anaesthesia when measured bladder volume was below 400 ml. He concluded, after examining 46 patients who went home without voiding, that discharge after spinal anaesthesia with short-acting local anaesthetics is safe without voiding when blad-der volume is below 400 ml [110].

Other authors agree that short-acting local anaesthetics should be used and bladder volumes should be monitored when patients are discharged without voiding. Some advice patients to return to the hospital when no voiding took place within 8 h of interval after discharge or until the evening of the day of surgery [3, 35, 38, 132]. After anaesthesia, overdistension of the bladder is not always clear for the patient [121]. Instructions when to return to the hospital based on measured bladder volumes seem a better option [38].

3. Conclusions

Effective anaesthesia, fast block regression and fast voiding are of uppermost importance in creating a good flow for spinal anaesthesia in day-case surgery. For this, we need a local anaesthetic with a favourable pharmacokinetic profile.

For years, lidocaine has been the drug of choice for spinal use in day-case surgery. The importance of quality of care and the demand for a fast turnover in our modern ambulatory practice has increased. Therefore, nowadays, the intrathecal use of lidocaine is criticised because of its high incidence of TNS.

Different aspects of spinal anaesthesia were studied in order to minimise side effects and to obtain short discharge times. Discharge time is mainly affected by the time to void and the occurrence of micturition problems.

Not only the local anaesthetic choice but also dose contributes to the optimal flow in a day-case setting. Other factors are also important, such as spinal anaesthetic technique, fluid policy and discharge criteria.

Author details

Margaretha Barbara Breebaart
Faculty of Medicine and Health Sciences, University of Antwerp, Wilrijk, Belgium

*Address all correspondence to: margaretha.breebaart@uza.be

References

[1] Joshi GP, Twersky RS. Fast tracking in ambulatory surgery. Ambulatory Surgery. 2000;**8**(4):185-190

[2] Zaric D et al. Transient neurologic symptoms (TNS) following spinal anaesthesia with lidocaine versus other local anaesthetics. Cochrane Database of Systematic Reviews. 2005;**19**(4): CD003006. DOI: 10.1002/14651858. CD003006.pub2

[3] Choi S, Mahon P, Awad IT. Neuraxial anesthesia and bladder dysfunction in the perioperative period: A systematic review. Canadian Journal of Anaesthesia. 2012;**59**(7):681-703. DOI: 10.1007/s12630-012-9717-5

[4] Pitkanen M, Rosenberg PH. Local anaesthetics and additives for spinal anaesthesia--characteristics and factors influencing the spread and duration of the block. Best Practice & Research. Clinical Anaesthesiology. 2003;**17**(3):305-322

[5] Elia N et al. Clonidine as an adjuvant to intrathecal local anesthetics for surgery: Systematic review of randomized trials. Regional Anesthesia and Pain Medicine. 2008;**33**(2):159-167. DOI: 10.1016/j.rapm.2007.10.008

[6] Mulroy MF, Alley EA. Management of bladder volumes when using neuraxial anesthesia. International Anesthesiology Clinics. 2012;**50**(1):101-1 10. DOI: 10.1097/AIA.0b013e318217754d

[7] Holmadahl M. Xylocaine : Its discovery and Gordh's contribution to its clinical use. Acta Anesthesiologica Scandinavica. 1998;**113**(Suppl):8-12

[8] Schneider M et al. Transient neurologic toxicity after hyperbaric subarachnoid anesthesia with 5% lidocaine. Anesthesia and Analgesia. 1993;**76**(5):1154-1157

[9] Hampl K, Schneider M. Transient radicular irritation after spinal anaesthesia with xylocain. Acta Anaesthesiologica Scandinavica. 1999;**43**(3):35 9-362

[10] Pollock JE et al. Prospective study of the incidence of transient radicular irritation in patients undergoing spinal anesthesia. Anesthesiology. 1996;**84**(6): 1361-1367

[11] Freedman JM et al. Transient neurologic symptoms after spinal anesthesia: An epidemiologic study of 1,863 patients. Anesthesiology. 1998;**89**(3):6 33-641

[12] Liu SS, McDonald SB. Current issues in spinal anesthesia. Anesthesiology. 2001;**94**(5):888-906 888-906

[13] Drasner K. Spinal anaesthesia: A century of refinement, and failure is still an option. British Journal of Anaesthesia. 2009;**102**(6):729-730. DOI: 10.1093/bja/aep085

[14] Gielen MJ. Fewer headaches following lumbar puncture when using an atraumatic needle; double-blind randomized study. Nederlands Tijdschrift voor Geneeskunde. 1995;**139**(13):694

[15] Turnbull DK, Shepherd DB. Post-dural puncture headache: Pathogenesis, prevention and treatment. British Journal of Anaesthesia. 2003;**91**(5): 718-729

[16] Pollock JE et al. Spinal nerve function in five volunteers experiencing transient neurologic symptoms after lidocaine subarachnoid anesthesia. Anesthesia and Analgesia. 2000;**90**(3): 658-665

[17] Ganapathy S et al. Transient neurologic symptom (TNS) following

intrathecal ropivacaine. Anesthesiology. 2000;**93**(6):1537-1539

[18] Zaric D, Pace NL. Transient neurologic symptoms (TNS) following spinal anaesthesia with lidocaine versus other local anaesthetics. Cochrane Database of Systematic Reviews. 2009;**15**(2):CD003006. DOI: 10.1002/14651858.CD003006.pub3

[19] Pollock JE et al. Dilution of spinal lidocaine does not alter the incidence of transient neurologic symptoms. Anesthesiology. 1999;**90**(2):445-450

[20] Lindh A, Andersson AS, Westman L. Is transient lumbar pain after spinal anaesthesia with lidocaine influenced by early mobilisation? Acta Anaesthesiologica Scandinavica. 2001;**45**(3):290-293

[21] Corbey MP, Bach AB. Transient radicular irritation (TRI) after spinal anaesthesia in day-care surgery. Acta Anaesthesiologica Scandinavica. 1998;**42**(4):425-429

[22] Etezadi F et al. The effect of needle type, duration of surgery and position of the patient on the risk of transient neurologic symptoms. Anesthesiology and Pain Medicine. 2013;**2**(4):154-158. DOI: 10.5812/aapm.6916

[23] Liu SS et al. A comparison of regional versus general anesthesia for ambulatory anesthesia: A meta-analysis of randomized controlled trials. Anesthesia and Analgesia. 2005;**101**(6):1634-1642. DOI: 10.1213/01.ANE.0000180829.70036.4F

[24] Symeonidis D et al. Prospective non-randomized comparison of open versus laparoscopic transabdominal preperitoneal (TAPP) inguinal hernia repair under different anesthetic methods. Surgery Today. 2014;**44**(5):906-913. DOI: 10.1007/s00595-013-0805-0

[25] Mehrabi S et al. General versus spinal anesthesia in percutaneous nephrolithotomy. Urology Journal. 2013;**10**(1):756-761

[26] Gonen M, Basaran B. Tubeless percutaneous nephrolithotomy: Spinal versus general anesthesia. Urology Journal. 2014;**11**(1):1211-1215

[27] Nouralizadeh A et al. Comparison of percutaneous nephrolithotomy under spinal versus general anesthesia: A randomized clinical trial. Journal of Endourology. 2013;**27**(8):974-978. DOI: 10.1089/end.2013.0145

[28] Bessa SS et al. Spinal versus general anesthesia for day-case laparoscopic cholecystectomy: A prospective randomized study. Journal of Laparoendoscopic & Advanced Surgical Techniques. Part A. 2012;**22**(6):550-555. DOI: 10.1089/lap.2012.0110

[29] Schuster M, Standl T. Cost drivers in anesthesia: Manpower, technique and other factors. Current Opinion in Anaesthesiology. 2006;**19**(2):177-184. DOI: 10.1097/01. aco.0000192790.78139.82

[30] Schuster M et al. Effect of different cost drivers on cost per anesthesia minute in different anesthesia subspecialties. Anesthesiology. 2004;**101**(6):1435-1443

[31] Camponovo C. Spinal 1% 2-Chloroprocaine versus general anesthesia for ultra-short outpatient procedures: A retrospective analysis. Acta Biomed. 2014;**85**(3):265-268

[32] Azmude A et al. Pregnancy outcome using general anesthesia versus spinal anesthesia for in vitro fertilization. Anesthesiology and Pain Medicine. 2013;**3**(2):239-242. DOI: 10.5812/aapm.11223

[33] Newman S et al. Postoperative cognitive dysfunction after noncardiac

surgery: A systematic review. Anesthesiology. 2007;**106**(3):572-590

[34] Shi HJ et al. Effects of different anesthesia methods on cognitive dysfunction after hip replacement operation in elder patients. International Journal of Clinical and Experimental Medicine. 2015;**8**(3):3883-3888

[35] Baldini G et al. Postoperative urinary retention: Anesthetic and perioperative considerations. Anesthesiology. 2009;**110**(5): 1139-1157. DOI: 10.1097/ALN.0b013e31819f7aea

[36] Hansen BS et al. Risk factors of post-operative urinary retention in hospitalised patients. Acta Anaesthesiologica Scandinavica. 2011;**55**(5):545-548. DOI: 10.1111/j.1399-6576.2011.02416.x

[37] Linares Gil MJ et al. Factors associated with delayed postsurgical voiding interval in ambulatory spinal anesthesia patients: A prospective cohort study in 3 types of surgery. American Journal of Surgery. 2009;**197**(2): 182-188. DOI: 10.1016/j. amjsurg.2007.12.064

[38] Souter KJ, Pavlin DJ. Bladder function after ambulatory surgery. Journal of Ambulatory Surgery. 2005;**12**:89-97

[39] Voelckel WG et al. Unilateral anesthesia does not affect the incidence of urinary retention after low-dose spinal anesthesia for knee surgery. Anesthesia and Analgesia. 2009;**109**(3):986-987. DOI: 10.1213/ane.0b013e3181af406e

[40] Kreutziger J et al. Urinary retention after spinal anaesthesia with hyperbaric prilocaine 2% in an ambulatory setting. British Journal of Anaesthesia. 2010;**104**(5):582-586. DOI: 10.1093/bja/aeq054

[41] Olschewski A et al. Blockade of Na+ and K+ currents by local anesthetics in the dorsal horn neurons of the spinal cord. Anesthesiology. 1998;**88**(1):172-179

[42] Hadzic A. Textbook of Regional Anesthesia and Acute Pain Management. New York: Mc Graw-Hill; 2007

[43] Urmey WF et al. Combined spinal-epidural anesthesia for outpatient surgery. Dose-response characteristics of intrathecal isobaric lidocaine using a 27-gauge Whitacre spinal needle. Anesthesiology. 1995;**83**(3):528-534

[44] Liam BL, Yim CF, Chong JL. Dose response study of lidocaine 1% for spinal anaesthesia for lower limb and perineal surgery. Canadian Journal of Anaesthesia. 1998;**45**(7):645-650. DOI: 10.1007/BF03012094

[45] Gaiser RR. Should intrathecal lidocaine be used in the 21st century? Journal of Clinical Anesthesia. 2000;**12**(6):476-481

[46] Salinas FV, Liu SS. Spinal anaesthesia: Local anaesthetics and adjuncts in the ambulatory setting. Best Practice & Research. Clinical Anaesthesiology. 2002;**16**(2):195-210

[47] Kamphuis ET et al. Recovery of storage and emptying functions of the urinary bladder after spinal anesthesia with lidocaine and with bupivacaine in men. Anesthesiology. 1998;**88**(2):310-316

[48] Tarkkila P, Huhtala J, Tuominen M. Home-readiness after spinal anaesthesia with small doses of hyperbaric 0.5% bupivacaine. Anaesthesia. 1997;**52**(12):1157-1160

[49] Pavlin DJ et al. Factors affecting discharge time in adult outpatients. Anesthesia and Analgesia. 1998;**87**(4):816-826

[50] Ben-David B et al. Spinal bupivacaine in ambulatory surgery: The effect of saline dilution. Anesthesia and Analgesia. 1996;**83**(4):716-720

[51] Liu SS et al. Dose-response characteristics of spinal bupivacaine in volunteers. Clinical implications for ambulatory anesthesia. Anesthesiology. 1996;**85**(4):729-736

[52] Nair GS et al. Systematic review of spinal anaesthesia using bupivacaine for ambulatory knee arthroscopy. British Journal of Anaesthesia. 2009;**102** (3):307- 315. DOI: 10.1093/bja/aen389

[53] Salazar F et al. Transient neurologic symptoms after spinal anaesthesia using isobaric 2% mepivacaine and isobaric 2% lidocaine. Acta Anaesthesiologica Scandinavica. 2001;**45**(2): 240-245

[54] Le Truong HH et al. Spinal anesthesia: A comparison of procaine and lidocaine. Canadian Journal of Anaesthesia. 2001;**48**(5):470-473. DOI: 10.1007/BF03028311

[55] Breebaart MB et al. Urinary bladder scanning after day-case arthroscopy under spinal anaesthesia: Comparison between lidocaine, ropivacaine, and levobupivacaine. British Journal of Anaesthesia. 2003;**90**(3):309-313

[56] Kumar SS et al. Comparison of the efficacy of Intrathecal isobaric Ropivacaine and bupivacaine in day care knee arthroscopy: A randomized controlled trial. Anesthesia, Essays and Researches. 2018;**12**(4):859-864. DOI: 10.4103/aer.AER_135_18

[57] Forster JG, Rosenberg PH. Revival of old local anesthetics for spinal anesthesia in ambulatory surgery. Current Opinion in Anaesthesiology. 2011;**24**(6):633-637. DOI: 10.1097/ ACO.0b013e32834aca1b

[58] Drasner K. Chloroprocaine spinal anesthesia: Back to the future? Anesthesia and Analgesia. 2005; **100**(2):549-552. DOI: 10.1213/01. ANE.0000143382.89888.C3

[59] Forster JG. Short-acting spinal anesthesia in the ambulatory setting. Current Opinion in Anaesthesiology. 2014;**27**(6):597-604. DOI: 10.1097/ ACO.0000000000000126

[60] Goldblum E, Atchabahian A. The use of 2-chloroprocaine for spinal anaesthesia. Acta Anaesthesiologica Scandinavica. 2013;**57**(5):545-552. DOI: 10.1111/aas.12071

[61] de Jong RH. The chloroprocaine controversy. American Journal of Obstetrics and Gynecology. 1981;**140** (3):237-239

[62] Hejtmanek MR, Pollock JE. Chloroprocaine for spinal anesthesia: A retrospective analysis. Acta Anaesthesiologica Scandinavica. 2011;**55**(3):267-272. DOI: 10.1111/j. 1399-6576.2010. 02371.x

[63] Lacasse MA et al. Comparison of bupivacaine and 2-chloroprocaine for spinal anesthesia for outpatient surgery: A double-blind randomized trial. Canadian Journal of Anaesthesia. 2011;**58**(4):384-391. DOI: 10.1007/ s12630-010-9450-x

[64] Breebaart MB et al. Intrathecal chloroprocaine vs. lidocaine in day-case surgery: Recovery, discharge and effect of pre-hydration on micturition. Acta Anaesthesiologica Scandinavica. 2014; **58**(2):206-213. DOI: 10.1111/aas.12247

[65] Saporito A et al. Does spinal chloroprocaine pharmacokinetic profile actually translate into a clinical advantage in terms of clinical outcomes when compared to low-dose spinal bupivacaine? A systematic review and meta-analysis. Journal of Clinical Anesthesia. 2019;**52**:99-104. DOI: 10.1016/j.jclina ne.2018.09.003

[66] Black AS et al. Spinal anaesthesia for ambulatory arthroscopic surgery of the knee: A comparison of low-dose prilocaine and fentanyl with bupivacaine and fentanyl. British Journal of Anaesthesia. 2011;**106**(2): 183-188. DOI: 10.1093/bja/aeq272

[67] Camponovo C et al. A prospective, double-blinded, randomized, clinical trial comparing the efficacy of 40 mg and 60 mg hyperbaric 2% prilocaine versus 60 mg plain 2% prilocaine for intrathecal anesthesia in ambulatory surgery. Anesthesia and Analgesia. 2010;**111**(2):568-572. DOI: 10.1213/ANE.0b013e3181e30bb8

[68] Hendriks MP et al. Plain articaine or prilocaine for spinal anaesthesia in day-case knee arthroscopy: A double-blind randomized trial. British Journal of Anaesthesia. 2009;**102**(2):259-263. DOI: 10.1093/bja/aen357

[69] Guntz E et al. ED50 and ED90 of intrathecal hyperbaric 2% prilocaine in ambulatory knee arthroscopy. Canadian Journal of Anaesthesia. 2014;**61**(9):801-807. DOI: 10.1007/s12630-014-0189-7

[70] Snoeck M. Articaine: A review of its use for local and regional anesthesia. Local and Regional Anesthesia. 2012;**5**:23-33. DOI: 10.2147/LRA.S16 682

[71] Forster JG et al. Chloroprocaine 40 mg produces shorter spinal block than articaine 40 mg in day-case knee arthroscopy patients. Acta Anaesthesiologica Scandinavica. 2013;**57**(7):91 1-919. DOI: 10.1111/aas.12107

[72] van der Griend BF, Ho D. The effect of temperature on baricity of local anaesthetic solutions. Anaesthesia. 2006;**61**(10):1016-1017. DOI: 10.1111/j.1365-2044.2006.04812.x

[73] Liu S et al. Comparison of 5% with dextrose, 1.5% with dextrose, and 1.5% dextrose-free lidocaine solutions for spinal anesthesia in human volunteers. Anesthesia and Analgesia. 1995;**81**(4):697-702

[74] Malinovsky JM et al. Intrathecal bupivacaine in humans: Influence of volume and baricity of solutions. Anesthesiology. 1999;**91**(5):1260-1266

[75] Fettes PD et al. Comparison of plain and hyperbaric solutions of ropivacaine for spinal anaesthesia. British Journal of Anaesthesia. 2005;**94**(1):107-111. DOI: 10.1093/bja/aei008

[76] Harbers JB et al. A double blind comparison of lidocaine 2% with or without glucose for spinal anesthesia. Acta Anaesthesiologica Scandinavica. 1995;**39**(7):881-884

[77] Warren DT, Kopacz DJ. Spinal 2-chloroprocaine: The effect of added dextrose. Anesthesia and Analgesia. 2004;**98**(1):95-101

[78] Hocking G, Wildsmith JA. Intrathecal drug spread. British Journal of Anaesthesia. 2004;**93**(4):568-578. DOI: 10.1093/bja/aeh204

[79] Hamber EA, Viscomi CM. Intrathecal lipophilic opioids as adjuncts to surgical spinal anesthesia. Regional Anesthesia and Pain Medicine. 1999;**24**(3): 255-263

[80] Varrassi G et al. Ventilatory effects of subarachnoid fentanyl in the elderly. Anaesthesia. 1992;**47**(7):558-562

[81] Chaney MA. Side effects of intrathecal and epidural opioids. Canadian Journal of Anaesthesia. 1995;**42**(10): 891-903. DOI: 10.1007/BF03011037

[82] Popping DM et al. Opioids added to local anesthetics for single-shot intrathecal anesthesia in patients undergoing minor surgery: A meta-analysis of randomized trials. Pain.

2012;**153**(4):784-793. DOI: 10.1016/j.pain.2011.11.028

[83] Ben-David B et al. A comparison of minidose lidocaine-fentanyl and conventional-dose lidocaine spinal anesthesia. Anesthesia and Analgesia. 2000;**91**(4):865-870

[84] Korhonen AM et al. Intrathecal hyperbaric bupivacaine 3 mg + fentanyl 10 microg for outpatient knee arthroscopy with tourniquet. Acta Anaesthesiologica Scandinavica. 2003;**47**(3):342-346

[85] Ben-David B et al. Intrathecal fentanyl with small-dose dilute bupivacaine: Better anesthesia without prolonging recovery. Anesthesia and Analgesia. 1997;**85**(3):560-565

[86] Kuipers PW et al. Intrathecal opioids and lower urinary tract function: A urodynamic evaluation. Anesthesiology. 2004;**100**(6):1497-1503

[87] Kamphuis ET et al. The effects of spinal anesthesia with lidocaine and sufentanil on lower urinary tract functions. Anesthesia and Analgesia. 2008;**107**(6):2073-2078. DOI: 10.1213/ane.0b013e318187bc0e

[88] Kairaluoma P et al. Hyperbaric articaine with or without fentanyl in spinal anaesthesia: Patient and observer blinded comparison. Acta Anaesthesiologica Scandinavica. 2013;**57**(1):118-125. DOI: 10.1111/j.1399-6576.2012.02794.x

[89] Goel S, Bhardwaj N, Grover VK. Intrathecal fentanyl added to intrathecal bupivacaine for day case surgery: A randomized study. European Journal of Anaesthesiology. 2003;**20**(4):294-297

[90] Eisenach JC, De Kock M, Klimscha W. Alpha(2)-adrenergic agonists for regional anesthesia. A clinical review of clonidine (1984-1995). Anesthesiology. 1996;**85**(3):655-674

[91] Moore JM et al. The effect of epinephrine on small-dose hyperbaric bupivacaine spinal anesthesia: Clinical implications for ambulatory surgery. Anesthesia and Analgesia. 1998;**86**(5):973-977

[92] Chiu AA et al. The effects of epinephrine on lidocaine spinal anesthesia: A cross-over study. Anesthesia and Analgesia. 1995;**80**(4):735-739

[93] Smith KN, Kopacz DJ, McDonald SB. Spinal 2-chloroprocaine: A dose-ranging study and the effect of added epinephrine. Anesthesia and Analgesia. 2004;**98**(1):81-88

[94] Hood DD, Eisenach JC, Tuttle R. Phase I safety assessment of intrathecal neostigmine methylsulfate in humans. Anesthesiology.1995;**82**(2):331-343

[95] Albrecht E et al. The analgesic efficacy and safety of neuraxial magnesium sulphate: A quantitative review. Anaesthesia. 2012;**68**:190-202. DOI: 10.1111/j.1365-2044.2012.07337.x

[96] Dayioglu H et al. Effects of adding magnesium to bupivacaine and fentanyl for spinal anesthesia in knee arthroscopy. Journal of Anesthesia. 2009;**23**(1):19-25. DOI: 10.1007/s00540-008-0677-4

[97] Urmey WF et al. The direction of the Whitacre needle aperture affects the extent and duration of isobaric spinal anesthesia. Anesthesia and Analgesia. 1997;**84**(2):337-341

[98] Schmittner MD et al. Randomized clinical trial of perianal surgery performed under spinal saddle block versus total intravenous anaesthesia. The British Journal of Surgery. 2010;**97**(1):12-20. DOI: 10.1002/bjs.6792

[99] Schmittner MD et al. Practicability and patients' subjective experiences of low-dose spinal anaesthesia using

hyperbaric bupivacaine for transanal surgery. International Journal of Colorectal Disease. 2009;**24**(7):827-836. DOI: 10.1007/s00384-009-0681-7

[100] Gudaityte J et al. Low-dose spinal hyperbaric bupivacaine for adult anorectal surgery: A double-blinded, randomized, controlled study. Journal of Clinical Anesthesia. 2009;**21**(7):474-481. DOI: 10.1016/j.jclinane.2008.11.014

[101] Gebhardt V et al. Dosage finding for low-dose spinal anaesthesia using hyperbaric prilocaine in patients undergoing perianal outpatient surgery. Acta Anaesthesiologica Scandinavica. 2013;**57**(2):249-256. DOI: 10.1111/aas.12031

[102] Akhtar MN et al. Comparison of haemodynamic changes in patients undergoing unilateral and bilateral spinal anaesthesia. Journal of the College of Physicians and Surgeons–Pakistan. 2012;**22**(12):747-750. DOI: 12.2012/JCPSP.747750

[103] Casati A, Fanelli G. Unilateral spinal anesthesia. State of the art. Minerva Anestesiologica. 2001;**67**(12):855-862

[104] Borghi B et al. Unilateral spinal block for outpatient knee arthroscopy: A dose-finding study. Journal of Clinical Anesthesia. 2003;**15**(5):351-356

[105] Imbelloni LE, Beato L, Gouveia MA. Low isobaric 0.5% bupivacaine doses for unilateral spinal anesthesia. Revista Brasileira de Anestesiologia. 2004;**54**(3):423-430

[106] Kim JT et al. The influence of spinal flexion in the lateral decubitus position on the unilaterality of spinal anesthesia. Anesthesia and Analgesia. 2013;**117**(4):1017-1021. DOI: 10.1213/ANE.0b013e3182a1ee53

[107] Al Malyan M et al. Role of patient posture during puncture on successful unilateral spinal anaesthesia in outpatient lower abdominal surgery. European Journal of Anaesthesiology. 2006;**23**(6):491-495. DOI: 10.1017/s0265021506000020

[108] Esmaoglu A et al. Bilateral vs. unilateral spinal anesthesia for outpatient knee arthroscopies. Knee Surgery, Sports Traumatology, Arthroscopy. 2004;**12**(2):155-158. DOI: 10.1007/s00167-003-0350-2

[109] Fry CH, Meng E, Young JS. The physiological function of lower urinary tract smooth muscle. Autonomic Neuroscience. 2010;**154**(1-2):3-13. DOI: 10.1016/j.autneu.2009.10.006

[110] Mulroy MF et al. Ambulatory surgery patients may be discharged before voiding after short-acting spinal and epidural anesthesia. Anesthesiology. 2002;**97**(2):315-319

[111] Bailey HR, Ferguson JA. Prevention of urinary retention by fluid restriction following anorectal operations. Diseases of the Colon and Rectum. 1976;**19**(3):250-252

[112] Orbey BC et al. Do we still need to restrict preoperative fluid administration in ambulatory anorectal surgery under spinal anaes-thesia? Techniques in Colo proctology. 2009;**13**(1):35-40. DOI: 10.1007/s10151-009-0456-8

[113] Yogendran S et al. A prospective randomized double-blinded study of the effect of intravenous fluid therapy on adverse outcomes on outpatient surgery. Anesthesia and Analgesia. 1995;**80**(4):682-686

[114] Ali SZ et al. Effect of supplemental pre-operative fluid on postoperative

nausea and vomiting. Anaesthesia. 2003;**58**(8):780-784

[115] Bakhshi KN, Igbal S, Wilkinson DJ. An open randomized study of the effects of intravenous fluid replacement during day case anaesthesia. Ambulatory Surgery. 1994;**2**:49-51

[116] Toyonaga T et al. Postoperative urinary retention after surgery for benign anorectal disease: Potential risk factors and strategy for prevention. International Journal of Colorectal Disease. 2006;**21**(7):676-682. DOI: 10.1007/s00384-005-0077-2

[117] Tammela T. Postoperative urinary retention--why the patient cannot void. Scandinavian Journal of Urology and Nephrology. Supplementum. 1995;**175**:75-77

[118] Keita H et al. Predictive factors of early postoperative urinary retention in the postanesthesia care unit. Anesthesia and Analgesia. 2005;**101**(2):592-596. DOI: 10.1213/01. ANE.0000159 165.90094.40

[119] Zaheer S et al. Urinary retention after operations for benign anorectal diseases. Diseases of the Colon and Rectum. 1998;**41**(6):696-704

[120] Luger TJ et al. Management of temporary urinary retention after arthroscopic knee surgery in low-dose spinal anesthesia: Development of a simple algorithm. Archives of Orthopaedic and Trauma Surgery. 2008;**128**(6):607-612. DOI: 10.1007/s00402-007-0481-x

[121] Pavlin DJ et al. Voiding in patients managed with or without ultrasound monitoring of bladder volume after outpatient surgery. Anesthesia and Analgesia. 1999;**89**(1):90-97

[122] Aldrete JA. Modifications to the postanesthesia score for use in ambulatory surgery. Journal of Perianesthesia Nursing. 1998;**13**(3):148-155

[123] Chung F, Chan VW, Ong D. A post-anesthetic discharge scoring system for home readiness after ambulatory surgery. Journal of Clinical Anesthesia. 1995;**7**(6):500-506

[124] Junger A et al. Factors determining length of stay of surgical day-case patients. European Journal of Anaesthesiology. 2001;**18**(5):314-321

[125] Gebhardt V, Weiss M, Schmittner C, Schmittner MD. Discharge times for knee arthroscopy in spinal vs. general anesthesia. Central European Journal of Medicine. 2014;**9**(3):446

[126] Pavlin DJ et al. Management of bladder function after outpatient surgery. Anesthesiology. 1999;**91**(1): 42-50

[127] Association of Anaesthetists of Great, B., Ireland, S. British Association of Day. Day case and short stay surgery: 2. Anaesthesia. 2011 ; **66**(5) : 417-434. DOI: 10.1111/j.1365-2044.2011.06651.x

[128] Apfelbaum JL et al. Practice guidelines for postanesthetic care: An updated report by the American Society of Anesthesiologists Task Force on Postanesthetic care. Anesthesiology. 2013;**118**(2):291-307. DOI: 10.1097/ALN.0b013e31827773e9

[129] Pertek JP, Haberer JP. Effects of anesthesia on postoperative micturition and urinary retention. Annales Françaises d'Anesthèsie et de Rèanimation. 1995;**14**(4):340-351

[130] Petros JG et al. Factors influencing postoperative urinary retention in patients undergoing elective inguinal

herniorrhaphy. American Journal of Surgery. 1991;**161**(4):431-433

[131] Fritz WT, George L, Krulll N, Krug J. Utilisation of a home nursing protocol allows ambulatory surgery patients to be discharged prior to voiding. Anesthesia and Analgesia. 1998;**84**(2S):S6

[132] Mulroy MF. Outpatients do not need to void after short neuraxial blocks. Anesthesiology. 2009;**111**(6): 1388. DOI: 10.1097/ALN.0b013e3181b fa8d3

11

New Application of Low-Molecular Weight Dextran as Local Anesthetic Adjuvant for Ultrasound-Guided Nerve Block

Masahiko Tsuchiya

Abstract

Advances in ultrasound technology and the increased risk of opioid overdose following surgery have expanded applications of nerve block for surgical cases, resulting in reevaluation of adjuvants used to potentiate local anesthetics. We have found that a mixture of local anesthetic with low-molecular weight dextran, one such local anesthetic adjuvant, greatly enhances analgesic duration and potency in patients receiving an interfascial compartment nerve block under ultrasound-guidance as well as those receiving a single peripheral nerve block. Notably, a compartment nerve block in the abdominal trunk with an extra-large amount of low-molecular weight dextran mixture, which results in a longer duration of the injected drugs at the injection site, provides good analgesia that is comparable to epidural anesthesia. Such a dextran mixture also suppresses systemic absorption of local anesthetics, thus reducing their systemic toxicity, which enhances regional anesthesia safety. Furthermore, it controls unintended spread of injected local anesthetics, thus increasing nerve block accuracy. In this chapter, recent find-ings regarding use of low-molecular weight dextran as a local anesthetic adjuvant obtained in our laboratory are presented.

Keywords: low-molecular weight dextran, ultrasound-guided nerve block, local anesthetics, adjuvant, regional anesthesia, anesthesia safety, toxicity

1. Introduction

Recent advances in ultrasound technology have improved the accuracy and reliability of nerve block procedures [1–3]. As a result, there has been a shift from general anesthesia alone to that in combination with a nerve block. In addition, important related issues are opioid abuse, which has become a matter of public concern [4], as well as possible reduction in the risk of cancer recurrence in patients undergoing surgery with regional anesthesia [5, 6]. Evidence suggesting that general anesthesia in combination with regional anesthesia is superior for intraoperative hemodynamic stability and postoperative recovery has been reported [7, 8] (**Figure 1**). Those findings further advanced the shift to application of nerve block with general anesthesia, thus techniques to modify the effects of local anesthetics including use of an adjuvant compound have also regained attention [9]. Dextran,

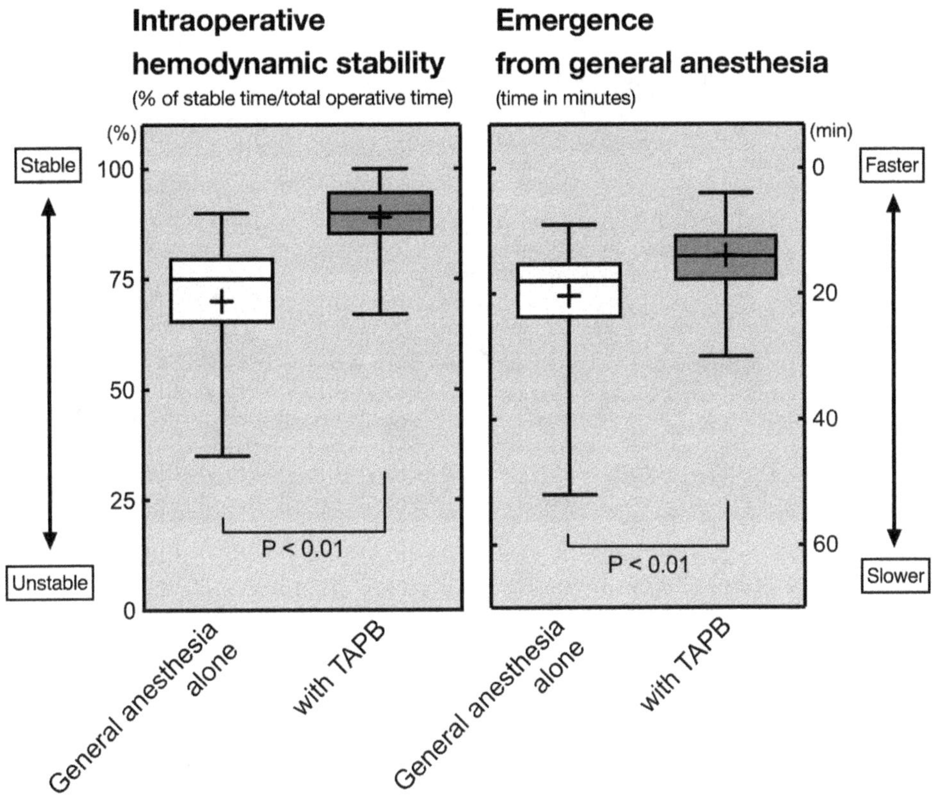

Figure 1.
Left panel: *Comparison of intraoperative hemodynamic stability between patients with general anesthesia alone (n = 35) and general anesthesia with a transversus abdominis plane block (TAPB) (n = 33) [8]. General anesthesia was maintained in the same manner with sevoflurane and remifentanil in both groups. The period during the operation when both systolic blood pressure and heart rate were within 70–110% of their pre-anesthesia value was defined as the hemodynamic stable time. The ratio of hemodynamic stable time to total operative time was used as an indicator of hemodynamic stability. The stability ratio was significantly higher in the group receiving general anesthesia with TAPB (91%, range 50–100%) as compared to general anesthesia alone (79%, range 40–91%), indicating greater hemodynamic stability with general anesthesia plus TAPB. Values are presented as the median and minimum-maximum range (mean value indicated by "+").* ***Right panel:*** *Comparison of anesthesia emergence time between the same groups shown in left panel. Anesthesia emergence time was defined as the time from completion of surgery to extubation. That was significantly shorter in the group receiving general anesthesia plus TAPB (14 minutes, range 4–30 minutes) as compared to general anesthesia alone (18 minutes, range 9–52 minutes). Values are presented as the median and minimum-maximum range (mean value indicated by "+").*

which is composed of complex branched polysaccharides derived from sucrose with various lengths and weights, is such a local anesthetic adjuvant and investigated many decades ago, though nearly forgotten in recent times.

Accumulated attention and increased need of regional anesthesia have resulted in development of new nerve block procedures, with transversus abdominis plane and quadratus lumborum blocks typically employed [8, 10] (**Figure 2**). However, these new types of nerve blocks require accurate injection of a sufficient quantity of local anesthetic into the targeted interfascial compartment. A compartment nerve block performed in this manner has potential to serve as a substitute for epidural anesthesia, the current gold standard method for surgical pain control. On the other hand, there is a risk of systemic toxicity of local anesthetics associated with this procedure because the drug is given in a large amount [11]. Furthermore, another weak point to be solved is insufficient analgesic duration for controlling postoperative pain when the nerve block is performed with a single injection.

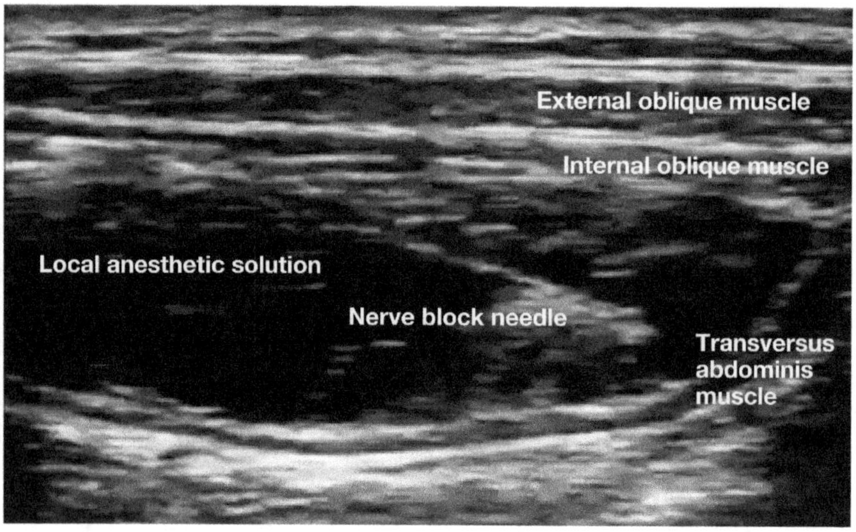

Figure 2.
Ultrasound image obtained during transversus abdominis plane block [8]. A local anesthetic solution was injected into the interfascial compartment between the internal oblique and transversus abdominis muscles.

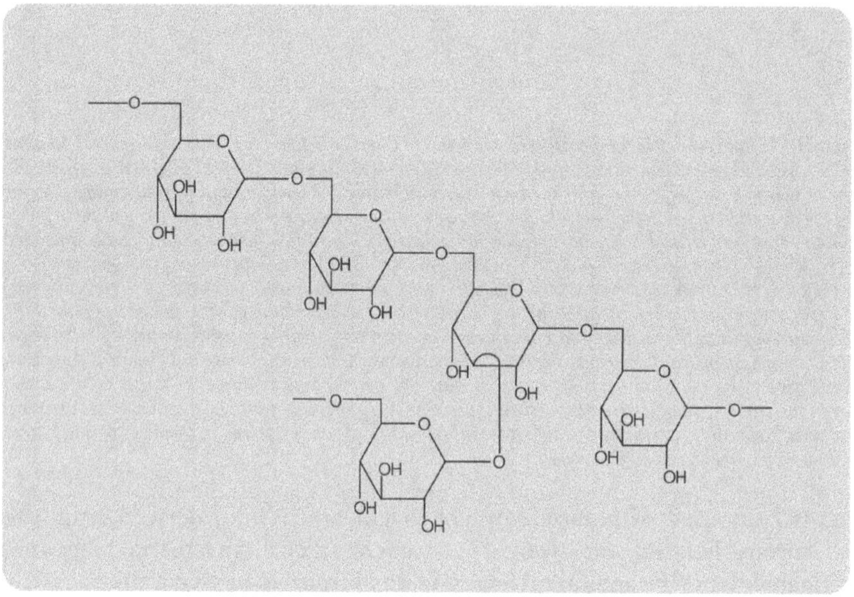

Figure 3.
Molecular structure of low-molecular weight dextran.

We recently performed a reinvestigation of dextran effects under modern clini-cal environments and found that low-molecular weight dextran, with an average molecular weight of 40,000 (**Figure 3**), used as a local anesthetic adjuvant resolves the disadvantages of a trunk nerve block by improving the potency and safety of the local anesthetic [10, 12–15]. In this chapter, effects and clinical applications of low-molecular weight dextran as a local anesthetic adjuvant are discussed based on recent findings obtained by our research team.

2. Toxicity of adjuvant adrenaline and prevention by low-molecular weight dextran

Adrenaline (epinephrine) is the oldest adjuvant given with local anesthetics and continues to be used. When used as an adjuvant it is typically applied with lidocaine, and known to induce vasoconstriction for reducing systemic absorption of the administered local anesthetic and enhancing the analgesia effects, and seems to be an optimal application. However, the combination of adrenaline and lidocaine does not always lead to good results.

Lidocaine has potent vasodilation effects, thus it can enhance the absorption of adrenaline into systemic circulation when a lidocaine-adrenaline mixture is administered. Wasa Ueda, presently professor emeritus and executive advisor of our research team, validated this issue in a clinical study, in which application of a lidocaine-adrenaline mixture for infiltration anesthesia was shown to significantly increase the plasma concentration of adrenaline in comparison with an infiltration injection of the same amount of a pure adrenaline solution [16] (**Figure 4**). An increase in adrenaline concentration in the circulation can increase blood pressure and heart rate, sometimes leading to severe lethal cardiac dysrhythmia. Such toxic effects of a lidocaine-adrenaline mixture are a significant problem for patients under general anesthesia using halothane, which has a characteristic property to increase sensitivity to adrenaline, whereas aggravating effects on circulation, such as increase in blood pressure, can still develop when the more recently introduced anesthetics desflurane and sevoflurane are used as an inhalant (**Figure 5**).

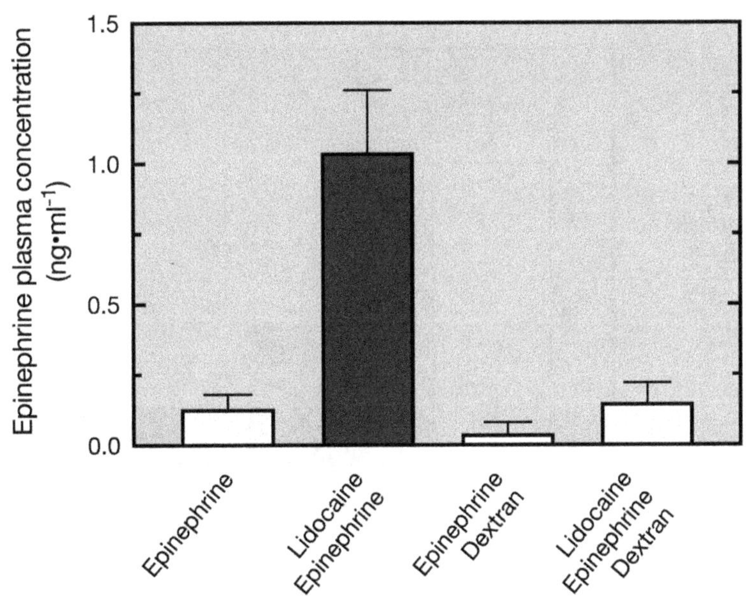

Figure 4.
Peak plasma concentration of adrenaline (epinephrine) following subcutaneous infiltrative injection of various adrenaline solutions in humans [16]. Each column indicates the following. (1) epinephrine: 1:200,000 adrenaline in normal saline solution. (2) lidocaine epinephrine: 1:200,000 adrenaline with 0.5% lidocaine in normal saline solution. (3) epinephrine dextran: 1:200,000 adrenaline with 10% low-molecular weight dextran in saline solution. (4) lidocaine epinephrine dextran: 1:200,000 adrenaline with 0.5% lidocaine and 10% low-molecular weight dextran in saline solution. The adrenaline concentration in the solutions was the same in all four groups. Values are expressed as the mean ± standard deviation. When adrenaline was subcutaneously injected with lidocaine (lidocaine epinephrine), the peak plasma adrenaline concentration showed an approximately 7-fold increase as compared with injection of the pure adrenaline solution (epinephrine). However, the presence of low-molecular weight dextran in the lidocaine adrenaline solution (lidocaine epinephrine dextran) suppressed the toxic increase in plasma adrenaline concentration.

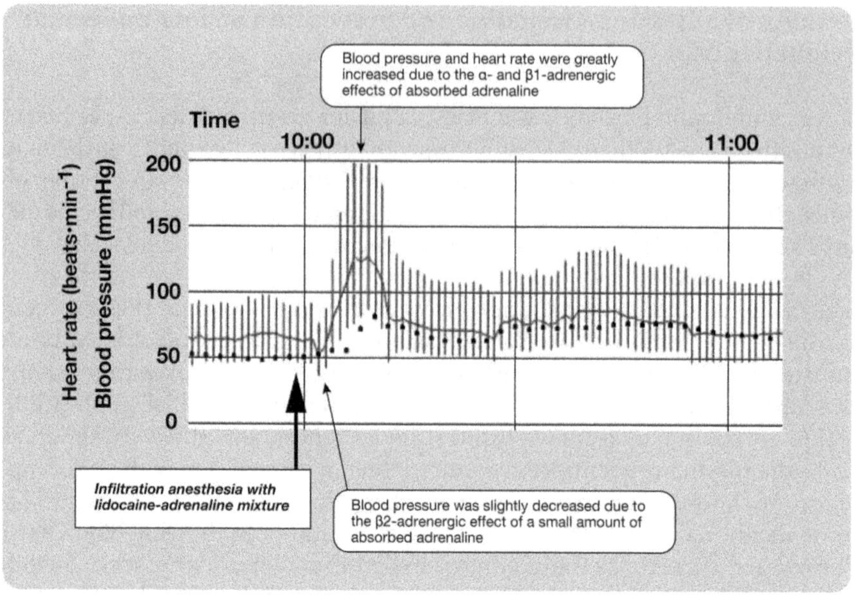

Figure 5.
Typical increases in blood pressure and heart rate with subcutaneous infiltration anesthesia using 20 ml of 0.5% lidocaine and 1:200,000 adrenaline in normal saline solution in patients receiving sevoflurane general anesthesia. Soon after injection of the lidocaine-adrenaline mixture, blood pressure was slightly decreased due to the β2-adrenergic effect of a small amount of absorbed adrenaline. Thereafter, blood pressure and heart rate were greatly increased due to the α- and β1-adrenergic effects of adrenaline.

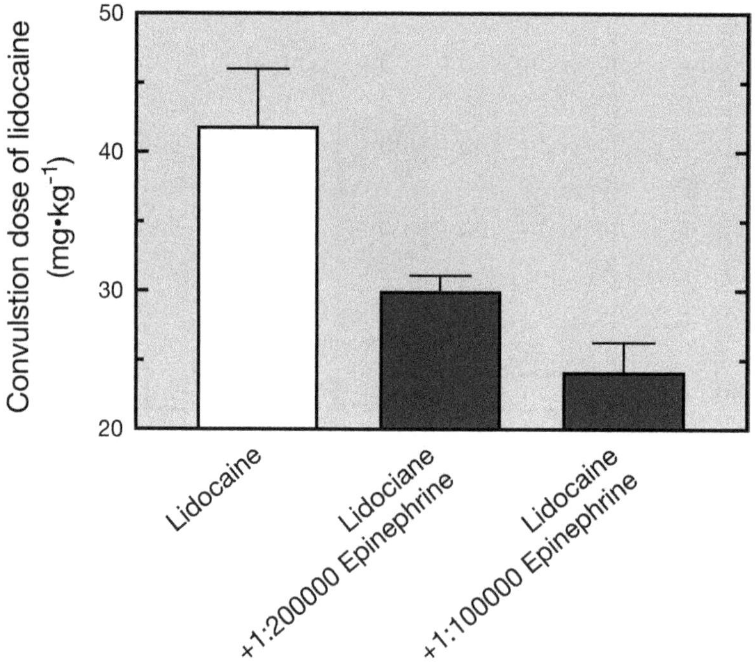

Figure 6.
Convulsion dose of plasma concentration of lidocaine in rat [17]. Male Wistar rats were divided into three groups and received continuous intravenous injections of 1.5% lidocaine, 1.5% lidocaine with 1:200,000 adrenaline (epinephrine), or 1.5% lidocaine with 1:100,000 adrenaline (epinephrine). Values are expressed as the mean ± standard deviation. The total lidocaine dose from the beginning of infusion of the lidocaine mixture to onset of generalized convulsions was analyzed. Addition of adrenaline to the lidocaine solutions significantly decreased the threshold of lidocaine-induced convulsions in a dose-dependent manner, indicating that adrenaline increased lidocaine systemic toxicity.

Furthermore, the presence of adrenaline decreases the threshold concentration of lidocaine to induce convulsions, leading to enhancement of the central nervous system toxicity of lidocaine [17] (**Figure 6**). Another study showed that concomitant administration of adrenaline with lidocaine increased the concentration of extracellular lidocaine in the brain [18], which may be another supporting mechanism by which adrenaline increases the toxicity of lidocaine for the central nervous system. Therefore, though this combination can be useful for regional anesthesia, a lidocaine-adrenaline mixture is not completely safe.

The Ueda research team found a solution to the hazardous risk of a lidocaine-adrenaline mixture, as addition of low-molecular dextran into the mixture was shown to suppress absorption of adrenalin into circulation [16]. The peak plasma adrenaline concentration with a lidocaine-adrenaline mixture with low-molecular weight dextran was 0.15 ± 0.07 ng•ml^{-1}, while that was 1.04 ± 0.22 ng•ml^{-1} with the standard lidocaine-adrenaline mixture (**Figure 4**). Thus, it was concluded that a lidocaine-adrenaline-dextran mixture is safe for application as regional anesthesia, which is now considered to be a landmark finding indicating an adjuvant function of low-molecular weight dextran to improve the safety of local anesthetic usage.

3. Early history of dextran as local anesthetic adjuvant and possible action mechanism

Apart from the effects of dextran on lidocaine-adrenaline mixtures, the first description of the adjuvant effects of dextran with local anesthetics can be traced back to the 1960s [19]. Thereafter, prolongation and enhancement of analgesia by dextran were studied, and some favorable results reported [20–22], with possible mechanisms for those actions also investigated. Dextran may form a water-soluble complex with local anesthetics that is slowly absorbed and remains at the injection site for a longer period with increased viscosity [23, 24]. Moreover, addition of dextran was shown to change the pH of a local anesthetic solution and that may further contribute to prolongation of action [25]. Despite these positive results, several studies that failed to find potential effects for analgesia with dextran have also been reported [26, 27]. As a result, along with the expanding applicability of general anesthesia for surgery, dextran has gone largely unnoticed and its adjuvant effects remain inclusive.

4. Adjuvant effects of low-molecular weight dextran with current nerve block techniques

Assuming an interaction of dextran with local anesthetics, its effectiveness as a local anesthetic adjuvant may be dependent on the type of nerve block employed and procedure used. Such nerve block dependency may induce inconsistent adjuvant effects, as shown in several previous studies. Because an interfascial compartment nerve block, such as a transversus abdominis plane block, is required to perform accurate injection of a large amount of local anesthetic solution into the targeted interfascial compartment, that is difficult to perform with a conventional landmark method. Fortunately, advancements in ultrasound guidance techniques have made this possible at a clinically acceptable quality. Consequently, an interfascial compartment nerve block has become popular. Maintaining the amount of injected local anesthetics in the compartment for a longer period is essential to induce sufficient analgesia in cases with such a compartment block, thus it is quite reasonable to assume that the possible fluid retention properties of dextran have a favorable impact. Based on findings obtained in previous studies reported by the

Ueda research team concerning use of a lidocaine-adrenaline mixture, we consider that low-molecular weight dextran is the most suitable local anesthetic adjuvant among the various dextran compounds available for interfascial compartment nerve block procedures currently used.

4.1 Pharmacokinetics and analgesia: transversus abdominis plane block and rectus sheath block cases

First, we investigated the adjuvant effects of low-molecular weight dextran when used for a transversus abdominis plane block and rectus sheath block [12]. Patients scheduled for a laparoscopic colectomy [age 66 ± 9.8 years, body weight 59 ± 11.7 kg, anesthesia time 322 ± 69 minutes (values shown as mean ± standard deviation)] received a combination of two bilateral interfascial compartment blocks, a transversus abdominis plane block and rectus sheath block. Following anesthesia induction, they received this two-block combination with either 0.2% levobupivacaine in a saline solution (control group: 20 ml × 4 injections = total 160 mg of levobupivacaine in saline; n = 27), or 0.2% levobupivacaine and 8% low-molecular weight dextran (LMWD) in a saline solution (LMWD group: 20 ml × 4 injections = total 160 mg of levobupivacaine in LMWD; n = 27). General anesthesia was maintained with sevoflurane and remifentanil, with 200 μg of fentanyl given at the end of surgery. Continuous intravenous infusions of fentanyl at 25 $\mu g \cdot hr.^{-1}$ and droperidol at 63 $\mu g \cdot hr^{-1}$ were postoperatively given for 24 hours as analgesia and antiemetic treatments.

There were no significant differences in regard to patient age, body weight, amount of intraoperative blood loss, or anesthesia time between the groups. Furthermore, no typical adverse effects, such as wound infection, delayed wound healing, tissue necrosis, or prolonged abnormal sensory disorder over the area of injection, or other systemic abnormalities were observed in either group. In the control group, the plasma concentration of levobupivacaine rose quickly just after performing the nerve block and reached a maximum at 51 ± 30 minutes (Tmax), while in the LMWD group, that rose in a more gradual manner with a significantly longer Tmax value (73 ± 25 minutes, $P < 0.05$ vs. control group) (**Figure** 7). The maximum concentration of levobupivacaine (Cmax) in the control group was 1410 ± 322 $ng \cdot ml^{-1}$, whereas that in the LMWD group was significantly lower at 1141 ± 287 $ng \cdot ml^{-1}$($P < 0.05$). Also, the area under the plasma concentration-time curve (AUC) from 0 to 240 minutes was significantly lower in the LMWD as compared to the control group (172,484 ± 50,502 vs. 229,124 ± 87,254 $ng \cdot min \cdot ml^{-1}$, $P < 0.05$). In contrast, the plasma levobupivacaine concentration in the LMWD group was higher than that seen in the control group after 1200 minutes. These results demonstrated that use of a low-molecular weight dextran mixture results in reduced systemic absorption of the local anesthetic from the injection compartment along with its longer retention in that compartment for more than 20 hours. Such a reduction in systemic absorption lowers the risk of local anesthetic systemic toxicity. In addition, the postopera-tive 24-hour numerical rating scale (NRS) for pain (0-no pain, 10-worst pain) demonstrated significantly better analgesia in patients with the local anesthetic mixture with low-molecular weight dextran as compared to those in the control group who received a standard local anesthetic solution (**Figure** 7). That result was considered to be due to extended presence of the injected local anesthetic in the injection compartment.

Together, our findings indicated that low-molecular weight dextran as a local anesthetic adjuvant provides great clinical advantages for enhancement of analgesia effect as well as reduction in systemic toxicity of a local anesthetic.

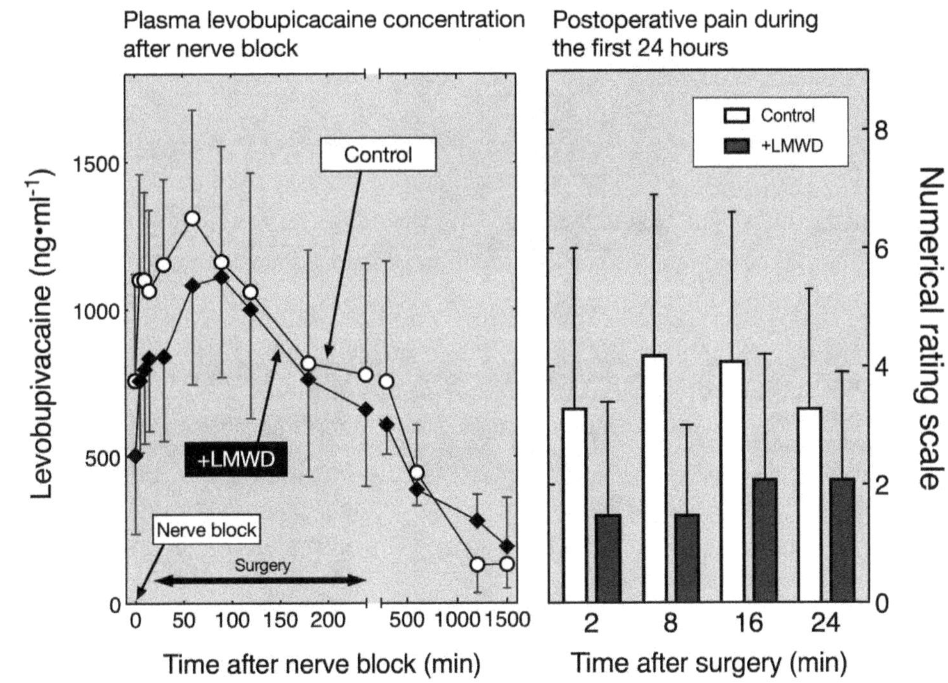

Figure 7.
Left panel: *Changes in levobupivacaine plasma concentration in patients receiving bilateral transversus abdominis plane blocks plus rectus sheath blocks with 160 mg of levobupivacaine [12]. For nerve blocks, the control group (n = 27) received nerve blocks using 80 ml of 0.2% levobupivacaine in a saline solution, while the +LMWD group (n = 27) received 80 ml of 0.2% levobupivacaine and 8% low-molecular weight dextran in a saline solution just before starting a laparoscopic colectomy. Values are expressed as the mean ± standard deviation. Addition of low-molecular weight dextran to the levobupivacaine solution was shown to lower the peak level of levobupivacaine plasma concentration, indicating that dextran suppresses systemic absorption of levobupivacaine from the injection site, which may prolong analgesic effects and decrease the systemic toxicity of levobupivacaine. After 1200 minutes, plasma levobupivacaine concentration in the +LMWD group was significantly higher than that in the control group, indicating longer retention of levobupivacaine at the injection site following its slow release.* ***Right panel:*** *Numerical rating scale (NRS) scores for postoperative pain in the same patients. Values are expressed as the mean ± standard deviation. NRS: 0, no pain, to 10, worst pain. NRS scores in the +LMWD group were significantly lower at each time point after surgery as compared to the control group (P < 0.01 at 2, 8, 16 hours; P = 0.035 at 24 hours).*

4.2 Extended retention time in injected area: quadratus lumborum block cases

To confirm the longer retention time of the local anesthetic and low-molecular weight dextran mixture at the injection site, a different group of cases that underwent a quadratus lumborum block, another type of interfascial compartment nerve block, were investigated [10]. A quadratus lumborum block using a low-molecular weight dextran mixture with ropivacaine was applied in 18 patients undergoing open abdominal surgery (age 67 ± 8.4 years, body weight 72.6 ± 4.6 kg, anesthesia time 429 ± 123 minutes) following anesthesia induction (**Figure 8**). One hundred ml of 0.1% ropivacaine and 8% low-molecular weight dextran in saline solution with 2 mg of morphine was injected into interfascial space posterior of the qua-dratus lumborum muscle (so-called QLB2 nerve block) on each side (total 200 ml in both sides). Anesthesia was maintained with desflurane and remifentanil. Postoperatively, intravenous flurbiprofen (50 mg) was given every 8 hours, with acetaminophen (15 mg•kg^{-1}) used as rescue treatment for pain.

No rescue drug was given to any of the patients on the first night after surgery and the NRS for pain (0-no pain, 10-worst pain) during that period was 2.2 ± 1.7.

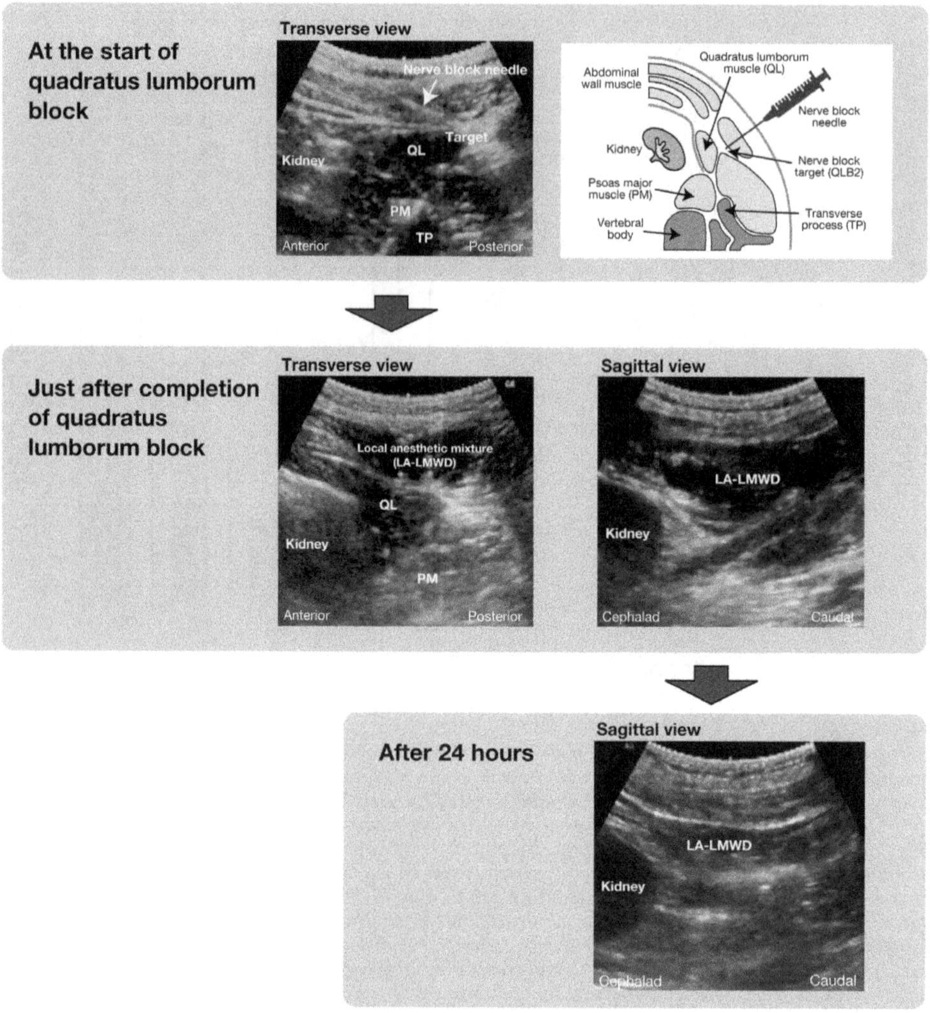

Figure 8.
Upper panel: *Transverse ultrasound image obtained just when nerve block needle reached target site in posterior quadratus lumborum block (so-called QLB2 nerve block) and related anatomical schema [10].* ***Middle panel:*** *Transverse and sagittal ultrasound images obtained just after completion of posterior quadratus lumborum block with 100 ml of 0.1% ropivacaine with 8% low-molecular weight dextran in a saline solution in the same patient shown in the upper panel. The injected local anesthetic mixture (LA-LMWD) was correctly and widely spread over the interfascial space posterior to the quadratus lumborum muscle.* ***Lower panel:*** *Sagittal ultrasound image obtained from the same injection site at 24 hours after completion of quadratus lumborum block in the same patient shown in the upper panel. Some of the local anesthetic mixture (LA-LMWD) remained. PM: psoas major muscle; QL: quadratus lumborum muscle; TP: transverse process.*

Each successfully walked more than 20 meters with less pain the next day. No local or systemic adverse effects from use of low-molecular weight dextran including tissue necrosis over the area of injection were observed. Ultrasound examinations performed after 24 hours indicated that some amount of local anesthetic mixture remained at the injected site (**Figure 8**). These findings well support the proposed mechanism of low-molecular weight dextran as an adjuvant that maintains the analgesic mixture at the injection site for an extended time, thus enabling longer lasting effects. The analgesia effect obtained with this method seems to be comparable with that with epidural anesthesia during the initial 24 hours follow surgery, thus is adequate for early postoperative pain control.

4.3 Guidance effect: erector spinae plane block cases

Findings obtained in transversus abdominis plane block, rectus sheath block, and quadratus lumborum block cases suggested that use of a mixture of local anesthetics and low-molecular weight dextran can provide good analgesia as part of an erector spinae plane (ESP) block in the same manner [14]. Thus, we applied such a block with a dextran mixture in patients undergoing video-assisted thoracic surgery (VATS) to confirm clinical feasibility and investigate the technical benefits of performing a nerve block with adjuvant dextran.

Five patients scheduled for video-assisted thoracic surgery for lung cancer (age 63 ± 7 years, body weight 59 ± 7 kg, anesthesia time 295 ± 94 minutes) received a unilateral erector spinae plane block just prior to starting surgery (**Figure 9**). Targeting the transverse process at the level of the thoracotomy incision, 40 ml of 0.3% ropivacaine and 7% low-molecular weight dextran in a saline solution were injected under ultrasound guidance. General anesthesia was maintained with

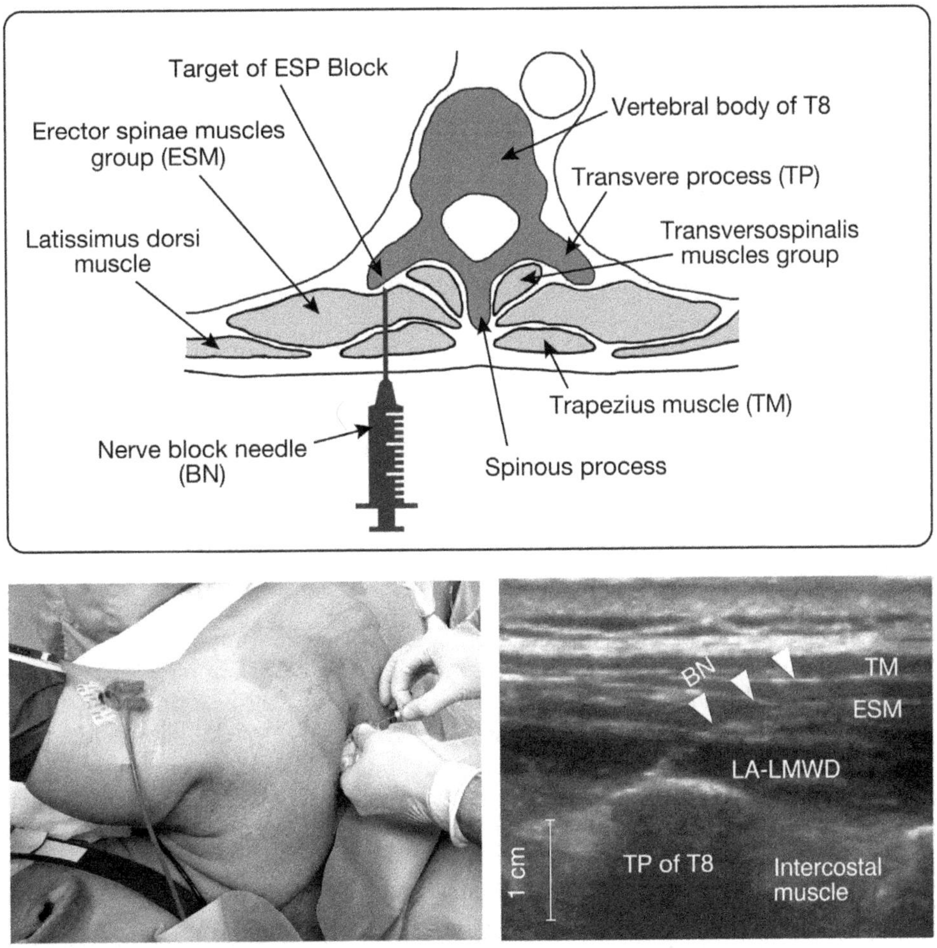

Figure 9.
Upper panel: *Anatomical scheme for erector spinae plane (ESP) block at T8 level of spine.* ***Lower left panel:*** *Positions of ultrasound linear probe and nerve block needle (BN) for ESP block targeting of the transverse process of T8 level of spine in patient positioned in a lateral decubitus position just prior to starting video-assisted thoracic surgery (VATS) for lung cancer [14].* ***Lower right panel:*** *Corresponding ultrasound image obtained during ESP block with use of linear ultrasound probe (8–13 MHz). A mixture of local anesthetic and low-molecular weight dextran (LA-LMWD) was shown spread on the compartment just above the transverse process. ESM: erector spinae muscles; TM: trapezius muscle; TP: transverse process.*

desflurane and remifentanil. Acetaminophen (15 mg•kg^{-1}) was also administrated at the end of surgery. For postoperative rescue analgesia, intravenous flurbiprofen (50 mg) was prepared.

During the first night after surgery, no additional rescue analgesic was given to any of the patients and the NRS pain score (0-no pain, 10-worst pain) was uniformly very low at 2.2 ± 1.1. No adverse effects were observed with use of the low-molecular weight dextran mixture, the same as seen in cases examined in our other nerve block studies that received a dextran mixture. As a control, we enrolled five patients who underwent our usual protocol for video-assisted thoracic surgery, general anesthesia combined with epidural anesthesia and 15 mg•kg^{-1} of acetaminophen, with postoperative continuous epidural anesthesia performed with 3 ml•hr.$^{-1}$ of 0.25% ropivacaine. The first night, NRS pain score (0-no pain, 10-worst pain) for those patients was 2.1 ± 1.2, indicating that an ESP block with a mixture of ropivacaine and low-molecular weight dextran has nearly the same analgesia effect as epidural anesthesia.

It should be noted that use of low-molecular weight dextran significantly increases the viscosity of the injection preparation. Should such a high-viscosity mixture be injected into the wrong portion of parenchymal tissue or an area outside of the target compartment, extra high pressure will likely develop. A large increase in injection pressure related to the site of injection can be a great help to avoid miss-injection, resulting in accurate compartment injection. This guidance effect may be related, at least in part, to the adjuvant effect of low-molecular weight dextran. In addition, the impact of injection pressure could be especially beneficial for novice practitioners learning nerve block procedures.

4.4 Inhibition of unintended spread: mandibular nerve block cases

Based on the above results obtained in our study of compartment nerve block cases, we also examined use of low-molecular weight dextran for cases with a single nerve block [15]. Patients undergoing a mandibular nerve block performed at a site close to the oval foramen from which the mandibular nerve appears were enrolled. In this target site, various nerves and vessels are closely assembled, thus accuracy is essential. However, a correct nerve block needle tip position alone is not sufficient for an accurate injection. In addition to that, spreading of the injected local anesthetic into the unintended surrounding area must be avoided for precision as well as safety, thus the high viscosity characteristic of a dextran solution may be best for such a procedure. Based on this speculation, we performed a study.

A mandibular nerve block was performed using a lateral extraoral approach with guidance using ultrasound imaging in 10 patients undergoing a parotidectomy under general anesthesia (age 60 ± 12 years, body weight 69.5 ± 14.6 kg, anesthesia time 227 ± 92 minutes). Following anesthesia induction, the head of the patient was turned according to the surgical site with the mouth open, then a convex ultrasound transducer was placed just below and parallel to the zygomatic bone (**Figure 10**). Next, a 23-gauge nerve block needle was inserted towards the dorsal edge of the plate, close to the mandibular nerve. When the needle touched the plate edge, 3 ml of a mixture of 0.3% ropivacaine and 7% low-molecular weight dextran in a saline solution was injected. The maxillary artery frequently appears in this section and should not be traumatized. Eighteen hours after surgery, the NRS pain score (0-no pain, 10-worst pain) was 1.2 ± 0.4 without use of a rescue drug, as compared to 2.7 ± 0.7 in our previous non-nerve block cases ($P < 0.01$). No side effects related to unintended spread of the injected ropivacaine were noted.

Performance of a mandibular nerve block using a mixture of ropivacaine and low-molecular weight dextran provided good postoperative analgesia, as well as

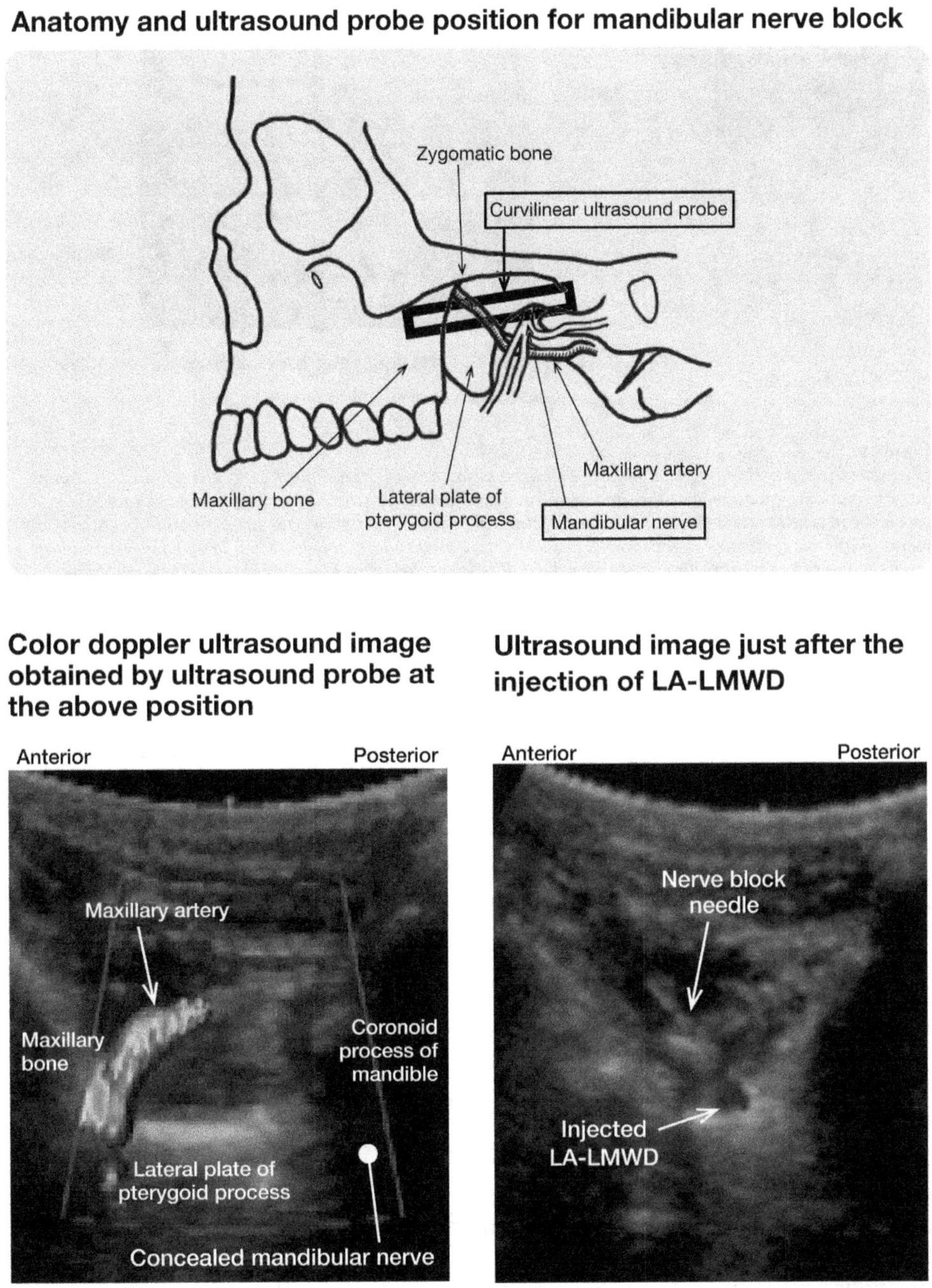

Figure 10.
Upper panel: *Anatomical relationships of mandibular nerve, lateral pterygoid plate, and maxillary artery. For a mandibular nerve block, the ultrasound probe is placed just below and parallel to the zygomatic bone [15].* ***Lower left panel:*** *Typical color Doppler ultrasound image obtained at 4.5 MHz with curvilinear ultrasound probe placed as shown in the upper panel. The maxillary artery is frequently visualized in such cases. The mandibular nerve could not be seen with this view due to acoustic shadows from surrounding bone.* ***Lower right panel:*** *Ultrasound image obtained at the moment when 3 ml of a mixture of ropivacaine and low-molecular weight dextran (LA-LMWD) was injected to the site close to the mandibular nerve emerging from the oval foramen.*

safety. These findings validated our speculation that such a dextran mixture enables an accurate single nerve block for enhancing analgesic potency of an injected local anesthetic without unintended spreading of the injectant.

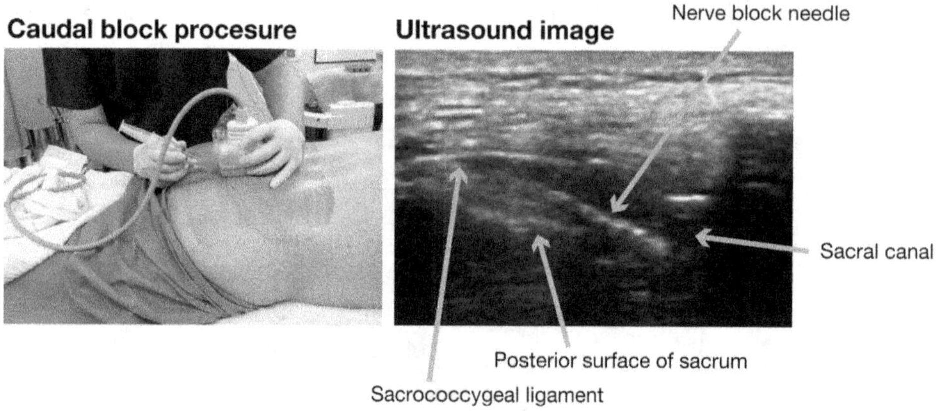

Figure 11.
Ultrasound probe positioning and block needle orientation during caudal block (left panel), and ultrasound longitudinal images obtained at the same moment (right panel) [2]. An ultrasound-guided caudal block procedure in adult patients is performed as follows. After prone positioning, the location and structure of the sacral hiatus are confirmed in ultrasound transverse and longitudinal images. Then, a 23-gauge nerve block needle is inserted in the direction of the sacral canal through the sacral hiatus while monitoring real-time ultrasound images. Next, the tip of the nerve block needle is inserted into the sacral canal approximately 0.5–1 cm ahead. After negative aspiration, a local anesthetic mixture is injected.

4.5 Advanced application of low-molecular weight dextran mixture

A local anesthetic and low-molecular weight dextran mixture can be used for a caudal block. Based on their experience, most anesthesiologists consider that a caudal block procedure in adults is generally not feasible and unreliable. However, an ultrasound-guidance technique makes such a procedure possible in adults and is rather easy to perform [2] (**Figure 11**). We consider that use of a block with a mixture that includes dextran can lead to a longer analgesia duration, thus is well applicable for gynecological, urological, and lower abdominal surgery procedures.

5. New local anesthetics with extended activities

Liposomal bupivacaine has recently become commercially available for use in cases with local infiltration anesthesia or a brachial plexus nerve block [28, 29]. Although this agent has shown excellent potential, it is quite expensive, and systemic or local toxicity occurring long after administration has yet to be determined. Low-molecular weight dextran was first used as an adjuvant more than half a century ago and its long history of clinical use, though recently limited in applica-tion, provides evidence of its therapeutic safety. Furthermore, it is inexpensive and approaches with it are easy to perform. Therefore, we consider that use of low-molecular weight dextran as a local anesthetic adjuvant remains beneficial even when compared with newer local anesthetics such as liposomal bupivacaine, with clinical condition a key factor for choosing the best method.

6. Conclusion

Findings obtained in our studies have demonstrated that low-molecular weight dextran functions as an effective adjuvant for potentiation of local anesthetic analgesia in patients undergoing an interfascial compartment nerve block, such as a transversus abdominis plane block, under ultrasound guidance. Notably, use of an abdominal trunk block with a large amount of a mixture of local anesthetic and low-molecular weight dextran, which allows the injected mixture to remain for a longer period at the injection site, provides good analgesia comparable to epidural anesthesia. The high viscosity of dextran can cause extra-high injection pressure when injected into the improper area or portion, alerting the practitioner regarding improper injection, a guidance effect and another practical advantage. Also, use of a dextran mixture may inhibit unintended spread of the injected solution and increase the accuracy of the intended nerve block. As a pharmacological safety aspect, use of a dextran mixture reduces the risk of systemic toxicity related to local anesthetics by suppressing their systemic absorption. All of these factors are significant clinical advantages gained by use of low-molecular weight dextran as a local anesthetic adjuvant when performing various nerve block procedures.

Abbreviations

ESP block	erector spinae plane block
LA-LMWD	local anesthetic and low-molecular weight dextran
LMWD	low-molecular weight dextran
NRS	numerical rating scale

Author details

Masahiko Tsuchiya[1,2]

1 Department of Anesthesia, Kishiwada Tokushukai Hospital, Kishiwada, Osaka, Japan

2 Department of Anesthesiology, Osaka City University Graduate School of Medicine, Osaka, Japan

*Address all correspondence to: oxymasa@ea.mbn.or.jp

References

[1] Tsuchiya M, Kyoh Y. Key points for intraoperative management of percutaneous endoscopic lumbar discectomy (PELD) for anesthesiologists. Minerva Anestesiol 2013; **79:** 1318-1319.

[2] Tsuchiya M, Kyoh Y, Mizutani K, Yamashita J, Hamada T. Ultrasound-guided single shot caudal block anesthesia reduces postoperative urinary catheter-induced discomfort. Minerva Anestesiol 2013; **79:** 1381-1388.

[3] Tsuchiya M, Mizutani K, Funai Y, Nakamoto T. In-line positioning of ultrasound images using wireless remote display system with tablet computer facilitates ultrasound-guided radial artery catheterization. J Clin Monit Comput 2016; **30:** 101-106. DOI: 10.1007/s10877-015-9692-9.

[4] Soffin EM, Lee BH, Kumar KK, Wu CL. The prescription opioid crisis: role of the anaesthesiologist in reducing opioid use and misuse. Br J Anaesth 2019; **122:** e198-e208. DOI: 10.1016/j.bja.2018.11.019.

[5] Exadaktylos AK, Buggy DJ, Moriarty DC, Mascha E, Sessler DI. Can anesthetic technique for primary breast cancer surgery affect recurrence or metastasis? Anesthesiology 2006; **105:** 660-664. DOI: 10.1097/00000542-200610000-00008.

[6] Grandhi RK, Lee S, Abd-Elsayed A. The Relatsionship Between Regional Anesthesia and Cancer: A Metaanalysis. Ochsner J 2017; **17:** 345-361.

[7] Bugada D, Ghisi D, Mariano ER. Continuous regional anesthesia: a review of perioperative outcome benefits. Minerva Anestesiol 2017; **83:** 1089-1100. DOI: 10.23736/S0375-9393.17.12077-8.

[8] Tsuchiya M, Takahashi R, Furukawa A, Suehiro K, Mizutani K, Nishikawa K. Transversus abdominis plane block in combination with general anesthesia provides better intraoperative hemodynamic control and quicker recovery than general anesthesia alone in high-risk abdominal surgery patients. Minerva Anestesiol 2012; **78:** 1241-1247.

[9] Wiles MD, Nathanson MH. Local anaesthetics and adjuvants--future developments. Anaesthesia 2010; **65 Suppl 1:** 22-37. DOI: 10.1111/j.1365-2044.2009.06201.x.

[10] Tsuchiya M, Mizutani K, Ueda W. Large volume of low concentration of local anesthetic dissolved with low-molecular weight dextran as adjuvant for ultrasound-guided posterior quadratus lumborum block greatly enhances and extends analgesic effects. Minerva Anestesiol 2018; **84:** 876-878. DOI: 10.23736/S0375-9393.18.12653-8.

[11] Oda Y. Local anesthetic systemic toxicity: proposed mechanisms for lipid resuscitation and methods of prevention. J Anesth 2019; **33:** 569-571. DOI: 10.1007/s00540-019-02648-y.

[12] Hamada T, Tsuchiya M, Mizutani K, Takahashi R, Muguruma K, Maeda K, Ueda W, Nishikawa K. Levobupivacaine-dextran mixture for transversus abdominis plane block and rectus sheath block in patients undergoing laparoscopic colectomy: a randomised controlled trial. Anaesthesia 2016; **71:** 411-416. DOI: 10.1111/anae.13408.

[13] Tsuchiya M, Mizutani K, Ueda W. Adding dextran to local anesthetic enhances analgesia. J Anesth 2019; **33:** 163. DOI: 10.1007/s00540-018-2573-x.

[14] Tsuchiya M, Mizutani K, Yabe M, Mori T. Possible use of low-molecular weight dextran as adjuvant for erector spinae plane block procedure. Saudi J Anaesth 2020; **14:** 576-577. DOI: 10.4103/sja.SJA_533_20.

[15] Tsuchiya M, Mizutani K, Yabe M, Mori T, Ueda W. Ultrasound-guided mandibular nerve block with local anesthetic and low-molecular weight dextran helps reduce anesthetic requirements for parotidectomy. Minerva Anestesiol 2019; **85:** 202-203. DOI: 10.23736/S0375-9393.18.12966-X.

[16] Ueda W, Hirakawa M, Mori K. Acceleration of epinephrine absorption by lidocaine. Anesthesiology 1985; **63:** 717-720. DOI: 10.1097/00000542-198512000-00034.

[17] Yokoyama M, Goto H, Ueda W, Hirakawa M, Arakawa K. Modification of intravenous lidocaine-induced convulsions by epinephrine in rats. Can J Anaesth 1993; **40:** 251-256. DOI: 10.1007/BF03037037.

[18] Takahashi R, Oda Y, Tanaka K, Morishima HO, Inoue K, Asada A. Epinephrine increases the extracellular lidocaine concentration in the brain: a possible mechanism for increased central nervous system toxicity. Anesthesiology 2006; **105:** 984-989. DOI: 10.1097/00000542-200611000-00020.

[19] Loder RE. A local-anaesthetic solution with longer action. Lancet 1960; **2:** 346-347. DOI: 10.1016/s0140-6736(60)91485-9.

[20] Ito E, Ichinohe T, Shibukawa Y, Aida H, Kaneko Y. Anesthetic duration of lidocaine with 10% dextran is comparable to lidocaine with 1:160 000 epinephrine after intraosseous injection in the rabbit. Oral Surg Oral Med Oral Pathol Oral Radiol Endod 2007; **104:** e26-e31. DOI: 10.1016/j.tripleo.2007.03.008.

[21] Kaplan JA, Miller ED, Jr., gallagher EG, Jr. Postoperative analgesia for thoracotomy patients. Anesth Analg 1975; **54:** 773-7. DOI: 10.1213/00000539-197511000-00025.

[22] Simpson PJ, Hughes DR, Long DH. Prolonged local analgesia for inguinal herniorrhaphy with bupivacaine and dextran. Ann R Coll Surg Engl 1982; **64:** 243-246.

[23] Aberg G, Friberger P, Sydnes G. Studies on the duration of local anaesthesia: a possible mechanism for the prolonging effect of dextran on the duration of infiltration anaesthesia. Acta Pharmacol Toxicol (Copenh) 1978; **42:** 88-92. DOI: 10.1111/j.1600-0773.1978.tb02174.x.

[24] Hassan HG, Renck H, Lindberg B, Akerman B, Hellquist R. Effects of adjuvants to local anaesthetics on their duration. I. Studies of dextrans of widely varying molecular weight and adrenaline in rat infraorbital nerve block. *Acta Anaesthesiol Scand* 1985; **29:** 375-379. DOI: 10.1111/j.1399-6576.1985.tb02218.x.

[25] Covino BG. Pharmacology of local anaesthetic agents. Br J Anaesth 1986; **58:** 701-716. DOI: 10.1093/bja/58.7.701.

[26] Armstrong DN, Kingsnorth AN. Local anaesthesia in inguinal herniorrhaphy: influence of dextran and saline solutions on duration of action of bupivacaine. Ann R Coll Surg Engl 1986; **68:** 207-208.

[27] Kingsnorth AN, Wijesinha SS, Grixti CJ. Evaluation of dextran with local anaesthesia for short-stay inguinal herniorraphy. Ann R Coll Surg Engl 1979; **61:** 456-458.

[28] Malik O, Kaye AD, Kaye A, Belani K, Urman RD. Emerging roles of liposomal bupivacaine in anesthesia practice. J Anaesthesiol Clin Pharmacol 2017; **33:** 151-156. DOI: 10.4103/joacp.JOACP_375_15.

[29] Skolnik A, Gan TJ. New formulations of bupivacaine for the treatment of postoperative pain: liposomal bupivacaine and SABER-Bupivacaine. Expert Opin Pharmacother 2014; **15:** 1535-1542. DOI: 10.1517/14656566.2014.930436.

12

Regional Anesthesia in the Prevention of Chronic Postoperative Pain

Brenda O. Lezcano Velazquez
and Guillermo A. Castorena Arellano

Abstract

Chronic postsurgical pain (CPSP) develops after a surgical procedure but increases its intensity and persists beyond the healing process without another cause to explain it. The incidence ranges from 5–85%, according to the type of surgery. Patients who develop CPSP may have a protracted ambulation, cardiac and pulmonary complications and increased morbidity and mortality. Several risk factors have been found related to the development of CPSP: female gender, young age, genetic predisposition, and psychosocial problems, hence prevention, early identification and treatment of these factors is essential. Several guidelines recommend the use of multimodal analgesia to treat postoperative pain, and the perioperative management seems to have a preventive role in the development of CPSP. Regional anesthesia (RA) either neuraxial or peripheral nerve blocks, by modulating signaling created by a surgical incision, play a key role in the prevention of CPSP. Local anesthetics have anti-inflammatory properties which decrease sensitization, reduce ectopic firing of neurons, cytokines expression and decrease neutrophil priming. RA reduces pain signals to the spinal cord and supraspinal and cortical nociceptive centers. RA along with other pharmacologic interventions can improve the CPSP as well as the physical and social functionality.

Keywords: acute pain, chronic pain, multimodal, regional analgesia, ultrasound

1. Introduction

Pain is a universal experience but unique for every individual. Any surgical intervention is a common pain source, that results from a planned incision at a specified point in time, often approached and managed sub optimally or without proper prevention, for this reason it should be prevented or controlled. However, there are many factors that contribute to the development and persistence of Chronic Postsurgical pain [CPSP], and only some of these are related to the surgery. As with nonsurgical chronic pain, psychological and social factors have an impor-tant influence [1].

Poor pain management will contribute to a worse experience of the disease for the patient, lower satisfaction, delayed ambulation, increased incidence of cardiac and pulmonary complications, and increased morbidity and mortality. It also has a negative impact on the health system by having short-term and long-term consequences such as late discharge and slow recovery and late rehabilitation [2].

All clinicians should have some knowledge on CPSP and how to manage established cases, which can persist for months or years after the procedure. As with many other chronic conditions, early intervention is likely to improve outcomes, so identifying patients at risk is crucial. The incidence of chronic postoperative pain varies according to the type of surgery and may be severe and disabling. Chronic pain is difficult to treat and is often permanent. For this reason, efforts to prevent its development after surgery are especially important [3].

An accurate clinical history and physical examination are essential to identify known risk factors leading to postoperative acute and chronic pain. The outcome improves with pharmacological and non-pharmacological multimodal analgesia, peripheral regional anesthesia or neuraxial techniques are some current tools that may reduce the incidence and severity of CPSP.

2. Postoperative pain

The International Association for the Study of Pain (IASP) describes pain as an unpleasant sensory and emotional experience associated with an actual or potential injury or described in terms of such injury [4].

Acute postoperative pain is a result of noxious stimulation of skin, subcutaneous tissues, viscera and neural structures. The 11th revision of the International Classification of Diseases defines CPSP as pain developing or increasing in intensity after a surgical procedure, in the area of the surgery, persisting beyond the healing process (at least 3 months) and not better explained by another cause such as infec-tion, malignancy, or a pre-existing pain condition [5].

The prevention of CPSP is an important goal, for this reason the IASP named 2017 as the Global Year Against Pain After Surgery [6, 7]. Substantial rates of chronic postoperative pain after a variety of surgical procedures, have revealed important demographic, genetic and psychosocial risk factors, which allow us in cases of elective surgery, to investigate or and prevent some of them that may influence pain chronicity. While traumatic injury is clearly not predictable [8].

2.1 Incidence

CPSP has been reported after almost all types of surgery with a high prevalence >20%, the incidence of CPSP varies depending on the surgical procedure ranging from a low of 5% to a high of 85% [9]. Some studies following limb amputation have reported incidences ranging from 50–85%, following mastectomy 11–57%, after thoracotomy 5–65%, and 5–63% following hernia repair [10, 11].

The high prevalence after these procedures may be attributed to the increased risk of nerve injury and central sensitization on this type of surgeries; but also, there could be other explanations, including persistence of a pre-existing pain in the operated area [12].

2.2 Risk factors for chronic postsurgical pain

Several studies have attempted to identify specific surgical factors that increase the risk of developing chronic postoperative pain. The surgical location, duration, and extent, as well as the experience of the surgical team, have been implicated [13, 14]. There are predictors for developing persistent pain, which are divided into preoperative, perioperative, or immediate postoperative and late postoperative.

Among the predictors in the preoperative period are patient factors including female gender, being a young adult, genetic predisposition, and psychosocial fac-tors like depression tendency to catastrophize, preexisting patient conditions, for example, pain present preoperatively, and any preexisting painful conditions [15, 16].

Perioperative factors include duration and type of surgery, extent of nerve damage intraoperatively, longer duration and an open vs. laparoscopic approach [15, 16]. Modifying surgical technique to minimize nerve damage and using minimally invasive approaches may decrease chronic postoperative pain risk [13].

In the postoperative period, the predictors will be related to the analgesic treatment, psycho-social factors, or patient factors such as chemotherapy or radiotherapy treatments, because they could be related to other states of hyperalgesia [17].

The time-point of chronic postoperative pain assessment, ranging from months to several years after surgery, may impact incidence estimates, with longer follow-up times corresponding to lower incidence rates [18].

2.3 Transition from acute to chronic pain

The intensity of acute pain is one of the strongest predictors of chronic postoperative pain, likely because acute pain itself is a product of biopsychosocial variables [19]. Pain is not only a sensation to protect the body from harm, but also a process where nociceptive information is transformed into a complex, subjective, unpleas-ant, sensory, and emotional experience with different factors that define it [20]. Acute pain responds to tissue damage, a certain pathology or abnormal function of a muscle or viscera. It is protective, adaptive and self-limited, its evolutionary function is to restrict behaviors that increase the risk of inadequate tissue recovery [21]. Nociception is a protective process that helps prevent further tissue damage by triggering reflex withdrawal responses and modification of behavior to avoid injury [22].

Tissue damage triggers profound changes in peripheral and predominantly central somatosensory circuits. Chronic pain does not have a specific function, it is related to inadequate and aberrant adaptation that can include some states of neuroplasticity [23].

Neuropathic pain is defined by the IASP as pain caused directly by an injury or disease that affects the somatosensory nervous system, it is characterized by spontaneous pain with abnormal sensory symptoms [24].

Persistent pain following surgery can have neuropathic characteristics, and many of the surgeries associated with persistent pain, such as thoracotomy, breast surgery and amputation, involve major nerves in the surgical field [13]. Following nerve injury, nociceptive neurons fire rapidly leading to changes in N-methyl-D-aspartate receptors NMDAR composition and activation. NMDARs are highly permeable to calcium, whose influx triggers neuron- specific cascades that underlie synaptic plasticity and, in extreme cases, cause excitotoxicity and neuronal death. In a neuropathic pain model, the conditional deletion of spinal NMDARs prevents calcium-dependent neuronal death and the transition from acute to persistent pain-like behaviors. This shows that glutamate, NMDARs, and calcium influx play an essential role in the development of chronic pan [25].

However, intra-operative nerve transection does not inevitably result in neuropathic pain and avoiding nerve transection does not necessarily prevent chronic pain [26]. Risk factors for persistent postoperative pain, other than nerve injury and ongoing inflammation, include pre-operative pain, younger age, female sex, genetic factors, and psychological vulnerability [13].

The pathophysiological mechanism is considered mostly neuropathic when finding an important association between persistent postoperative pain and sensory abnormalities, the evidence indicates that there are other components involved such as inflammatory processes, central sensitization, damage to nerves or somatic/visceral structures, or a combination of the above [27].

3. Multimodal analgesia

Some risk factors for postoperative chronic pain can be modifiable especially if surgery is elective, like body-mass index, preoperative pain, and some comorbidities, whereas others like demographics, genetics, and pain sensitivity are not. The site, timing and intensity of surgical damage are predictable. An analgesic regimen can be designed to anticipate, prevent, or modify the nociceptive barrage, thereby preventing central sensitization [28].

Multimodal analgesia has become an important concept in the field of modern pain management. The use of multimodal analgesia is highly recommended for postoperative pain management. It is defined as the use of a variety of drugs and combined techniques, with different mechanisms of action at the central and/or peripheral nervous system level and may have an additive effect or synergism. Some of these agents include $alpha_2$ agonists, NMDA receptor antagonists, gabapenti-noids, dexamethasone, NSAIDs, acetaminophen, and duloxetine [29].

Advantages include superior analgesia secondary to the synergistic effects of multiple agents acting via different pain pathways, the ability to limit parenteral opioid administration, and minimizing opioid-related side effects [28].

The site, timing and intensity of surgical damage are predictable. An analgesic regimen can be designed to anticipate, prevent, or modify the nociceptive barrage, thereby preventing central sensitization. Pain management plays a fundamental role in enhanced recovery after surgery (ERAS) pathways. The concept of multimodal analgesia in providing a balanced and effective approach to perioperative pain management is widely accepted and practiced, with regional anesthesia playing a main role [30].

There are evidence-based guidelines for the management of postoperative pain, like the American Society for pain management, the European guidelines PROSPECT (Procedure Specific Postoperative Management) and ERAS guidelines (Enhanced Recovery After Surgery), all of them have similar objectives; an early mobilization, a reduction in hospital stay times, a decrease in morbidity and mortality, an increase in patient satisfaction and the use of multimodal analgesia, specially regional anesthesia [30–32]. A multidisciplinary team-based approach for defining the goals is essential, based on each patient's needs, and incorporating patient, surgical, and social factors.

4. Regional anesthesia

The guidelines on postoperative pain management created by multiple societies advocate for the use of site-specific regional anesthetic techniques as part of a multimodal analgesic regimen, which is effective in several surgical procedures including thoracotomy, joint replacement surgery, and cesarean sections. Central neuraxial blocks alone or in combination with catheter techniques are performed in order to decrease stress surgically induced and inflammation, and they could improve pulmonary functions, and reduce the period of hospitalization with better pain control [30].

Effective regional anesthesia may prevent central sensitization by blocking nociceptive input into the spinal cord. Epidural anesthesia and paravertebral blocks reduce the risk of persistent pain after open thoracotomy and breast cancer surgery, respectively [33]. These findings are interesting also in view of the apparent beneficial effect of regional anesthesia in reducing tumor recurrence [34]. Regional anesthesia has been advocated in oncological surgery to reduce the risk of cancer recurrence, based on some evidence by the inhibition of tumor cell seeding and growth by various pathways. These include effective suppression of the adrenergic and inflammatory response to surgery, preservation of immune function and direct action of systemic local anesthetics on tumor cell apoptosis, and indirectly through reduction in the use of opioids which may have their own pro-metastatic effects [35].

Improvement in ultrasound technology may increase clinical applications not only for epidural and paravertebral blocks but also for peripheral nerve and truncal blocks. The use of real time of ultrasound while performing the block may reduce the complications, performance time, and local anesthetic requirements. The rate of success may increase with clinical experience. Peripheral nerve blocks seem to lack systemic side effect related to sympathetic blockade and lesser incidence of minor complications including urinary retention when compared with central neuraxial blocks or catheter applications. For what they seem to be safer than either central neuraxial blocks or general anesthesia, especially in patients with severe coexisting disease [36].

The potential beneficial effect of local anesthesia on inflammation and immune function has long been suggested [37]. Local anesthetics have anti-inflammatory properties which may also decrease sensitization. The clinical anti-inflammatory effect of intravenous lidocaine is today reasonably well documented. The exact mechanisms of action are not clear but seem to involve a reversible interaction with membrane proteins and lipids, thus regulating cell metabolic activity, migration, exocytosis, and phagocytosis [38].

The shift toward peripheral and regional anesthetic techniques has largely been driven by the advent of ultrasound-guided regional anesthesia, it provides real-time visualization and targeting of major nerves that were previously located with landmark-based “blind” techniques, therefore, it has made regional anesthesia safer, more efficient, and more accessible to general anesthesiologists [39]. There is a growing interest in the potential preventative impact of regional anesthesia on chronic postoperative pain, especially with ongoing development of new techniques.

5. Conclusions

The role of regional anesthesia in peri-operative care and acute pain management is more important now than it has ever been. Postoperative pain management continues to be a challenge for the health professional, due to the combination of factors that produce it. If not treated correctly, postoperative pain may become chronic which can cause functional limitation and psychological distress to patients. We should identify the risk factors in a patient undergoing surgery and institute appropriate preventive measures.

When seeking satisfaction in the patient, it must be understood that suboptimal pain management may be due to the lack of an updated and multidisciplinary approach. The use of regional techniques in the pre, intra and postoperative period, based on the recommendations of the multimodal therapy guidelines, implemented according to the setting and the availability of the health center, hence it can make a difference in terms of acute postoperative pain and long-term preventable consequences.

The ability of regional anesthesia to target many areas of the surgically induced pain pathways makes it a powerful tool in reducing neural activation from surgical injury, making it the centerpiece of a well-rounded multimodal approach. Several ongoing studies addressing innovative blocks will likely continue to inform preven-tative treatment options. Successful approaches to decrease chronic postoperative pain incidence should start at the time of pre-operative planning and extend into the recovery period.

Adoption of ultrasound guidance as the gold standard has been key to this; recently new techniques have been developed. Fascial plane blocks have been an important step in increasing the reach of regional anesthesia, although more research is needed to clarify their role in peri-operative pain management, reason why is particularly important to continue investing into regional anesthesia education. Advances in technology, technique development and pharmacology over the last decade have significantly improved efficacy and safety of regional anesthesia.

Abbreviations

CPSP	Chronic Postsurgical pain
RA	Regional anesthesia
IASP	International Association for the Study of Pain
NMDARs	N-methyl-D- aspartate receptors
PROSPECT	Procedure Specific Postoperative Management
ERAS	Enhanced Recovery After Surgery

Author details

Brenda O. Lezcano Velazquez[1*] and Guillermo A. Castorena Arellano[2]

1 Department of Pain Clinic, Instituto Nacional de Cancerlogía (INCAN), México

2 Anesthesia, Hospital Médica Sur, México

*Address all correspondence to: brendadelonge@hotmail.com

References

[1] Fletcher D, Stamer UM, Pogatzki-Zahn E, et al. Chronic post-surgical pain in Europe: an observational study. Eur J Anaesthesiol 2015; 32: 725-734. DOI: 10.1097/EJA.0000000000000319

[2] Rawal N. Current issues in postoperative pain management. Eur J Anaesthesiol 2016; 33 (3):160-171. DOI: 10.1097/EJA.0000000000000366

[3] Dworkin RH, McDermott MP, Raja SN. Preventing chronic post- operative pain: how much of a difference makes a difference? Anesthesiology 2010; 112: 516-518. DOI:10.1097/ALN.0b013e3181cf4253

[4] Part III: Pain Terms, A Current List with Definitions and Notes on Usage. Classification of Chronic Pain, Second Edition, IASP Task Force on Taxonomy, edited by H. Merskey and N. Bogduk, IASP Press, Seattle. (pp 209-214)

[5] Treede RD, Rief W, Barke A, et al. A classification of chronic pain for ICD-11. Pain 2015; 156: 1003-1007. DOI: 10.1097/j.pain.0000000000000160

[6] Nugraha B, Gutenbrunner C, Barke A, et al. The IASP classification of chronic pain for ICD-11: functioning properties of chronic pain. Pain 2019; 160: 88-94. DOI: 10.1097/j.pain.0000000000001433

[7] Werner MU, Kongsgaard UEI. Defining persistent post-surgical pain: is an update required?, British Journal of Anaesthesia 2014; 113: 1-4. DOI: 10.1093/bja/aeu012

[8] Kehlet H, Jensen TS, Woolf CJ. Persistent postsurgical pain: risk factors and prevention. Lancet 2006; 367: 1618-1625. DOI:10.1016/S0140-6736(06)68700-X

[9] Gan TJ, Habib AS, Miller TE, White W, Apfelbaum JL, Incidence, patient satisfaction, and perceptions of post- surgical pain: Results from a US national survey. Curr Med Res Opin 2014. 30:149-160. DOI: 10.1185/03007995.2013.860019

[10] Schug SA, Bruce J. Risk stratification for the development of chronic postsurgical pain. Pain Reports 2017; 2: e627. DOI: 10.1097/PR9.0000000000000627

[11] Schug SA, Pogatzki-Zahn EM. Chronic pain after surgery or injury. In: Pain: clinical updates. Washington, D.C., International Association for the Study of Pain 2011, p 19.

[12] Roth RS, Qi J, Hamill JB, et al. Is chronic postsurgical pain surgery-induced? A study of persistent postoperative pain following breast reconstruction. Breast 2018; **37:** 119-125. DOI: 10.1016/j.breast.2017.11.001

[13] Katz J, Ze S. Transition from acute to chronic postsurgical pain: risk factors and protective factors. Expert Review of Neurotherapeutics 2009; 9: 723-744. DOI:10.1586/ern.09.20

[14] Thapa P, Euasobhon P. Chronic postsurgical pain: current evidence for prevention and management. Korean Journal of Pain 2018; 31: 155-173. DOI: 10.3344/kjp.2018.31.3.155

[15] Sommer M, de Rijke JM, van Kleef M, et al. Predictors of acute postoperative pain after elective surgery. Clin J Pain 2010, 26: 87-94. DOI: 10.1097/AJP.0b013e3181b43d68

[16] Saxena AK, Chilkoti GT, Chopra AK, Banerjee BD, Sharma T. Chronic persistent post-surgical pain following staging laparotomy for carcinoma of ovary and its relationship to signal transduction genes. Korean J Pain 2016; 29: 239-248. DOI:10.3344/kjp.2016.29.4.239

[17] Wu CL, Raja SN. Treatment of acute postoperative pain. Lancet 2011; 377: 2215-2225. DOI: 10.1016/ S0140-6736 (11)602456.

[18] Schug SA, Lavand'homme P, Barke A, Korwisi B, Rief W, Treede RD. The IASP classification of chronic pain for ICD-11: chronic postsurgical or posttraumatic pain. Pain 2019; 160: 45-52. DOI: 10.1097/j.pain.000000 0000001413

[19] Katz J, Jackson M, Kavanagh BP, Sandler AN. Acute pain after thoracic surgery predicts long-term post-thoracotomy pain. Clinical Journal of Pain 1996; 12: 50-55. DOI:10.1097/ 00002508-199603000-00009

[20] Sjövall S, et al. Laparoscopic Surgery: A Narrative Review of Pharmacotherapy in Pain Management. Drugs 2015, 75 (16), 1867-1889. DOI: 10.1007/s40265-015-0482-y

[21] Radnovich R, Chapman CR, Gudin JA, Panchal SJ, Webster LR, Pergolizzi JV Jr. Acute pain: effective management requires comprehensive assessment. Postgrad Med 2014; 126(4):59-72. DOI: 10.3810/pgm. 2014.07.2784

[22] Latremoliere A, Woolf CJ. Central sensitization: a generator of pain hypersensitivity by central neural plasticity. The Journal of Pain 2009; 10: 895-926 DOI:10.1016/j.jpain.2009. 06.012

[23] Petrenko AB, Yamakura T, Baba H, Shimoji K. The role of N-methyl-D-aspartate (NMDA) receptors in pain: a review. Anesth Analg 2003; **97:** 1108-1116. DOI:10.1213/01.ane.00000 81061.12235.55

[24] Colloca L, Ludman T, Bouhassira D, Baron R, Dickenson A H, Yarnitsky D, Freeman R, Truini A, Attal N, Finnerup N B, Eccleston C, Kalso E, Bennett D L, Dworkin R H, & Raja S N. Neuropathic pain. 2017, Nature reviews 3, 17002. DOI:10.1038/nrdp.2017.2

[25] Inquimbert P, Moll M, Latremoliere A, et al. NMDA receptor activation underlies the loss of spinal dorsal horn neurons and the transition to persistent pain after peripheral nerve injury. Cell Rep 2018; 23: 2678-2689. DOI: 10.1016/ j.celrep.2018.04.107

[26] Macrae WA. Chronic post-surgical pain: 10 years on. Brit J of Anaesth 2008; 101:77-86. DOI: 10.1093/bja/aen099

[27] Haroutiunian S, Nikolajsen L, Finnerup NB, Jensen T. The neuropathic component in persistent postsurgical pain. A systematic literature review. Pain 2013; 154:95-102. DOI: 10.1016/j. pain.2012. 09.010

[28] Jin F, Chung F. Multimodal analgesia for postoperative pain control. J Clin Anesth 2001;13:524-539.

[29] Antonella Paladini and Giustino Varrassi: Multimodal Pharmacological Analgesia in Pain Management. In Pain Management - Practices. Novel Therapies and Bioactives, Viduranga Yashasvi Waisundara, Ines Banjari and Jelena Balkić, IntechOpen, 2020, DOI: 10.5772/ intechopen.93620.

[30] Chou R, Gordon DB, de Leon-Casasola OA, Rosenberg JM, Bickler S, Brennan T, et al. Management of postoperative pain: a clinical practice guideline from the American Pain Society, the American Society of Regional Anesthesia and Pain Medicine, and the American Society of Anesthesiologists' Committee on Regional Anesthesia, executive committee, and administrative council. J Pain 2016; 17: 131-157. DOI:10.1016/j. jpain.2015.12.008

[31] Kehlet H, Wilkinson RC, Fischer HB, Camu F; Prospect Working Group. PROSPECT: evidence-based, procedure-specific postoperative pain

management. Best Pract Res Clin Anaesthesiol 2007 Mar;21(1):149-159. DOI: 10.1016/j.bpa.2006.12.001

[32] Nelson G, Altman AD, Nick A, Meyer LA, Ramirez PT, Achtari C, Antrobus J, Huang J, Scott M, Wijk L, Acheson N, Ljungqvist O, Dowdy SC. Guidelines for postoperative care in gynecologic/oncology surgery: Enhanced Recovery After Surgery (ERAS®) Society recommendations--Part II. Gynecol Oncol 2016 Feb;140(2):323-332. DOI:10.1016/j.ygyno.2015.12.019..

[33] Andreae MH, Andreae DA. Regional anaesthesia to prevent chronic pain after surgery: a Cochrane systematic review and meta-analysis. Br J Anaesth 2013 Nov;111(5):711-720. DOI: 10.1093/bja/aet213.

[34] Snyder GL, Greenberg S. Effect of anaesthetic technique and other perioperative factors on cancer recurrence. Br J Anaesth 2010 Aug;105(2):106-115. DOI:10.1093/bja/aeq164.

[35] Cata JP. Outcomes of regional anesthesia in cancer patients. Current Opinion in Anaesthesiology 2018; 31: 593-600. DOI: 10.1097/ACO.0000000000000636

[36] Kettner S C, Willschke H, and Marhofer P. Does regional anaesthesia really improve outcome?, Brit J of Anaesth 2011 vol. 107, no. 1, pp. i90–i95. DOI: 10.1093/bja/aer340.

[37] Picardi S, Cartellieri S, Groves D, Hahnenkamp K, Gerner P, Durieux ME, Stevens MF, Lirk P, Hollmann MW. Local anesthetic-induced inhibition of human neutrophil priming: the influence of structure, lipophilicity, and charge. Reg Anesth Pain Med 2013 Jan-Feb;38(1):9-15. DOI: 10.1097/AAP.0b013e31827a3cbe.

[38] Cassuto J, Sinclair R, Bonderovic M. Anti-inflammatory properties of local anesthetics and their present and potential clinical implications. Acta Anaesthesiol Scand 2006 Mar;50(3): 265-282. DOI:10.1111/j.1399-6576.2006.00936.x.

[39] Albrecht E, Chin KJ. Advances in regional anaesthesia and acute pain management: a narrative review. Anaesthesia 2020; 75 Suppl 1: 101-110. DOI: 10.1111/anae.14868

13

Tackling Local Anesthetic Failure in Endodontics

Krishnamachari Janani, Kavalipurapu Venkata Teja, Harini K, Kaligotla Apoorva Vasundhara and Jerry Jose

Abstract

Achieving anesthesia in a hot tooth or tooth with inflamed pulp is challenging, especially during endodontic treatment. In the presence of symptomatic irreversible pulpitis, mainly in mandibular teeth, pose even more challenge to attain profound anesthesia. Tetradoxin resistant channel is a class of sodium channel that is found to be increased in such condition and is found to resist local anesthesia. The pH also determines the success of local anesthesia. In inflammatory conditions, the surrounding area's pH, which eventually decreases the amount of base form of local anesthetic penetration into the nerve membrane, thereby causing anesthetic failure. In such conditions, the excitability threshold is reduced, leading to failure in achieving anesthesia. This chapter highlights and discusses the cause of anesthetic failure and its management in obtaining profound anesthesia during endodontic treatment.

Keywords: Local Anesthesia, Endodontic Treatment, Pain, Irreversible Pulpitis Pulpal Inflammation

1. Introduction

Pain is an unpleasant sensation that can range from slight discomfort to excruciating agony and can be linked to actual or potential tissue damage [1]. It is a multimodal and biopsychosocial event with an individual objective and subjective occurrences, resulting in significantly diverse perceptions of pain between the individuals. One of the most common reasons for a patient to visit an endodontist is dental pain. Managing dental pain and anxiety during and after treatment is still a difficult task, which depends on the clinician's skill and knowledge [2].

2. Pulpal inflammation

In symptomatic pulp tissue diagnosed with irreversible pulpitis, extracellular levels of Substance P are elevated. When comparing pulp tissue diagnosed with irreversible pulpitis to clinically normal pulp tissue, an 8-fold rise in Substance P was found [3]. As a result, irreversible pulpitis is linked to high peptidergic system activation. It is generally known that root canal preparation causes inflammation in the periapical tissues, explaining why root canal therapy causes post-treatment pain (such as symptomatic apical periodontitis). SP is released in the periodontal ligaments as a result of varied canal preparation approaches, which was found to be quite interesting. However, the amount of released SP differs among procedures. Inflammation in the periapical tissues could be triggered by an elevation in SP [4]. This might thus be considered a key mediator of neurogenic inflammation and related hyperalgesia, and hence a prospective target for therapeutics targeted at regulating pain and minimizing the harmful effects of tissue injury [5].

When a carious lesion gets close to the pulp, the pulp's inflammatory alterations get worse. An acute exacerbation of chronic inflammation occurs at this stage, with an influx of neutrophils and the release of inflammatory mediators (prostaglandins and interleukins), proinflammatory neuropeptides and mediators (substance P, Bradykinin, and calcitonin gene related peptide) [6]. These mediators can increase pain perception and neuronal excitability by stimulating peripheral nociceptors within the pulp of the affected tooth. This causes moderate-to-severe discomfort. Conventional procedures may not provide sufficient anesthesia. As a result, endodontists must achieve profound anesthesia in order to alleviate the pain [7].

3. Local anesthetics

The use of local anesthetic agents in pain management plays a vital role. It is the safest and most effective medications to prevent and manage pain during dental treatment [8]. Today's availability of a variety of local anesthetic agents allows dentists to choose an anesthetic with specific properties such as time of onset and duration, hemostatic control, and degree of cardiac side effects that are suited for each individual patient and dental operation [9]. 2 percent lignocaine (Xylotox, Adcock Ingram; Xylesthesin, 3 M) with 1:80000 adrenaline content, 3 percent mepivacaine (Carbocaine) without a vasoconstrictor and 4 percent articaine (Ubistesin 3 M) with either 1:100000 or 1:200000 adrenaline concentration is currently the most commonly used local anesthetic agents in general dentistry [10]. Each local anesthetic has its own maximum recommended dose (MDR) measured in mg/kg body weight. Unfortunately, the literature7 shows that the mg/kg MDR for each drug ranges from 4.4 mg/kg 8 to 6.6 mg/kg [11, 12].

4. Evaluate the anesthesia before treatment

When dealing with a tooth that has been diagnosed with irreversible pulpitis or "Hot" tooth, it's critical to determine whether enough local anesthetic has been attained. Subjective and objective testing has historically been used to validate successive inferior alveolar nerve block (IANB). Signs such as lip numbness, probing the gingiva surrounding the tooth to be treated, and so forth are examples of subjective tests [13]. Patients should not suffer discomfort throughout therapy if they respond favorably to the subjective results. These approaches, however, are not confirmatory test for detecting pulpal anesthesia.

5. Failure of local anesthesia

5.1 Anatomic factors

While it's possible that the operator's inability to deposit anesthetic solution close to the targeted nerve would result in an insufficient blockade in both normal and non-inflamed states, it's also possible that a partial blockade would suffice in neurons that inflammatory mediators did not sensitize. It's crucial to understand the nerve supply to the anesthetized tissue and the anatomy of the injection site and any changes [14].

During a local infiltration at the root apex, however, the cortical bone of the body of the mandible can effectively block the anesthetic. The maxillary cortical bone is often thinner. Anesthetic diffusion is more easily achieved through this bone. Therefore, infiltration anesthesia, which is routinely used in the maxilla, would be less affected by anatomic variance. Block anesthesia is advised in the mandible because it is more predictable. Still, it demands a deeper awareness of the deep anatomy of the jaw and is more technique sensitive, which is why anesthetic failures in the mandible are more common. Inadequate local anesthetic has also been linked to accessory innervation of the mandibular teeth from various sources. The nerve to the mylohyoid muscle, in particular, has been linked to the transport of afferent fibers from the mandibular teeth [14]. The clinician has many alternatives for overcoming accessory innervations from the mylohyoid nerve, including using a blocking technique that deposits anesthetic solution higher in the pterygomandibular space.

5.2 Inflammation and tissue pH

The pH of the anesthetic solution determines the ratio of RN to RNH^+. According to the Henderson–Hasselbalch equation, there are equal amounts of half-charged and half-uncharged molecules when the acid dissociation constant Pka equals the pH of the solution. In a cartridge of local anesthetic solution, both charged (RNH^+) and uncharged (RN) molecules exist in equilibrium. The deionized lipid-soluble (RH) form penetrates the neuronal membrane and takes up H^+. RNH^+ within the nerve, resulting in RNH^+, which enters the sodium channel and blocks conduction. To produce anesthesia, the body buffers the pH-injected anesthetic solution to the physiological pH [15].

This becomes potentially critical since inflammation-induced tissue acidosis can cause local anesthetics to get "ion trapped." According to this theory, the low tissue pH causes a higher proportion of the local anesthetic to be held in the charged acid form of the molecule, preventing it from passing through cell membranes. This theory has been proposed as a primary cause of local anesthetic failures in situa-tions like endodontic pain [16].

5.3 Central sensitization

Local anesthetic failures may be exacerbated by central sensitization. Increased sensitivity may enhance incoming sensory nerve impulses. There is a significant response to peripheral stimuli in central sensitization, and as a result, the IANB may allow adequate signaling to occur, leading to the experience of pain [16].

5.4 Central core theory

According to this hypothesis, the nerves on the exterior of the nerve bundle supply the molar teeth, while the nerves on the inside supply the anterior teeth. Even if the anesthetic solution is placed in the right location, it may not disperse enough into the nerve trunk to reach all nerves and cause a sufficient block. This concept may only apply to the increased failure rates associated with IANB in the anterior teeth, not the posterior teeth [17].

5.5 Tetrodoxin resistant channels (TTXr)

The Tetrodoxin resistant channels (TTXr) family of sodium channels have been demonstrated to be resistant to the effects of local anesthesia. Anesthetic failures in a hot tooth are caused by increased expression of sodium channels in the pulp. The TTXr channels are resistant to lidocaine, resulting in insufficient anesthetic [18]. TTXr channels are expressed on nociceptors, and their activation with Prostaglandin E2 is relatively resistant to lidocaine. Because they are less susceptible to lidocaine, sodium channels that are resistant to TTX. As the concentration of lidocaine rises, the sodium channels get blocked [19].

5.6 Altered membrane excitability of peripheral nociceptors

Inflamed tissue nerves have a lower excitability threshold and an altered resting potential. Lower excitability thresholds are responsible for impulse transmission [20].

5.7 Psychological factors

Anxiety in the patient may also play a role in the local anesthetic failure. Clinicians who have worked with anxious patients know that they have a lower pain threshold and are more likely to complain about an unpleasant dental experience. The sight of a needle and the sound of the dental handpiece are frequently reported as causes of anxiety in patients. Furthermore, patients may be particularly appre-hensive about root canal therapy.

5.8 Effect of inflammation on blood flow

Inflammation has several additional consequences on the physiology of local tissues. Inflammatory mediators cause peripheral vasodilation, which increases the rate of systemic absorption, lowering the concentration of local anesthetics. Local anesthetics, in most circumstances, need formulation with vasoconstrictor drugs. Thus, this is a potentially relevant mechanism. Although regional variations in blood flow occur in inflamed dental pulp, little is known regarding inflammation-induced vascular alterations in periradicular tissue [21]. Furthermore, this vasodilation is likely to be confined and not seen at distant injection sites. As a result, compared to nerve block anesthesia, this concept may be more useful in understanding issues with infiltration anesthesia.

5.9 Effect of inflammation on nociceptors

Inflammation alters the production of many proteins in nociceptors, resulting in a rise in neuropeptides such substance P and calcitonin gene-related peptide. These neuropeptides have an essential role to perform have a role in regulating pulpal inflammation. Furthermore, tissue damage can change the composition, distribution, and activity of sodium channels expressed on the nociceptors. Inflammation's effect on these sodium channels might substantially impact local anesthetic failures [22].

5.10 Tachyphylaxis

Tachyphylaxis is a condition in which a receptor agonist medication causes a reduction in responsiveness to a subsequent dose of the drug. Because local anesthetics are frequently used in conjunction with vasoconstrictors, the medication may remain in the tissue long enough to trigger tachyphylaxis at the sodium channel. This has been suggested as a factor in decreased anesthetic efficacy, particularly after many administrations [21].

6. Factors influence the efficiency of local anesthesia

6.1 Anesthetic agent

Contrary to popular belief, most moderate-duration anesthetics are equally efficient in inducing deep pulpal anesthetic for root canal treatment. Understanding the anatomical, local, and psychological aspects of each patient against the type of anesthetic utilized is critical to success. Most dentists prefer to employ a combination of anesthetics and a vasoconstrictor. When some types of anesthetic drugs are used, it is possible that the patients would experience more pain. Because of the acidic nature of local anesthetics, lower pH values are considered to produce a burning sensation during injection [23].

6.2 Site of injection

The injection location might influence injection discomfort. According to one study, maxillary buccal injections with plain 2% lidocaine Was found to be considerably less discomfort than 2% lidocaine with 1:80000 epinephrine. However, using the same anesthetic drugs, no difference in injection discomfort was recorded at the palatal location [12]. The type of anesthetic solution has little effect on injection discomfort when a location with less connective tissue (such as the palatal site in the maxilla) is injected. Faster injection speed leads to increased drug distribution. It has been proposed that a speed of injection exposes a larger portion of a nerve to the anesthetic solution, resulting in a higher rate of local anesthesia success. The rapid injections, on the other hand, produced more pain and discomfort during the procedure [23–25].

6.3 Preoperative pain

In individuals with symptomatic irreversible pulpitis, the degree of preoperative pain might impact anesthetic success. The activation of nociceptors during inflammation might be one reason for the lower success rate of inflamed pulp. The peripheral and central pain pathways are altered and modulated by the barrage of painful stimuli, as well as tissue destruction. Another reason for failure is that nerves from inflamed tissue have reduced excitability thresholds and altered resting potentials [26].

6.4 Pre emptive medication

Inflamed pulps may have more tetrodotoxin-resistant sodium channels, which are resistant to local anesthetics. Prostaglandins, which can influence tetrodotoxin-resistant receptors and reduce nerve responses to anesthetic drugs, have also risen considerably in inflamed pulps [27]. As a result, premedication with nonsteroidal anti-inflammatory medicines (NSAIDs) and corticosteroids to increase anesthetic success appear to be a viable option. However, the findings of such research do not agree on the effectiveness of premedication on anesthetic success [28, 29]. However, if the patient does not have spontaneous pain, pre-treatment with particular types of NSAIDs may improve the effectiveness of anesthesia when treat-ing irreversible pulpitis [30]. Premedication with corticosteroids before anesthesia with an inferior alveolar nerve block (IANB) injection resulted in a considerably better success rate.

6.5 Gender and genetic factor

Genetics may play a role in predisposing specific individuals to problems such as discomfort, delayed healing, and abscess development. A range of genetic variations influences pain perception and behavior. Pain becomes significantly more common in women, and various explanations have been proposed, including hormonal and genetically driven sex variations in brain neurochemistry [27].

7. Pain management

7.1 Supplementary anesthesia

7.1.1 Intraligamentary anesthesia

Intraligamentary anesthesia is a technique wherein local anesthetic solution administered via the periodontal ligament to reach the pulpal nerve supply. The use of conventional or customized syringes can be used for this technique. At the mesiobuccal aspect, the needle is placed as deeply between the root surface and alveolar bone at a 30° angle to the long axis of the tooth. The needle can be placed with the bevel pointing in either direction, and 0.2 ml of the solution should be injected per root using back pressure. For 5 to 10 seconds, the needle is held in place [31]. The anesthetic action begins almost immediately and lasts for around 15–20 minutes [32].

In comparison to other anesthetic techniques, Intraligamentary anesthesia allows for a substantial reduction in the overall volume of anesthetic solution and vasoconstrictor supplement. At the same time, the unintentional intravascular application is avoided [33]. Furthermore, the effectiveness of Intraligamentary anesthesia is limited in cases of severe marginal periodontitis or teeth with a sclerotic periodontal gap, and alternate anesthetic methods such as inferior alveolar nerve block can be advised [32].

7.1.2 Intraosseous anesthesia

Intraosseous Anesthesia is more invasive and necessitates the use of specialist equipment, such as a perforator (e.g., Stabident, X-Tip). The gingiva must first be sedated for the perforator to penetrate without discomfort. A slow-speed handpiece is used to move the perforator into the anesthetic gingiva and bone until the cancellous bone is felt like a sharp dip. The perforator is then withdrawn, and a small 27-gauge needle is introduced through the perforation, injecting approximately 1 mL of solution over 2 minutes. It's one of the most effective supplemental methods available [34]. The intraosseous injection permits the local anesthetic solution to be injected directly into the cancellous bone adjacent to the tooth that has to be sedated [35]. The intraosseous anesthetic onset of anesthesia is immediate and lasts for around 15 to 30 minutes, and was found to be more efficient than intraligamentary anesthesia [36].

7.1.3 Buccal infiltration

After a failed IANB, buccal infiltration has been utilized as a supplemental anesthetic for anesthetizing mandibular molar teeth, especially in symptomatic irreversible pulpitis. A mandibular buccal infiltration injection of 4% articaine with 1:100,000 epinephrine as an additional injection to improve the effectiveness of the IANB injection has recently been investigated. The usage of the articaine solution was shown to be better than the lidocaine solution in asymptomatic individuals (88 percent vs. 71 percent, respectively) [37]. Only 58% anesthesia was achievable with buccal infiltration injection when used as a supplement to the IANB in case of symptomatic irreversible pulpitis [38].

7.1.4 Intrapulpal anesthesia

Intrapulpal anesthesia is one of the supplementary anesthesia that is beneficial, especially in a hot tooth. The most crucial aspect of this technique is to pump the fluid into the pulp forcefully. If the physician does not feel pressure or resistance to injection, the solution is not reaching the pulp and is most likely running out of the pulp chamber and back into the access cavity [39]. However, this type of anesthesia is excruciating and should only be used as the last option during endodontic therapy. Intrapulpal anesthesia has the drawback of having a limited duration of effect. As a result, it's critical to remove the pulp from all of the root canals as soon as possible after injection to avoid repeated injection [40]. It is necessary that the patient should be informed that the type of anesthesia will cause moderate to severe discomfort in the beginning.

7.2 Buffered anesthesia

Buffered local anesthesia technique to one of the techniques to improve the efficiency of the local anesthetics. Alkalinization accelerates the dissociation of the LA molecule, increasing in the uncharged base form that penetrates the nerve membrane and acts in the intraneuronal location. The addition of sodium bicarbonate is the most frequent technique for buffering LAs. The addition of sodium bicarbon-ate to local anesthetics reacts to form sodium chloride water and carbon dioxide. Alkalinization with sodium bicarbonate raise the pH of the solution. Carbon dioxide produces an independent anesthetic effect by changing the local anesthetic inside the nerve direct depressant effect of carbon dioxide on the nerve axon [41]. 50 mEq is the maximum dose of sodium bicarbonate. 20 ml of 1 or 2% lignocaine is recommended to be added with 2 ml of 8.4 percent sodium bicarbonate. The ratio of lignocaine to bicarbonate should be between 5:1 and 10:1 for best effects. If the bicarbonate level exceeds this ratio, precipitation may occur. In individuals with metabolic acidosis and hypocalcemia, this method is contraindicated [15].

8. Conclusion

Pain being the most common symptom, every effort should be made to manage it during and after root canal treatment and should be informed priorly the type of anesthesia administered to the patient. Although various anesthetic agents and techniques are available, the choice of them is specific and customized to each patient and their preoperative status and clinical condition. So, ultimately, the clinician should critically decide on a specific agent or a technique for the clinical condition of the patient. It is necessary to provide appropriate pulpal anesthesia when treating teeth with irreversible pulpitis.

Author details

Krishnamachari Janani[1], Kavalipurapu Venkata Teja[2*], Harini K[3], Kaligotla Apoorva Vasundhara[4] and Jerry Jose[2]

1 Department of Conservative Dentistry and Endodontics SRM Dental College, Ramapuram, Chennai, Tamilnadu, India

2 Department of Conservative Dentistry and Endodontics, Saveetha Dental College and Hospitals, Saveetha Institute of Medical and Technical Sciences, Saveetha University, Chennai, Tamilnadu, India

3 Centre for Food Technology, Anna University, Guindy, Chennai, Tamilnadu, India

4 Private Practitioner MDS, Prosthodontist and Oral Implantologist, Andhra Pradesh, India

*Address all correspondence to: venkatatejak.sdc@saveetha.com

References

[1] Sadaf D, Ahmad MZ. Factors associated with postoperative pain in endodontic therapy. Int J Biomed Sci IJBS. 2014;10(4):243-7.

[2] Perković I, Romić MK, Perić M, Krmek SJ. The level of anxiety and pain perception of endodontic patients. Acta Stomatol Croat. 2014;48(4):258-67. https://doi.org/10.15644/asc48/4/3

[3] Bowles WR, Withrow JC, Lepinski AM, Hargreaves KM. Tissue levels of immunoreactive substance P are increased in patients with irreversible pulpitis. J Endod. 2003;29(4):265-7. https://doi.org/10. 1097/00004770-20 0304000-00009

[4] Bamini L, Sherwood IA, Abbott PV, Uthandakalaipandian R, Velu V. Influence of anti-inflammatory irrigant on substance P expression for single-visit root canal treatment of teeth with irreversible pulpitis. Aust Endod J. 2020;46(1):73-81. doi: 10.1111/aej.12353.

[5] Caviedes-Bucheli J, Azuero-Holguin MM, Gutierrez-Sanchez L, Higuerey-Bermudez F, Pereira-Nava V, Lombana N, et al. The effect of three different rotary instrumentation systems on substance P and calcitonin gene-related peptide expression in human periodontal ligament. J Endod. 2010;36(12):1938-42. doi: 10.1016/j. joen.2010.08.043.

[6] Abdulkhaleq LA, Assi MA, Abdullah R, Zamri-Saad M, Taufiq-Yap YH, Hezmee MNM. The crucial roles of inflammatory mediators in inflammation: A review. Vet World. 2018;11(5):627-35. doi: 10.14202/vetworld.2018.627-635.

[7] Byers MR, Närhi MV. Dental injury models: experimental tools for understanding neuroinflammatory interactions and polymodal nociceptor functions. Crit Rev Oral Biol Med Off Publ Am Assoc Oral Biol. 1999;10(1):4-39. doi: 10.1177/10454411990100010101.

[8] Zanjir M, Lighvan NL, Yarascavitch C, Beyene J, Shah PS, Azarpazhooh A. Efficacy and safety of pulpal anesthesia strategies during endodontic treatment of permanent mandibular molars with symptomatic irreversible pulpitis: A systematic review and network meta-analysis. J Endod. 2019;45(12):1435-1464.e10. doi: 10.1016/j.joen.2019.09. 002.

[9] Vijayalakshmi B. Knowledge of students about local anaesthetics used during oral surgical procedures. J Pharm Sci. 2015;7:4.

[10] Moodley DS. Local anaesthetics in dentistry - Part 2: Choice of local anaesthetic agent. South Afr Dent J. 2017;72(3):128-30.

[11] Weaver JM. Calculating the maximum recommended dose of local anesthetic. J Calif Dent Assoc. 2007;35(1):61-3. PMID: 17269289

[12] Meechan JG. Why does local anaesthesia not work everytime? Dent Update. 2005;32(2):66-8, 70-2. doi: 10.12968/denu.2005.32.2.66.

[13] Claffey E, Reader A, Nusstein J, Beck M, Weaver J. Anesthetic efficacy of articaine for inferior alveolar nerve blocks in patients with irreversible pulpitis. J Endod. 2004;30(8):568-71. doi: 10.1097/01.don.0000125317. 21892.8f.

[14] Hargreaves KM, Keiser K. Local anesthetic failure in endodontics: Endod Top. 2002;1(1):26-39. https://doi.org/10. 1034/j.1601-1546.2002. 10103.x

[15] Senthoor P, Janani K, Ravindran C. A prospective, randomized double-blinded study to evaluate the efficacy of

buffered local anesthetics in infected and inflamed pulp and periapical tissues. J Maxillofac Oral Surg. 2020 Jun;19(2):246-250. doi: 10.1007/s12663-019-01188-y. Epub 2019 Feb 1. PMID: 32346235; PMCID: PMC7176779.

[16] Boopathi T, Sebeena M, Sivakumar K, Harikaran J, Karthick K, Raj A. Supplemental pulpal anesthesia for mandibular teeth. J Pharm Bioallied Sci. 2013;5(Suppl 1):S103-8. doi: 10.4103/0975-7406.113307.

[17] Fernandez C, Reader A, Beck M, Nusstein J. A prospective, randomized, double-blind comparison of bupivacaine and lidocaine for inferior alveolar nerve blocks. J Endod. 2005;31(7):499-503 . doi: 10.1097/01.don.0000167395.61075.38.

[18] Kistner K, Zimmermann K, Ehnert C, Reeh PW, Leffler A. The tetrodotoxin-resistant Na+ channel Na (v)1.8 reduces the potency of local anesthetics in blocking C-fiber nociceptors. Pflugers Arch. 2010;459(5): 751-63. doi: 10.1007/s00424-010- 0785-5

[19] Pinto V, Derkach VA, Safronov BV. Role of TTX-sensitive and TTX-resistant sodium channels in Adelta- and C-fiber conduction and synaptic transmission. J Neurophysiol. 2008; 99(2):617-28. doi: 10.1152/jn.00944.2007

[20] Byers MR, Taylor PE, Khayat BG, Kimberly CL. Effects of injury and inflammation on pulpal and periapical nerves. J Endod. 1990;16(2):78-84. doi: 10.1016/S0099-2399(06)81568-2

[21] Vandermeulen E. [Pain perception, mechanisms of action of local anesthetics and possible causes of failure]. Rev Belge Med Dent. 2000;55(1):29-40.

[22] Coward K, Plumpton C, Facer P, Birch R, Carlstedt T, Tate S, et al. Immunolocalization of SNS/PN3 and NaN/SNS2 sodium channels in human pain states. Pain. 2000;85(1-2):41-50. doi: 10.1016/s0304-3959(99)00251-1

[23] Kanaa MD, Whitworth JM, Corbett IP, Meechan JG. Articaine and lidocaine mandibular buccal infiltration anesthesia: a prospective randomized double-blind cross-over study. J Endod. 2006;32(4):296-8. doi: 10.1016/j.joen.2005.09.016.

[24] Whitworth JM, Kanaa MD, Corbett IP, Meechan JG. Influence of injection speed on the effectiveness of incisive/mental nerve block: a randomized, controlled, double-blind study in adult volunteers. J Endod. 2007;33(10):1149-54. doi: 10.1016/j. joen.2007.07.016

[25] Aggarwal V, Singla M, Rizvi A, Miglani S. Comparative evaluation of local infiltration of articaine, articaine plus ketorolac, and dexamethasone on anesthetic efficacy of inferior alveolar nerve block with lidocaine in patients with irreversible pulpitis. J Endod. 2011;37(4):445-9. doi: 10.1016/j.joen.2011.01.016.

[26] Aggarwal V, Singla M, Subbiya A, Vivekanandhan P, Sharma V, Sharma R, et al. Effect of preoperative pain on inferior alveolar nerve block. Anesth Prog. 2015;62(4):135-9.doi: 10.2344/15-00019.1.

[27] Rosenberg PA. Clinical strategies for managing endodontic pain. Endodontic Topics. 2002;3(1):78-92. https://doi.org/10.1034/j.1601-1546.2002. 30108.x

[28] Parirokh M, Ashouri R, Rekabi AR, Nakhaee N, Pardakhti A, Askarifard S, et al. The effect of premedication with ibuprofen and indomethacin on the success of inferior alveolar nerve block for teeth with irreversible pulpitis. J Endod. 2010;36(9):1450-4. doi: 10.1016/j.joen.2010.05.007.

[29] Jena A, Shashirekha G. Effect of preoperative medications on the efficacy

of inferior alveolar nerve block in patients with irreversible pulpitis: A placebo-controlled clinical study. J Conserv Dent JCD. 2013;16(2):171-4.doi: 10.4103/0972-0707.108209.

[30] Parirokh M, V. Abbott P. Various strategies for pain-free root canal treatment. Iran Endod J. 2014;9(1): 1-14. doi:10.22037/IEJ.V9I1.5126

[31] Subbiya A, Pradeepkumar AR, Vivekanandhan P, Karthick A. Comparative efficacy evaluation of articaine as buccal infiltration and lignocaine as IANB in the mandibular first molar with irreversible pulpitis. Indian J Multidiscip Dent. 2011 1;2(1):370.

[32] Burtscher D, Dalla Torre D. Intraligamentary anesthesia–A brief review of an underestimated anesthetic technique. Oral Health. 2019;4:1-3. doi:10.15761/OHC.1000177

[33] Kämmerer PW, Adubae A, Buttchereit I, Thiem DGE, Daubländer M, Frerich B. Prospective clinical study comparing intraligamentary anesthesia and inferior alveolar nerve block for extraction of posterior mandibular teeth. Clin Oral Investig. 2018;22(3):1469-75. doi: 10.1007/s00784-017-2248-2

[34] Pradeepkumar AR. Pain management in endodontics. J Oper Dent Endod. 2016;1(2):76-81.

[35] Bigby J, Reader A, Nusstein J, Beck M, Weaver J. Articaine for supplemental intraosseous anesthesia in patients with irreversible pulpitis. J Endod. 2006;32(11):1044-7. doi: 10.1016/j.joen.2006.06.006.

[36] Idris M, Sakkir N, Naik KG, Jayaram NK. Intraosseous injection as an adjunct to conventional local anesthetic techniques: A clinical study. Journal of conservative dentistry: J Conserv Dent 2014;17(5):432. doi: 10.4103/0972-0707.139828.

[37] Haase A, Reader A, Nusstein J, Beck M, Drum M. Comparing anesthetic efficacy of articaine versus lidocaine as a supplemental buccal infiltration of the mandibular first molar after an inferior alveolar nerve block. J Am Dent Assoc 1939. 2008;139(9):1228-35. doi: 10.14219/jada. archive.2008.0338.

[38] Matthews R, Drum M, Reader A, Nusstein J, Beck M. Articaine for supplemental buccal mandibular infiltration anesthesia in patients with irreversible pulpitis when the inferior alveolar nerve block fails. J Endod. 2009;35(3):343-6. doi: 10.1016/j.joen.2008.11.025.

[39] VanGheluwe J, Walton R. Intrapulpal injection: factors related to effectiveness. Oral Surg Oral Med Oral Pathol Oral Radiol Endod. 1997;83(1):38-40. doi: 10.1016/s1079-2104(97)90088-3.

[40] Evans G, Nusstein J, Drum M, Reader A, Beck M. A prospective, randomized, double-blind comparison of articaine and lidocaine for maxillary infiltrations. J Endod. 2008;34(4):389-93. doi: 10.1016/j.joen.2008.01.004.

[41] Saatchi M, Khademi A, Baghaei B, Noormohammadi H. Effect of sodium bicarbonate-buffered lidocaine on the success of inferior alveolar nerve block for teeth with symptomatic irreversible pulpitis: a prospective, randomized double-blind study. J Endod. 2015;41 (1):33-5. doi:10.1016/j.joen.2014.09.011.

14

Fast Track Arthroplasty Using Local Infiltration Analgesia

Timothy Cordingley, Daniel Chepurin, Ghada Younis, Islam Nassar and David Mitchell

Abstract

Fast track arthroplasty is a holistic approach to patients who undergo total hip and knee arthroplasty, a journey or care that begins with setting patient's expecta-tion, optimising medical status, using intraoperative local anaesthetic infiltra-tion, decreasing narcotics usage either in spinal or post-operative medication, discourag-ing usage of patient controlled analgesia or urinary catheters, encouraging day of operation mobilisation and optimising post-operative physiotherapy protocols. The use of local infiltration analgesia (LIA) is a good alternative compared to other traditional pain management techniques. The purpose of adoption of LIA technique is to provide comfort from the trauma associated with hip and knee arthroplasty particularly for the first 36 h post-operatively, during the time of high post-operative pain, to facilitate increased post-operative mobilisation and function. LIA is safe and effective to achieve good outcomes, early mobilisation and decreasing length of stay without jeopardising clinical outcomes. This chapter discusses LIA and its multimodal approach to analgesia, regional anaesthesia and early mobilisa-tion that improves overall patient experience and satisfaction. The chapter discusses LIA techniques, wound catheter placement, and postoperative protocol to achieve fast track hip and knee arthroplasty.

Keywords: local infiltration analgesia, fast track arthroplasty, rapid recovery arthroplasty, enhanced recovery after surgery, total hip arthroplasty, total knee arthroplasty

1. Introduction

Hip and knee joint arthroplasty are effective in reducing pain and improving function and quality of life in patients with osteoarthritis or other destructive joint disease [1, 2]. This brings an increasing demand on healthcare systems to facilitate smooth recovery, not troubled by nausea or the adverse effects of narcotics. Acute pain leads to decreased mobility, increased length of stay, and an increased need for inpatient rehabilitation, chronic pain, subsequently leading to dissatisfied patients and increasing burden on healthcare resources [3–5]. Utilising an optimum anal-gesic protocol is challenging; outweighing the benefits and risks of each protocol is key in improving clinical outcomes and patient satisfaction.

Rapid recovery following elective hip and knee arthroplasty has been adopted with consistent patient satisfaction without jeopardising clinical outcomes [6–9]. Several modalities for peri-operative analgesia have been used such as patient-controlled analgesia (PCA), systemic opioids, spinal anaesthetic, epidural catheter, and local anaesthetic blocks. These all carry associated risks and benefits which must be weighed.

The use of local infiltration analgesia (LIA) is a technique adopted in lower limb arthroplasty to improve post-operative pain. LIA is a technique described initially in literature by Kerr and Kohan who used a multimodal approach to relieve pain [10]. A cocktail of locally injected anaesthetic and direct acting analgesics create a prolonged analgesic effect post-operatively reduces the requirement of opioid analgesia and thus reducing nausea and increasing mobility.

This chapter discusses LIA and its multimodal approach to analgesia, regional anaesthesia and early mobilisation that improves overall patient experience and satisfaction. The chapter discusses LIA techniques, wound catheter placement, and postoperative protocol to achieve fast track hip and knee arthroplasty.

2. Local infiltration analgesia mixture

The local anaesthetic cocktail usually comprises of multiple active ingredients. The dose and volume of this cocktail is dependent on many factors including body mass index (BMI), renal function and patient's specific comorbidities. Local anaesthetic mixture has been validated in previous studies which showed that LIA is safe and effective in total hip and knee arthroplasty [11–13].

The anaesthetic mixture initially described by Kerr & Kohen in 2008 contained 2.0 mg/mL ropivacaine, 30 mg ketorolac and 10 µg/mL of adrenaline totalling 150–170 mL in knee arthroplasty and 150-200 mL in hip arthroplasty [10]. Ropivacaine was reduced to 250 mg if a patient was less than 55 kg, older than 85 years or had an American Society of Anaesthesiology (ASA) class of 3 or more. In this description, ketorolac was omitted in patients with poor renal function.

According to a study conducted in Ballarat, Victoria in 2020, they used a LIA cocktail derived from Kerr's protocol. Their mixture consisted of 350 mg of ropivacaine, 30 mg ketorolac, 4 mg dexamethasone and 0.5 mg adrenaline [14]. The catheter top-up was injected in the morning post-operative with dose of 20 mL including 100 mg ropivacaine, 4 mg dexamethasone, 30 mg ketorolac, 0.5 mg adrenaline (adrenaline given for total hip arthroplasty (THA) only and not total knee arthroplasty (TKA)) and normal saline. The study showed shorter length of stay, decreased incidence of discharge to rehabilitation, and reduction in healthcare cost without negative impact on patient outcomes when compared to the national average outcomes published in Royal Australasian College of Surgeons Variance Report in 2017. PCA (patient-controlled analgesia) was not used.

In a THR study, Busch et al. used a 100 mL mixture of local anaesthetic comprised of 400 mg of ropivacaine, 30 mg of ketorolac, 5 mg of morphine and 0.6 mL of epinephrine [15]. They found that their patients who received LIA, when compared to those who did not receive, had better pain and satisfaction scores, their PCA use was minimised, and their length of stay (LOS) decreased. Krenzel et al. performed a double-blinded randomised control study for patients with TKA that compared a 20 mL solution of 100 mg ropivacaine against 20 mL of saline placebo [16]. They found that patients received LIA had better pain scores and straight leg raise earlier. The systematic review conducted by Marques et al. used a combination of a local anaesthetic (ropivacaine or bupivacaine), ketorolac and epinephrine [17].

The factors that might impact LIA mixture include surgeon and anaesthetist preferences, low BMI, age, comorbidities, and allergies. Pantoprazole, a proton pump inhibitor, offsets the multiple risks that contribute to gastrointestinal bleeding or peptic ulcer disease in the perioperative period. These factors should be discussed and altered pre-operatively, and still enlist fast track protocol.

2.1 Safety of local anaesthetic

Local anaesthetic agents are toxic at certain levels in systemic circulation. With any use of local anaesthetic, care must be taken to ensure LIA mixture is not injected directly into the patient's circulation. Local anaesthetic will inevitably be transported into circulation at a small concentration. However, it has been shown that the volume of local anaesthetic used in LIA technique is safe, and their levels in blood tests show sub-toxic concentration [18–20].

Fenten et al. took multiple plasma samples after LIA and torniquet release for TKA (at 20, 40, 60, 90, 120, 240, 360 minutes and 24 hours) [18]. The mix comprised of 200 mL 0.2% ropivacaine and 0.75 mg epinephrine 1:1000. Maximum ropivacaine concentration (total and unbound serum concentration) remained well below the assumed toxic threshold at all serum plasma samples. Stringer et al. studied LIA with the use of pain pump infusions for 48 hours post-operatively and measured ropivacaine concentration in THA and TKA patients [20]. The mixture contained 350-400 mg ropivacaine and defined their safe threshold concentration of 1–3 microg/mL intravascularly. Their intra-articular pain pump infusion commenced 12 hours post-operatively. Ropivacaine concentration was below 2 microg/mL with LIA intraoperatively. Once intra-articular pain pump infusion commenced, peak ropivacaine concentration reached 0.65–4.36 microg/mL, however none of their patients experienced clinical signs of toxicity.

2.2 Adrenaline

The inclusion of adrenaline in LIA cocktail is safe, but it is not well understood whether including it improves outcomes. Adrenaline works as vasoconstrictive agent which prolongs the local anaesthetic effect [21]. However, there is a concern in the recent literature for the usage of adrenaline and its impacts on vasoconstriction and skin necrosis [21, 22].

Van Der Zwaard et al. studied 502 TKA and unicondylar knee replacements, and compared one group of LIA with ropivacaine only with the other group of ropivacaine and epinephrine [23]. They found there was no difference in pain scores between the two groups. The authors of this chapter found the usage of adrenaline in a staged injection technique has benefits. Adrenaline prolongs the effect of local anaesthetic and decrease bleeding which mitigates swelling and haematoma forma-tion, subsequently facilities early mobilisation. We recommend proximal infiltra-tion deep to the deep fascia rather than injecting the skin and subcutaneous in TKR to avoid skin necrosis.

2.3 Corticosteroids

Inclusion of corticosteroids in the local mix is controversial. Periprosthetic infection is a dreaded complication with significant implications for the patient and is of concern with use of corticosteroids given the drug's immunosuppres-sive properties. Steroids prolong the duration and efficacy of the local mix [24]. A randomised control trial (RCT) showed that adding corticosteroid to the local anaesthetic cocktail improved 24 hour post-operative pain with no increased complications for 12-months, including deep infections [25].

3. Comparative regional anaesthesia options

Several pain management methods are used after TKR and THR such as PCA, narcotics, epidural analgesia, and peripheral nerve block. However, those methods are associated with complications; continuous epidural infiltration and femoral and/or sciatic nerve block improve postoperative pain control and reduce consumption of narcotics but at the expense of other potential problems such as epidural bleeding (with prophylactic anticoagulation therapy), infection, urinary retention, diminished muscle control and nerve damage [26–31]. PCA administration of opioids is often associated with nausea and vomiting, respiratory depression, drowsiness, pruritus, reduced gut motility, and urinary retention. Continuous intra-articular infusion of analgesics is associated with large effusion of surgical wound [15, 26]. Even though those pain management methods have reduced the acute phase of postoperative pain to some extent, they do not address the major concerns of venous thromboembolism (VTE) and hospital-acquired infections.

3.1 Intrathecal morphine

Intrathecal morphine has emerged as an alternative approach to managing post-operative pain following THA and TKA. Intrathecal administration of morphine would manage pain experienced by a patient with lower limb surgery and is commonly used for other procedures such as intra-abdominal and caesarean operations. However, the risks might be respiratory depression, bradycardia and hypotension, seizures, and urinary retention [32].

Both intrathecal morphine and LIA minimise the need for systemic opioid usage and improve patient outcomes. A large meta-analysis performed by Qi et al. compared intrathecal morphine to LIA in patients with THA and TKA [33]. Patients receiving LIA required less systemic opioids (13.52 mg) and had better visual analogue score at rest and mobility at 72 hours, and lower incidence of nausea or vomiting post-operatively.

3.2 Epidural anaesthesia

The epidural catheter is another option for managing pain in THA and TKA patients. Although less commonly used, it is a good way to manage pain and avoid use of oral opioids. While effective, it also carries certain risks including urinary retention, neurological deficits and epidural hematoma, and has a number of contraindications [34]. Berninger et al. in their study found that no difference in pain among different combination of anaesthesia and nerve blocks, however they found that the group that included LIA had higher mobilisation and better muscle strength in the early post-operative phase [35].

3.3 Peripheral nerve block

Peripheral nerve blocks are another widely accepted method for analgesia peri-operatively and post-operatively for THA and TKA. The blocks minimise pain experienced by the patient whilst being more specific than systemic opioids or intrathecal/epidural analgesia. Peripheral nerve blocks however can cause some delays peri-operatively compared to LIA. A sterile field, commonly with ultrasound needs to be prepared and is performed before or after operation, as compared to LIA which is performed intra-operatively.

A large meta-analysis found that pain six hours post-operatively was better when LIA is used compared to peripheral nerve block, but there was no difference between the two for pain later, opioid consumption, length of stay and complications such as deep infection and VTE [36]. Berninger et al. found that the LIA group had better mobility than those who had peripheral nerve blocks, but other parameters were no different [35]. It can be argued that better pain relief acutely and better mobility post-operatively can reduce risk of complications, such as VTE, and would improve patient satisfaction and outcomes [35].

Two common peripheral nerve blocks used for TKA are femoral nerve block and adductor canal block. Kim et al. in their randomised trial, patients underwent TKA received either an adductor canal block or a femoral nerve block, and measured quadricep strength and pain scores at different time frames [37]. They found that the adductor canal group had better quadriceps strength in the 6-to-8-hour post-operative window compared to the patients receiving femoral nerve block, and pain was no different. Quadriceps strength and pain was no different after 24 hours post-operatively. A key fundamental to Fast Track Arthroplasty is early mobilisation and return to function; avoiding motor blockade would assist a patient to functionally progress earlier.

3.4 Complementary patient-controlled analgesia (PCA)

PCA is a commonly used pain management technique that individualises patient need for analgesia and aims to give patients control over their pain management; this helps determine the required oral analgesia. Pandazi et al. performed a ran-domised controlled trial; two of the included groups were LIA with PCA as rescue versus PCA alone in patients receiving THA [38]. The LIA group was shown to have significantly better pain scores at rest and when mobilising, and had less overall morphine consumption, with no difference in adverse events.

PCA combined with LIA can help manage pain post-operatively for patients with THA and TKA. For some patients however, adding another intravenous line can impede mobility – the enhanced recovery after surgery (ERAS) aims to mobilise patients as soon as possible. A multi-modal approach to analgesia should be utilised, with LIA providing a useful option in a patient's management.

4. Fast track hip and knee arthroplasty is not a new idea

The use of fast track or rapid recovery arthroplasty has been successfully implemented within multiple health systems in many different countries globally over the past 10–15 years [14, 39–43]. To successfully implement fast track arthroplasty, the care pathway involved is complex and multidisciplinary. Goals include ensuring correct indication for surgery and candidate selection, pre-operative optimisation, safe and evidence-based peri-operative management, good functional outcome and high patient satisfaction [44]. According to the Enhanced Recovery After Surgery (ERAS) Society, there are about 20 components of care involved for implementation of effective protocols, which is undertaken in a multidisciplinary fashion including expertise from anaesthetics, surgery, physical therapy, nursing and nutrition [7]. These protocol has been successfully implemented into multiple surgical specialities including gynaecological oncology, urology, vascular and thoracic surgeries [7]. Along with individual studies, systematic reviews and meta-analysis highlighted the benefits of fast-track arthroplasty for lower limb [6, 7, 9].

Malviya et al. implemented a rapid recovery protocol for hip and knee arthroplasty in May 2008 in the United Kingdom. They found the median LOS decreased from

6 days to 3 days and requirement for blood transfusion reduced from 23% to 9.8%, which was statistically significant. Most notably there was a reduction in 30-day mortality from 0.5% to 0.1% along with reduction in 90-day mortality of 0.8% to 0.2%. [42]

A retrospective study conducted by Auyong et al. on 252 patients who underwent rapid recovery protocol, showed a reduced length of stay, improved mobility, reduced overall opioid consumption with no difference in readmission rates or complication rates. [39]

In Australia, Christelis et al. in their study on 709 patients compared a pre-ERAS and post-ERAS cohort. They found the ERAS group had a reduced LOS with no change in complication rates by 6 weeks post operatively, no increase in hospital readmission along with similar pain scores, and higher patient satisfaction at the 6 weeks post-operative mark. [40]

Same day discharge arthroplasty has emerged recently that showed cost-effectiveness without jeopardising clinical outcomes [45]. Basques et al. identified several patient characteristics which favoured same day discharge including decreased age, male, lower ASA class, less obese along with lower rates of respiratory disease and hypertension [46].

5. Author's LIA technique

LIA is an effective method of post-operative pain control in hip and knee arthroplasty [11, 14]. This, combined with low- or no-dose opioid spinal anaesthesia, allows virtually avoids urinary catheters and ensures earlier mobilisation. This multi-modal opioid-sparing approach is central to the rapid recovery model of care, allowing safe early mobilisation with minimal pain. With the use of LIA there is the advantage of having no motor blockade [8], allowing the patient to be mobilised day of surgery.

The purpose of adoption of LIA technique is to provide comfort from the trauma associated with hip and knee arthroplasty particularly for the first 36 h post-operatively, during the time of high post-operative pain, to facilitate increased post-operative mobilisation and function. Further benefits for the use of LIA include no motor blockade also enabling mobilisation, along with reducing the requirement for systemic agents including opioids with associated negative side effects like nausea, vomiting and drowsiness [8, 14]. We have not observed local anaesthetic toxicity, impaired wound healing or increased risk of infection with the use of post-operative pain catheters inserted intra-articularly [8]. Further detail on evidence surround local anaesthetic toxicity is addressed in Section 2 however, nor have other authors found increased infections in hip and knee arthroplasty [13, 19].

The use of bolus injections via 0.22um filter and wound catheter into the joint on the morning after surgery possibly extravasates into surrounding tissues, especially in hip arthroplasty. However, dispersing the injection over a larger area is probably advantageous relative to local anaesthetic infusion, which may be concentrated at the tip of the wound catheter. Furthermore, it avoids "extra baggage" for the patient to carry.

Our LIA technique augments our multimodal therapy approach. Patients routinely receive paracetamol 1 g qid, meloxicam 7.5 mg bd, for more painful operations (TKA, or posterior approach THA) buprenophine 5ug/hr. patch, and tramadol 50 mg 3/24 prn.

5.1 Intra-operative considerations

LIA administration intraoperatively there are four aspects which need consideration; the components of the drug mixture, the injection of the mixture, the catheter placement and, application of compression bandage for TKA [14]. The details of the drug mixture are discussed in Section 2. Before wound closure, a catheter is inserted either intra-articular or periarticular for post-operative continuous or bolus application of LIA mixture.

The commonly used catheter is a 16G Tuohy needle, an 18G epidural catheter, and a 0.22-u high-performance antibacterial flat epidural filter (Portex, Smiths Medical) [10, 14, 19]. The use of a antibacterial filter has laboratory experiments show sustained efficacy of their use for 48 h continuous infusion [47] with efficacy in antimicrobial filtration for up to 60 days with low volume and low injection pressures [48]. To date the use of antibacterial filters have been used in several applications like epidural catheters and within LIA for post-operative delivery of anaesthesia with no reported increase in infections.

5.2 Total hip arthroplasty injection technique

A standard approach can be undertaken to local anaesthesia administration intraoperatively can be adopted regardless of approach used (anterior/posterior/lateral). The primary purpose is to provide anaesthesia to all area affected by the trauma of the surgery. The total volume used intraoperatively of anaesthetic mixture is 150-200 mL where three main stages of administration are involved.

- After skin incision typically 50 mL of mixture is used within the subcutaneous tissue and proximal gluteus maximus (posterior approach) or for 25 ml injected in the region of the lateral femoral cutaneous nerve (anterior approach). Administration is undertaken using a 'moving needle' technique.

- After cup implantation injection of 25 ml infero-medial capsule (where innervated by obturator nerve), and a further 25-50 mL injected through the capsule superiorly and anteriorly (posterior approach) or postero-superiorly (anterior approach) is performed. Once the definitive implantation of femoral components, injection of the periarticular tissue is performed with about 50 mL of mixture. Intra-articular epidural catheter is placed through skin and deep fascia with the use of a Tuohy needle where a small volume is injected to ensure no blockages prior to closing the deep structures. 5-10 cm of the catheter is placed intra-articularly. The exit position of the catheter through the skin within 2 cm of the incision allows it to be secured by the wound dressing. Note that particular care must be made during closure to ensure the catheter does not become inadvertently sutured.

This epidural catheter is then attached to either an antibacterial filter if the intention is post-operative bolus application of anaesthetic mixture or continuous elastomeric pain pump.

5.3 Total knee arthroplasty injection technique

As with hip arthroplasty, in knee arthroplasty the aim is to infiltrate local anaesthetic mixture into areas affected by the surgery. General principals can be broken into four main stages.

- Prior to skin incision, a block 10 cm proximal to the patella, just deep to the deep fascia, injection 25 ml from lateral to medial, and a second 25 ml injection medially in the region deep to sartorius. Administration is undertaken using a 'moving needle' technique.

- After femoral bone cuts are made injection through the posterior capsule of the knee with about 25 mL of mixture each side, aiming proximally, and away from the popliteal artery. Once the definitive implants are inserted structures around medial collateral ligaments, quadriceps, and tibial portion of the iliotibial band. The epidural catheter is placed through the skin, fascia, quadriceps, and joint capsule using a Tuohy needle, then inserting the tip of the wound catheter posterior to the medial femoral condyle. Also, as was mentioned with hip arthroplasty, care must be taken when closing the wound not to catch catheter with sutures which will impede catheter removal.

- The remaining mixture is used for infiltration into the synovium and capsule along with surrounding tissue in layers during closure.
- Compression bandages are then applied once the wound is dressed.

An alternate catheter placement can be within the adductor canal, performed intraoperatively. Adductor canal catheter placement may be performed under direct visualisation on subvastus approach. In recovery, ice pack should be applied hourly for 20-minute intervals for the first four hours to prevent swelling and assist in pain control.

5.4 Post-operative

5.4.1 Continuous infusion vs. bolus in LIA

The evidence favouring continuous, or bolus post-operative catheter regimes is limited. Early development by Kerr & Kohen used a bolus protocol in THA and TKA, along with other published protocols [10, 14, 42, 49]. Ballarat experience in their study published in ANZ Journal of Surgery in 2020 supported that bolus injection demonstrated better outcome. However, there is also evidence to support the use of continuous infusions of anaesthetic mixture delivered by elastomeric pump devices post operatively which has also shown success [50–52]. Typically, the infusion rate of 5 ml per hour for 48 hours if continuous infusion is used.

Our preference is 25 ml LIA cocktail without adrenaline is injected in the morning after surgery as a bolus.

5.4.2 Post-operative bandage

Compressive bandage applied post-operatively prolongs the local anaesthetic within the peri-articular tissues after TKA. An elastic binder compressing a sponge on the hip wound could be used but is not common practice and there is no evidence for efficacy. The bandage should be placed to have enough venous compression but not arterial compression [10].

A compression bandage is applied post operatively over the whole leg, from toes to high thigh, in three layers; one layer of soft padding, one layer of crepe bandage, and outer layer of elastic adhesive bandage as recommended by Kerr and Kohan in 2008 [10]. Another study confirmed the benefits of the compression bandage in TKA and demonstrated the improvement of LIA with compression bandage [53]. The compression dressing is removed 24–48 hours post operatively.

6. Pillars of fast track Arthroplasty

In recent times, many health care systems globally have undergone revision of their hip and knee arthroplasty pathways [40, 54]. The concept of ERAS, 'rapid recovery' or 'fast-tracking' aims to reduce operation-related physiological and psychological stress as well as enhance early mobilisation and reduce recovery time [44]. Implementation of this rapid recovery model has resulted in reduced length of stay with no increase in hospital re-admissions [40, 43]. In recent times, many health care systems globally have undergone revision of their hip and knee arthroplasty pathways [40, 54]. The concept of ERAS, 'rapid recovery' or 'fast-tracking' aims to reduce operation-related physiological and psychological stress as well as enhance early mobilisation and reduce recovery time [44]. Implementation of this rapid recovery model has resulted in reduced length of stay with no increase in hospital re-admissions [40, 43].

Three stages are identified in a patient's journey: pre-operative, peri-operative and post-operative. Pre-operative patient education is a recognised cornerstone in rapid recovery programs [54], with particular attention paid to patient expectation management regarding post-operative pain and LOS. Simultaneously, pre-operative anaesthetic review allows assessment and modification of patient risk factors that have been shown to reduce length of stay in hip and knee arthroplasty patients [55].

6.1 Preoperative

Rapid recovery protocol begins at the pre-admission stage. On presentation to pre-admission clinic, patients require education on appropriate expectations regarding their operation and post-operative course. An assessment tool in assisting prediction on length of stay and discharge destination (i.e. home or rehabilitation facility) is the Risk Assessment and Prediction Tool (RAPT) which has been previously validated [56, 57]. This tool is a score from 0 to 12, the higher the score the better, where points are given based on age, gender, average walking distance, requirement for walking aids, commu-nity, and home supports. With RAPT score < 6 the patient will likely require rehabilita-tion, between 6 and 9 the patient will likely be discharged home and with a score greater than 9 the patient will likely be discharged post-operative day 1 [57].

There is minimal evidence relating to the impact of preoperative patient educa-tion where a Cochrane review by McDonald et al. found preoperative education had no measurable impact on preoperative anxiety or surgical outcomes including pain, function and adverse events [58]. McDonald et al. however noted that there was much heterogeneity and low-level evidence within included studies and preoperative education may benefit patients with depression, unrealistic expectations, anxiety or those with limited social support [58]. The authors believe that setting expectations preoperatively is extremely important for patients prior to their day of surgery where they understand arthroplasty will involve pain which cannot be completely removed, they will be mobilised day of operation, and the primary goal will be discharged home once they are deemed safe. Patients should be prepared to go home post-operative day one.

Pre-admission optimisation is another essential factor when preparing for hip and knee arthroplasty. Assessment and optimisation of risk factors including smoking, alcohol consumption, anaemia, nutritional and metabolic status, and low physical activity has been shown to have a positive impact on length of stay and post-operative complications [59]. Smoking has been shown to increase early post-opera-tive complications, however there is level 2 evidence showing that cessation 4 weeks or greater preoperatively can improve post-operative complications especially related to wound healing [8]. Preoperative optimisation within fast-track protocols has also been shown to reduce the number of patients with a delayed recovery [59].

6.2 Perioperative

There are several factors that are considered in fast-track arthroplasty regarding preparation for surgery including fasting duration and carbohydrate loading.

Although now relatively common practice, anaesthetic guidelines no longer recommend prolonged fasting status, rather a 2 hour clear and 6 hour solid fasting status prior to surgery [60]. Although a component of fast-track/ERAS protocol, carbohydrate has mixed evidence on impact of clinical outcomes in hip and knee arthroplasty even though there some studies have shown positive impact on post-operative hunger, pain, glucose metabolism and insulin resistance [8].

Standardised anaesthesia is another component included in ERAS protocols with mixed evidence regarding superiority between neuraxial anaesthesia/regional and general anaesthesia [7, 8, 11]. Several studies showed the benefit of neuraxial/regional anaesthesia including reduced pulmonary compromise, pulmonary embolism, need for transfusion, renal injury, infection, length of stay and 30-day mortality [61, 62]. Alternatively, a systematic review and meta-analysis by Johnston et al. found no difference between neuraxial and general anaesthesia [63]. In general, the aim with fast-track arthroplasty is to reduce systemic opioid use. This avoids associated side effects of opioid analgesia which can inhibit engagement in post-operative recovery by adopting effective multimodal analgesia and anaesthesia.

6.2.1 Tranexamic acid

There is potential for large blood loss with hip and knee arthroplasty which in turn can prolong hospital stay, increase risk of transfusion, renal failure and increase risk of deep infection. The inclusion of tranexamic acid in hip and knee arthroplasty is effective and safe medication which reduces blood loss with no increased risk of thromboembolic events [7, 8].

6.2.2 Post-operative nausea and vomiting

Post-operative nausea and vomiting (PONV) can be extremely distressing for patients which consequently impact their post-operative course. Risk factors include narcotics, inhalational anaesthesia, female sex, non-smoking status, history of motion sickness or previous PONV and predicted requirement for post-operative opioids [7]. Active screening and prophylactic treatment for at risk individuals is recommended, but our experience with Total Intravenous Anaesthesia (TIVA) or at least minimising inhalational anaesthesia suggests nausea and vomiting to be less common than it once was.

6.2.3 Active intraoperative warming

Maintaining normothermia must be a component of anaesthetic care for joint arthroplasty. When normothermia is maintained, it reduces infection, cardiac complications, transfusion requirements and coagulopathy [7]. With joint arthroplasty, aggressive warming has been shown to reduce intraoperative blood loss in total hip arthroplasty and reduce opioid requirements along with improved patient satisfaction in total knee arthroplasty [7]. Several techniques have been described to assist in maintain normothermia including warm IV fluids and irrigation fluid, prewarming and humidification of anaesthetic gases along with forced air-warming blankets and devices [8].

6.2.4 Avoid urinary catheters

With the use of low dose or no opioid spinal anaesthetic, urinary catheters are unnecessary for the majority of patients, avoiding bacteraemia which may increase risk of prosthetic joint infection [64]. A large RCT performed within a hip and knee arthroplasty ERAS program showed that increasing a catheterisation threshold from 500 ml to 800 ml over halved the incidence of catheterisation without increase in urological complications [64]. Routine use of urinary catheters is not recom-mended as per ERAS consensus statement for hip and knee arthroplasty and if used should be removed within 24 hours of insertion [8]. The catheter adds another line or attachment to the patient which increases risk of fall and does not facilitate early mobilisation. Lines should be removed as soon as possible to improve patients' psychological state and avoid any impediment to mobilisation. This not only pertains to urinary catheters but also applies to PCA and other IV lines unless required.

6.2.5 Surgical factors

Surgical approaches may play a role in ERAS THA and TKA however, the advantages or shortcomings between different approaches in both hip and knee arthroplasty in controversial in the literature. This will not be discussed in details, however, there is no conclusive evidence that surgical approach affect post-operative outcomes [8].

Tourniquet free TKR has recently gained popularity, a systematic review with meta-analysis conducted by Smith and Hing showed tourniquet does reduce intraop-erative blood loss however increases rates of haematoma, blisters, superficial wound complications, VTE and pulmonary embolism [65]. Furthermore, the use of knee tourniquet has been shown to negatively affect strength with no impact on range of motion [8]. We do not use a tourniquet. We do not apply but not inflate the tourniquet as this technique often creates a venous tourniquet, making surgery more difficult.

The use of the routine post-operative drain shows no improvement for complications including wound infections, haematomas and healing complications [8] and may increase blood loss and transfusion rate [66]. We do not use drain tubes for primary arthroplasty.

6.3 Post-operative

During the post-operative period, the primary aim is to ensure the patient is at full function as soon as possible. This is assisted by ensuring there is adequate analgesia, and the patient is mobilised at the day of operation. Patients are deemed safe for discharge when satisfy the following criteria.

- Medically stable and well; bladder and bowels working and tolerating food and drink
- Pain controlled
- Safe mobilising which is assessed by physiotherapy
- Safe discharge destination with appropriate support
- Medications arranged
- Appropriate follow-up arranged.

Appropriate education for ongoing rehabilitation is crucial to ensure that they will continue to progress their mobility, strength and range of motion [8].

6.3.1 Block (wound) catheter management

The use of the wound catheter post operatively has varied between different protocols in the literature [11, 12]. The method initially described by Kerr & Kohen was a 50 mL top-up of the anaesthetic mixture used intraoperatively 15–20 hours post operatively with 15 mL injected primarily then the remaining injected as the catheter was removed [10]. Nassar et al. describe a top-up with their anaesthetic mixture 18–24 hours post operatively where 20 mL was injected then the catheter was removed [14].

Alternative protocols which have been used include continuous infusion of 250 mL ropivacaine 0.2% over 48 hrs at which case the catheter is removed. If bolus regimes are used the doses involved the first bolus 12 hours post-operatively and the last (second) bolus at 24 hours post-operatively, each under aseptic technique then removal of the catheter where each injection contains 10 ml of 1% ropivacaine, made up to 20mLs with 0.9% saline.

6.3.2 Mobilisation and function

Early mobilisation is a core component to fast-track arthroplasty protocols. Multiple studies have shown that early (ideally day of operation) mobilisation post-operatively reduced length of stay, thromboembolic risk, and mortality [42, 67]. A systematic review and meta-analysis of 5 RCTs performed by Guerra et al. showed that early mobilisation was associated with reduced length of stay by 1.8 days with no increased incidence of negative events or complications [68]. Consequently, all patients should be mobilised with physiotherapy on the day of their operation and if this is not possible due to a late return to ward, at a minimum they must be transferred to sit out of bed. With the use of LIA there is the advantage of having no motor blockade [8] which further facilitates early mobilisation. In fact, day of surgery mobilisation in TKA has been shown to reduce LOS and improve the likelihood of discharge home rather than to a rehabilitation facility [69]. A haemoglobin level is not required prior to mobilisation, and mobilisation must not be delayed awaiting routine blood results. If there are symptomatic concerns, then an urgent medical review should be requested. To further encourage mobilisation simulating home life is encouraged by having all meals, including the first meal, sitting out of bed along with mobilising to bathroom to open bladder or bowels instead of using bedpans or commodes.

The use of corticosteroids is controversial due to the theoretical risk of infection. As mentioned in Section 2.3 there is no increased risk associated with corticosteroid use of periarticular injection. A systematic review and meta-analysis by Yue et al. showed corticosteroid (dexamethasone 0.1 mg/kg) had reduced PONV and pain within 24 hours post operatively [70]. They also showed systemic steroid use had faster functional rehabilitation with no increased risk of infection however, there was increased rates of high serum glucose levels post-operative [70]. Thus, improved patient well-being and analgesia will encourage early mobilisation and facilitate in early discharge and improved post-operative function.

Early mobilisation does not include sitting. We strongly reinforce to our patients that if not mobilising, it is better to lay down than to sit down. Sitting and using a footstool is not helpful, the wound is too low relative to the heart, the veins are potentially occluded in the groin. We recommend patients minimise sitting to 5-10 minutes at a time - it is better to lay on the bed or lounge suite than allow the leg to become swollen. We use 20 mmHg compression stocking during daylight hours. This approach we expect will diminish the readmisssions after arthroplasty caused by swelling, pain, and potentially thrombosis.

6.3.3 Post-operative analgesia

Multimodal analgesia is a well proven analgesia technique within hip and knee arthroplasty [7, 8, 11, 12]. It targets pain through multiple different mechanisms of action to reduce sensation of pain while also reducing the side effects of any one agent. This has also been shown to limit requirement on opioid analgesia which reduces risk of short term side effects like nausea, vomiting, respiratory depression along with long term addiction and development of chronic pain [8]. This involves the use of paracetamol and non-steroidal anti-inflammatory drugs (NSAIDs) along with supplementary opioid analgesia [7, 8], although some of us (DJM) prefer tramadol 50 mg 3/24prn avoiding oxycodone in the vast majority of patients. There has also been evidence for the use of gabapentinoids post operatively that reduce post-operative opioid consumption, pruritus and nausea after joint arthroplasty along with improving sleep however no clear evidence on their role in post-operative pain [8].

6.3.4 VTE prophylaxis

The rate of symptomatic VTE after total hip and knee arthroplasty is approximately 1.9%, with a significant increase of greater than 40% in times where no chemical thromboprophylaxis was used [71, 72]. The National Institute for Health and Care Excellence (NICE) guidelines certifies the use of aspirin, low molecular weight heparin (LMWH), dabigatran, apixaban and rivaroxaban for reducing the incidence of VTE after total knee arthroplasty [73]. In THR, these guidelines support the use of LMWH, dabigatran, apixaban or rivaroxaban [73], with aspirin is not inferior to the other chemical VTE prophylactic agents [74].

Combination of chemical and mechanical thromboprophylaxis is required post-operatively. Ultimately, early mobilisation is significantly influential in reducing the risk of VTE after lower limb total joint arthroplasties, as well as reducing the use of indwelling catheters [75, 76].

We stratify our patients - in easily mobilised patients without other indica-tions for anticoagulants, or past history of thromboembolic disease, we use aspirin 100 mg EC daily, and early mobilisation.

6.3.5 Aim to discharge directly home

Patients will be encouraged to discharge home rather than to inpatient rehabilitation unless indicated by medical issues or limited social supports as per RAPT score. In TKA, home discharge is not inferior to discharge to inpatient rehabilitation which is does not improve functional or patient-reported outcomes [77]. Similarly, inpatient rehabilitation after THA does not reflect any improvement in patient-reported hip pain and function compared to those discharged directly home [78].

7. Keys to success

7.1 Preoperative

- Setting patient expectations
- Use Risk Assessment and Prediction Tool (RAPT) to help predict discharge destination
- Medical optimisation

7.2 Perioperative

- Standardised practice
- Spinal with no (or low) intrathecal morphine
- No blocks that may affect quads, no fascia Iliaca block or femoral block.
- LIA cocktail infiltration
- Wound intra-articular catheter for postoperative cocktail administration

7.3 Post-operative

- Minimal attachments: no urinary catheter or no PCA & all drips and lines out within 24 hrs
- Day of operation mobilisation
- Multimodal opioid sparing analgesia

8. Conclusion

LIA is a good alternative compared to other traditional pain management techniques. LIA is safe and effective to achieve good outcomes, early mobilisation and decreasing length of stay without jeopardising clinical outcomes. Fast track arthroplasty is a holistic approach to patients who undergo total hip and knee arthroplasty, a journey or care that starts with setting patient's mind and expectation, optimising medical status, intraoperative LIA infiltration, decrease the usage of narcotics either in spinal or post-operative medication, discourage usage of PCA or IDC, encourage day of operation mobilisation and optimising post-operative physiotherapy protocols, post-operative exercise protocol.

Author details

Timothy Cordingley[1], Daniel Chepurin[1], Ghada Younis[2], Islam Nassar[1*] and David Mitchell[3]

1 Orthopaedic Department, Central Coast Local Health District, Gosford, NSW, Australia

2 El-Saraya Hospital, Alexandria, Egypt

3 Ballarat Orthopaedics and Sports Medicine, Novar Musculoskeletal Research Institute, Australia

*Address all correspondence to: drnassarislam@gmail.com

References

[1] Baker P, Van der Meulen J, Lewsey J, Gregg P. The role of pain and function in determining patient satisfaction after total knee replacement: data from the National Joint Registry for England and Wales. The Journal of Bone and Joint Surgery British Volume. 2007;89(7): 893-900.

[2] Learmonth ID, Young C, Rorabeck C. The operation of the century: total hip replacement. The Lancet. 2007;370(9597):1508-1519.

[3] Horlocker TT. Pain management in total joint arthroplasty: a historical review. Orthopedics. 2010;33(9):14-19.

[4] Parvizi J, Miller AG, Gandhi K. Multimodal pain management after total joint arthroplasty. The Journal of Bone & Joint Surgery. 2011;93(11): 1075-1084.

[5] Wylde V, Gooberman-Hill R, Horwood J, Beswick A, Noble S, Brookes S, et al. The effect of local anaesthetic wound infiltration on chronic pain after lower limb joint replacement: a protocol for a double-blind randomised controlled trial. BMC Musculoskeletal Disorders. 2011;12(1):1-10.

[6] Deng Q-F, Gu H-Y, Peng W-y, Zhang Q, Huang Z-D, Zhang C, et al. Impact of enhanced recovery after surgery on postoperative recovery after joint arthroplasty: results from a systematic review and meta-analysis. Postgraduate Medical Journal. 2018; 94(1118):678-693.

[7] Soffin E, YaDeau J. Enhanced recovery after surgery for primary hip and knee arthroplasty: a review of the evidence. British Journal of Anaesthesia. 2016;117(suppl_3):iii62-iii72.

[8] Wainwright TW, Gill M, McDonald DA, Middleton RG, Reed M, Sahota O, et al. Consensus statement for perioperative care in total hip replacement and total knee replacement surgery: Enhanced Recovery After Surgery (ERAS®) Society recommendations. Acta Orthopaedica. 2020;91(1):3-19.

[9] Zhu S, Qian W, Jiang C, Ye C, Chen X. Enhanced recovery after surgery for hip and knee arthroplasty: a systematic review and meta-analysis. Postgraduate Medical Journal. 2017;93(1106):736-742.

[10] Kerr DR, Kohan L. Local infiltration analgesia: a technique for the control of acute postoperative pain following knee and hip surgery: A case study of 325 patients. Acta Orthopaedica. 2008; 79(2):174-183.

[11] Andersen L, Kehlet H. Analgesic efficacy of local infiltration analgesia in hip and knee arthroplasty: a systematic review. British Journal of Anaesthesia. 2014;113(3):360-374.

[12] McCarthy D, Iohom G. Local infiltration analgesia for postoperative pain control following total hip arthroplasty: a systematic review. Anesthesiology Research and Practice. 2012;2012.

[13] Seangleulur A, Vanasbodeekul P, Prapaitrakool S, Worathongchai S, Anothaisintawee T, McEvoy M, et al. The efficacy of local infiltration analgesia in the early postoperative period after total knee arthroplasty: a systematic review and meta-analysis. European Journal of Anaesthesiology. 2016;33(11):816-831.

[14] Nassar I, Fahey J, Mitchell D. Rapid recovery following hip and knee arthroplasty using local infiltration analgesia: length of stay, rehabilitation protocol and cost savings. ANZ Journal of Surgery. 2020;90(3):355-359.

[15] Busch CA, Whitehouse MR, Shore BJ, MacDonald SJ, McCalden RW, Bourne RB. The efficacy of periarticular

multimodal drug infiltration in total hip arthroplasty. Clinical Orthopaedics and Related Research®. 2010;468(8):2152-9.

[16] Krenzel BA, Cook C, Martin GN, Vail TP, Attarian DE, Bolognesi MP. Posterior capsular injections of ropivacaine during total knee arthroplasty: a randomized, double-blind, placebo-controlled study. The Journal of Arthroplasty. 2009;24(6 Suppl):138-143.

[17] Marques EM, Jones HE, Elvers KT, Pyke M, Blom AW, Beswick AD. Local anaesthetic infiltration for peri-operative pain control in total hip and knee replacement: systematic review and meta-analyses of short- and long-term effectiveness. BMC Musculoskeletal Disorders. 2014;15:220.

[18] Fenten MG, Bakker SM, Touw DJ, van den Bemt BJ, Scheffer GJ, Heesterbeek PJ, et al. Pharmacokinetics of 400 mg ropivacaine after periarticular local infiltration analgesia for total knee arthroplasty. Acta Anaesthesiologica Scandinavica. 2017;61(3):338-345.

[19] Kerr DR. Local infiltration analgesia: a technique to improve outcomes after hip, knee or lumbar spine surgery: CRC Press; 2016.

[20] Stringer BW, Singhania AK, Sudhakar JE, Brink RB. Serum and wound drain ropivacaine concentrations after wound infiltration in joint arthroplasty. The Journal of Arthroplasty. 2007;22(6):884-892.

[21] Schotanus MGM, Bemelmans YFL, van der Kuy PHM, Jansen J, Kort NP. No advantage of adrenaline in the local infiltration analgesia mixture during total knee arthroplasty. Knee Surgery, Sports Traumatology, Arthroscopy. 2017;25(9):2778-2783.

[22] Toftdahl K, Nikolajsen L, Haraldsted V, Madsen F, Tønnesen EK, Søballe K. Comparison of peri-and intraarticular analgesia with femoral nerve block after total knee arthroplasty: a randomized clinical trial. Acta Orthopaedica. 2007;78(2):172-179.

[23] Van Der Zwaard BC, Roerdink RL, Van Hove RP. Increase in early wound leakage in total knee arthroplasty with local infiltrative analgesia (LIA) that includes epinephrine: a retrospective cohort study. Acta Orthopaedica. 2020;91(6):756-760.

[24] Tran J, Schwarzkopf R. Local infiltration anesthesia with steroids in total knee arthroplasty: A systematic review of randomized control trials. Journal of Orthopaedics. 2015;12(Suppl 1):S44-S50.

[25] Tsukada S, Wakui M, Hoshino A. The impact of including corticosteroid in a periarticular injection for pain control after total knee arthroplasty: a double-blind randomised controlled trial. The Bone & Joint Journal. 2016;98(2):194-200.

[26] Busch CA, Shore BJ, Bhandari R, Ganapathy S, MacDonald SJ, Bourne RB, et al. Efficacy of periarticular multimodal drug injection in total knee arthroplasty: a randomized trial. The Journal of Bone & Joint Surgery. 2006;88(5):959-963.

[27] DeWeese FT, Akbari Z, Carline E. Pain control after knee arthroplasty: intraarticular versus epidural anesthesia. Clinical Orthopaedics and Related Research®. 2001;392:226-31.

[28] Fischer H, Simanski C, Sharp C, Bonnet F, Camu F, Neugebauer E, et al. A procedure-specific systematic review and consensus recommendations for postoperative analgesia following total knee arthroplasty. Anaesthesia. 2008; 63(10):1105-1123.

[29] Hebl JR, Horlocker TT, Schroeder DR. Neuraxial anesthesia and analgesia in patients with preexisting central nervous system disorders. Anesthesia & Analgesia. 2006;103(1): 223-228.

[30] Horlocker TT, Cabanela ME, Wedel DJ. Does postoperative epidural analgesia increase the risk of peroneal nerve palsy after total knee arthroplasty? Anesthesia & Analgesia. 1994;79(3): 495-500.

[31] Horlocker TT, Hebl JR, Kinney MA, Cabanela ME. Opioid-free analgesia following total knee arthroplasty [mdash] a multimodal approach using continuous lumbar plexus (psoas compartment) block, acetaminophen, and ketorolac. Regional Anesthesia & Pain Medicine. 2002;27(1):105-108.

[32] Cummings A, Orgill BD, Fitzgerald BM. Intrathecal Morphine. [Updated 2021 May 4]. In: StatPearls [Internet]. Treasure Island (Fl): StatPearls Publishing; 2021 Jan-.

[33] Qi BC, Yu J, Qiao WS. Comparison of intrathecal morphine versus local infiltration analgesia for pain control in total knee and hip arthroplasty: A meta-analysis. Medicine. 2020;99(36): e21971.

[34] Bosch JC, Smith F, Becker P. Analgesia after total hip replacement: epidural versus psoas compartment block. Southern African Journal of Anaesthesia and Analgesia. 2007;13(2): 21-25.

[35] Berninger MT, Friederichs J, Leidinger W, Augat P, Bühren V, Fulghum C, et al. Effect of local infiltration analgesia, peripheral nerve blocks, general and spinal anesthesia on early functional recovery and pain control in total knee arthroplasty. BMC Musculoskeletal Disorders. 2018;19(1): 232.

[36] Yun X-D, Yin X-L, Jiang J, Teng Y-J, Dong H-T, An L-P, et al. Local infiltration analgesia versus femoral nerve block in total knee arthroplasty: a meta-analysis. Orthopaedics & Traumatology: Surgery & Research. 2015;101(5):565-569.

[37] Kim DH, Lin Y, Goytizolo EA, Kahn RL, Maalouf DB, Manohar A, et al. Adductor canal block versus femoral nerve block for total knee arthroplasty: a prospective, randomized, controlled trial. Anesthesiology. 2014;120(3):540-550.

[38] Pandazi A, Kanellopoulos I, Kalimeris K, Batistaki C, Nikolakopoulos N, Matsota P, et al. Periarticular infiltration for pain relief after total hip arthroplasty: a comparison with epidural and PCA analgesia. Archives of Orthopaedics and Trauma Surgery. 2013;133(11):1607-1612.

[39] Auyong DB, Allen CJ, Pahang JA, Clabeaux JJ, MacDonald KM, Hanson NA. Reduced Length of Hospitalization in Primary Total Knee Arthroplasty Patients Using an Updated Enhanced Recovery After Orthopedic Surgery (ERAS) Pathway. The Journal of Arthroplasty. 2015;30(10):1705-1709.

[40] Christelis N, Wallace S, Sage CE, Babitu U, Liew S, Dugal J, et al. An enhanced recovery after surgery program for hip and knee arthroplasty. Medical Journal of Australia. 2015;202(7):363-368.

[41] Courtney PM, Froimson MI, Meneghini RM, Lee G-C, Della Valle CJ. Can total knee arthroplasty be performed safely as an outpatient in the Medicare population? The Journal of Arthroplasty. 2018;33(7):S28-S31.

[42] Malviya A, Martin K, Harper I, Muller SD, Emmerson KP, Partington PF, et al. Enhanced recovery program for hip and knee replacement reduces death rate: a study of 4,500 consecutive primary hip and knee replacements. Acta Orthopaedica. 2011;82(5):577-581.

[43] Stambough JB, Nunley RM, Curry MC, Steger-May K, Clohisy JC. Rapid recovery protocols for primary total hip arthroplasty can safely reduce length of stay without increasing

readmissions. The Journal of Arthroplasty. 2015;30(4):521-526.

[44] Berg U, Berg M, Rolfson O, Erichsen-Andersson A. Fast-track program of elective joint replacement in hip and knee—patients' experiences of the clinical pathway and care process. Journal of Orthopaedic Surgery and Research. 2019;14(1):1-8.

[45] McClatchy SG, Rider CM, Mihalko WM, Pharr ZK, Toy PC. Defining outpatient hip and knee arthroplasties: a systematic review. Journal of the American Academy of Orthopaedic Surgeons. 2021;29(8): e410-e4e5.

[46] Basques BA, Tetreault MW, Della Valle CJ. Same-day discharge compared with inpatient hospitalization following hip and knee arthroplasty. The Journal of Bone & Joint Surgery. 2017;99(23): 1969-1977.

[47] Sener A, Erkin Y, Sener A, Tasdogen A, Dokumaci E, Elar Z. In vitro comparison of epidural bacteria filters permeability and screening scanning electron microscopy. Brazilian Journal of Anesthesiology (English Edition). 2015;65(6):491-496.

[48] De Cicco M, Matovic M, Castellani Guiseppe T, Basaglia G, Santini G, Del Pup C, et al. Time-dependent Efficacy of Bacterial Filters and Infection Risk in Long-term Epidural Catheterization. Anesthesiology. 1995;82(3):765-771.

[49] Andersen LJ, Poulsen T, Krogh B, Nielsen T. Postoperative analgesia in total hip arthroplasty: a randomized double-blinded, placebo-controlled study on peroperative and postoperative ropivacaine, ketorolac, and adrenaline wound infiltration. Acta Orthopaedica. 2007;78(2):187-192.

[50] Bianconi M, Ferraro L, Traina G, Zanoli G, Antonelli T, Guberti A, et al. Pharmacokinetics and efficacy of ropivacaine continuous wound instillation after joint replacement surgery. British Journal of Anaesthesia. 2003;91(6):830-835.

[51] Gómez-Cardero P, Rodríguez-Merchán EC. Postoperative analgesia in TKA: ropivacaine continuous intraarticular infusion. Clinical Orthopaedics and Related Research®. 2010;468(5):1242-7.

[52] Ong JC, Lin CP, Fook-Chong SM, Tang A, Ying YK, Keng TB. Continuous infiltration of local anaesthetic following total knee arthroplasty. Journal of Orthopaedic Surgery. 2010;18(2):203-207.

[53] Andersen LØ, Husted H, Otte KS, Kristensen BB, Kehlet H. A compression bandage improves local infiltration analgesia in total knee arthroplasty. Acta Orthopaedica. 2008;79(6):806-811.

[54] Husted H. Fast-track hip and knee arthroplasty: clinical and organizational aspects. Acta Orthopaedica. 2012; 83(sup346):1-39.

[55] Bernstein DN, Liu TC, Winegar AL, Jackson LW, Darnutzer JL, Wulf KM, et al. Evaluation of a preoperative optimization protocol for primary hip and knee arthroplasty patients. The Journal of Arthroplasty. 2018;33(12): 3642-3648.

[56] Dauty M, Schmitt X, Menu P, Rousseau B, Dubois C. Using the Risk Assessment and Predictor Tool (RAPT) for patients after total knee replacement surgery. Annals of Physical and Rehabilitation Medicine. 2012;55(1):4-15.

[57] Hansen VJ, Gromov K, Lebrun LM, Rubash HE, Malchau H, Freiberg AA. Does the risk assessment and prediction tool predict discharge disposition after joint replacement? Clinical Orthopaedics and Related Research®. 2015;473(2):5 97-601.

[58] McDonald S, Page MJ, Beringer K, Wasiak J, Sprowson A. Preoperative

education for hip or knee replacement. Cochrane Database of Systematic Reviews. 2014(5).

[59] Hansen TB, Bredtoft HK, Larsen K. Preoperative physical optimization in fast-track hip and knee arthroplasty. Danish Medical Journal. 2012;59(2): A4381.

[60] Smith I, Kranke P, Murat I, Smith A, O'Sullivan G, Søreide E, et al. Perioperative fasting in adults and children: guidelines from the European Society of Anaesthesiology. European Journal of Anaesthesiology.2011;28(8): 556-569.

[61] Hu S, Zhang Z-Y, Hua Y-Q, Li J, Cai Z-D. A comparison of regional and general anaesthesia for total replacement of the hip or knee: a meta-analysis. The Journal of Bone & Joint Surgery British Volume. 2009;91(7):935-942.

[62] Memtsoudis SG, Sun X, Chiu Y-L, Stundner O, Liu SS, Banerjee S, et al. Perioperative Comparative Effectiveness of Anesthetic Technique in Orthopedic Patients. Anesthesiology.2013;118(5): 1046-1058.

[63] Johnson R, Kopp S, Burkle C, Duncan C, Jacob A, Erwin P, et al. Neuraxial vs general anaesthesia for total hip and total knee arthroplasty: a systematic review of comparative-effectiveness research. British Journal of Anaesthesia. 2016;116(2):163-176.

[64] Bjerregaard LS, Hornum U, Troldborg C, Bogoe S, Bagi P, Kehlet H. Postoperative urinary catheterization thresholds of 500 versus 800 ml after fast-track total hip and knee arthroplasty: a randomized, open-label, controlled trial. Anesthesiology.2016;124(6):1256-1264.

[65] Smith TO, Hing CB. Is a tourniquet beneficial in total knee replacement surgery?: a meta-analysis and systematic review. The Knee. 2010;17(2):141-147.

[66] Kelly EG, Cashman JP, Imran FH, Conroy R, O'Byrne J. Systematic review and meta-analysis of closed suction drainage versus non-drainage in primary hip arthroplasty. Surgical Technology International. 2014;24:295-301.

[67] Husted H, Otte KS, Kristensen BB, Ørsnes T, Wong C, Kehlet H. Low risk of thromboembolic complications after fast-track hip and knee arthroplasty. Acta Orthopaedica. 2010;81(5):599-605.

[68] Guerra ML, Singh PJ, Taylor NF. Early mobilization of patients who have had a hip or knee joint replacement reduces length of stay in hospital: a systematic review. Clinical Rehabilitation. 2015;29(9):844-854.

[69] Yakkanti RR, Miller AJ, Smith LS, Feher AW, Mont MA, Malkani AL. Impact of early mobilization on length of stay after primary total knee arthroplasty. Annals of Translational Medicine. 2019;7(4).

[70] Yue C, Wei R, Liu Y. Perioperative systemic steroid for rapid recovery in total knee and hip arthroplasty: a systematic review and meta-analysis of randomized trials. Journal of Orthopaedic Surgery andResearch. 2017;12(1):1-11.

[71] Almegren MO, Alhedaithy AA, Alomri AS, Albawardy NF, Mesmar RS, Al Qahtani MA. Venous thrombo-embolism after total knee and hip arthroplasty: A retrospective study. Saudi Medical Journal. 2018;39(11):1096.

[72] Baser O. Prevalence and economic burden of venous thromboembolism after total hip arthroplasty or total knee arthroplasty. American Journal of Managed Care. 2011;17(1):S6.

[73] National Guideline Centre (UK). Venous thromboembolism in over 16s: Reducing the risk of hospital-acquired deep vein thrombosis or pulmonary embolism. London: National Institute

for Health and Care Excellence (UK); 2018 Mar. PMID: 29697228.

[74] Anderson DR, Dunbar M, Murnaghan J, Kahn SR, Gross P, Forsythe M, et al. Aspirin or rivaroxaban for VTE prophylaxis after hip or knee arthroplasty. New England Journal of Medicine. 2018;378(8):699-707.

[75] Chandrasekaran S, Ariaretnam SK, Tsung J, Dickison D. Early mobilization after total knee replacement reduces the incidence of deep venous thrombosis. ANZ Journal of Surgery. 2009; 79(7-8):526-529.

[76] Chua MJ, Hart AJ, Mittal R, Harris IA, Xuan W, Naylor JM. Early mobilisation after total hip or knee arthroplasty: A multicentre prospective observational study. PLOS One. 2017;12(6):e0179820-e.

[77] Padgett DE, Christ AB, Joseph AD, Lee Y-Y, Haas SB, Lyman S. Discharge to Inpatient Rehab Does Not Result in Improved Functional Outcomes Following Primary Total Knee Arthroplasty. The Journal of Arthroplasty. 2018;33(6):1663-1667.

[78] Naylor JM, Hart A, Mittal R, Harris IA, Xuan W. The effectiveness of inpatient rehabilitation after uncomplicated total hip arthroplasty: a propensity score matched cohort. BMC Musculoskeletal Disorders. 2018;19(1): 236-.

Permissions

All chapters in this book were first published by InTech Open; hereby published with permission under the Creative Commons Attribution License or equivalent. Every chapter published in this book has been scrutinized by our experts. Their significance has been extensively debated. The topics covered herein carry significant findings which will fuel the growth of the discipline. They may even be implemented as practical applications or may be referred to as a beginning point for another development.

The contributors of this book come from diverse backgrounds, making this book a truly international effort. This book will bring forth new frontiers with its revolutionizing research information and detailed analysis of the nascent developments around the world.

We would like to thank all the contributing authors for lending their expertise to make the book truly unique. They have played a crucial role in the development of this book. Without their invaluable contributions this book wouldn't have been possible. They have made vital efforts to compile up to date information on the varied aspects of this subject to make this book a valuable addition to the collection of many professionals and students.

This book was conceptualized with the vision of imparting up-to-date information and advanced data in this field. To ensure the same, a matchless editorial board was set up. Every individual on the board went through rigorous rounds of assessment to prove their worth. After which they invested a large part of their time researching and compiling the most relevant data for our readers.

The editorial board has been involved in producing this book since its inception. They have spent rigorous hours researching and exploring the diverse topics which have resulted in the successful publishing of this book. They have passed on their knowledge of decades through this book. To expedite this challenging task, the publisher supported the team at every step. A small team of assistant editors was also appointed to further simplify the editing procedure and attain best results for the readers.

Apart from the editorial board, the designing team has also invested a significant amount of their time in understanding the subject and creating the most relevant covers. They scrutinized every image to scout for the most suitable representation of the subject and create an appropriate cover for the book.

The publishing team has been an ardent support to the editorial, designing and production team. Their endless efforts to recruit the best for this project, has resulted in the accomplishment of this book. They are a veteran in the field of academics and their pool of knowledge is as vast as their experience in printing. Their expertise and guidance has proved useful at every step. Their uncompromising quality standards have made this book an exceptional effort. Their encouragement from time to time has been an inspiration for everyone.

The publisher and the editorial board hope that this book will prove to be a valuable piece of knowledge for researchers, students, practitioners and scholars across the globe.

List of Contributors

Jeffrey M. Carness
United States Naval Hospital, Bremerton, Washington, USA

Mark J. Lenart
Naval Medical Center, Portsmouth, Virginia, USA

Enrique Hernández-Cortez
Department of Anesthesia, Federación Mexicana de Colegios de Anestesiología, A.C., León, México

Cecilia G. Sandoval Larios
Anesthesia and Cardiovascular Anesthesia, Airway Committee Federación Mexicana de Colegios de Anestesiologia AC, Hospital Angeles León, México

Juan Carlos Flores-Carrillo
Anesthesia and Critical Care Medicine, Hospital Angeles Tijuana, México

Javier Marcos Michel-Levy
Hospital Obrero N°8, Caja Nacional de Salud, Trinidad-Beni, Bolivia

Basak Keskin Yalcin
Cerrahpasa Vocational School of Health Services, Istanbul University, Turkey

Yazmín Guillén-Dolores
Instituto Nacional de Cardiología Ignacio Chávez, México City, México

João Abrão and Marcelo Antunes
Medical School of Ribeirão Preto, University of São Paulo, Ribeirão Preto, SP, Brazil

Luis Vicente Garcia
Educational Hospital of the Medical School of Ribeirão Preto, University of São Paulo, Ribeirão Preto, SP, Brazil

Divya Garg, Shikha Soni and Rakesh Karnawat
Department of Anaesthesia and Critical Care, Dr. S.N. Medical College, Jodhpur, Rajasthan, India

Nandita Mehta and Sayyidah Aasima tu Nisa Qazi
Department of Anaesthesia and Critical Care, ASCOMS Jammu, J&K, India

Víctor M. Whizar-Lugo
Institutos Nacionales de Salud, Lotus Medical Group, Tijuana BC, México

Karen L. Íñiguez-López
Centro Médico Nacional Siglo XXI, Instituto Mexicano del Seguro Social, México City, México

Ana C. Cárdenas-Maytorena
Lotus Med Group, Tijuana BC, México

Cristian D. Ramírez-Puerta
School of Medicine, Campus Tijuana, Universidad Autónoma de Baja California, Tijuana BC, México

Margaretha Barbara Breebaart
Faculty of Medicine and Health Sciences, University of Antwerp, Wilrijk, Belgium

Masahiko Tsuchiya
Department of Anesthesia, Kishiwada Tokushukai Hospital, Kishiwada, Osaka, Japan
Department of Anesthesiology, Osaka City University Graduate School of Medicine, Osaka, Japan

Brenda O. Lezcano Velazquez
Department of Pain Clinic, Instituto Nacional de Cancerlogía (INCAN), México

Guillermo A. Castorena Arellano
Anesthesia, Hospital Médica Sur, México

Krishnamachari Janani
Department of Conservative Dentistry and Endodontics, SRM Dental College, Ramapuram, Chennai, Tamil Nadu, India

Kavalipurapu Venkata Teja and Jerry Jose
Department of Conservative Dentistry and Endodontics, Saveetha Dental College and Hospitals, Saveetha Institute of Medical and Technical Sciences, Saveetha University, Chennai, Tamil Nadu, India

Harini K
Centre for Food Technology, Anna University, Guindy, Chennai, Tamil Nadu, India

Kaligotla Apoorva Vasundhara
Prosthodontist and Oral Implantologist, Andhra Pradesh, India

Timothy Cordingley, Daniel Chepurin and Islam Nassar
Orthopaedic Department, Central Coast Local Health District, Gosford, NSW, Australia

Ghada Younis
El-Saraya Hospital, Alexandria, Egypt

David Mitchell
Ballarat Orthopaedics and Sports Medicine, Novar Musculoskeletal Research Institute, Australia

Index

www.ingramcontent.com/pod-product-compliance
Lightning Source LLC
LaVergne TN
LVHW062130200926
848484LV00007B/1792